Deutsches Krebsforschungszentrum

# Current Cancer Research

1986

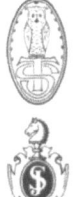

Springer-Verlag Berlin Heidelberg GmbH

Cover photograph:
Demonstration of papillomavirus sequences in a human genital cancer cell line by in situ hybridization. The clusters of grains characterize the localization of the sequences in metaphase chromosomes and in an interphase nucleus (below left).

Photograph:
Dr. Antoaneta Mincheva
Department of Genome Alterations and Carcinogenesis
Institute of Virus Research
Deutsches Krebsforschungszentrum

**Additional material to this book can be downloaded from http://extras.springer.com.**
ISBN 978-3-7985-0712-8      ISBN 978-3-662-21737-5 (eBook)
DOI 10.1007/978-3-662-21737-5

ISSN 0-177-0853

Editorial responsibility:
Press and Public Relations Office
Hilke Stamatiadis-Smidt, M.A.

Translated from the German by
David John Williams, B.Sc.
Brückenstraße 47
D-6900 Heidelberg

Text arrangement:
Heidi Hnatek

Photos:
Josef Wiegand

Photos in the reports of results by the authors or by members of the staff of the respective institutes and from the Central Photographic Department.

Figures from the teletext program "Cancer Encyclopedia", text and design:
Dr. Rudolf Süss and Dr. Margarete Malter

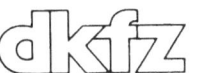

| Chapter | | Page |
|---|---|---|

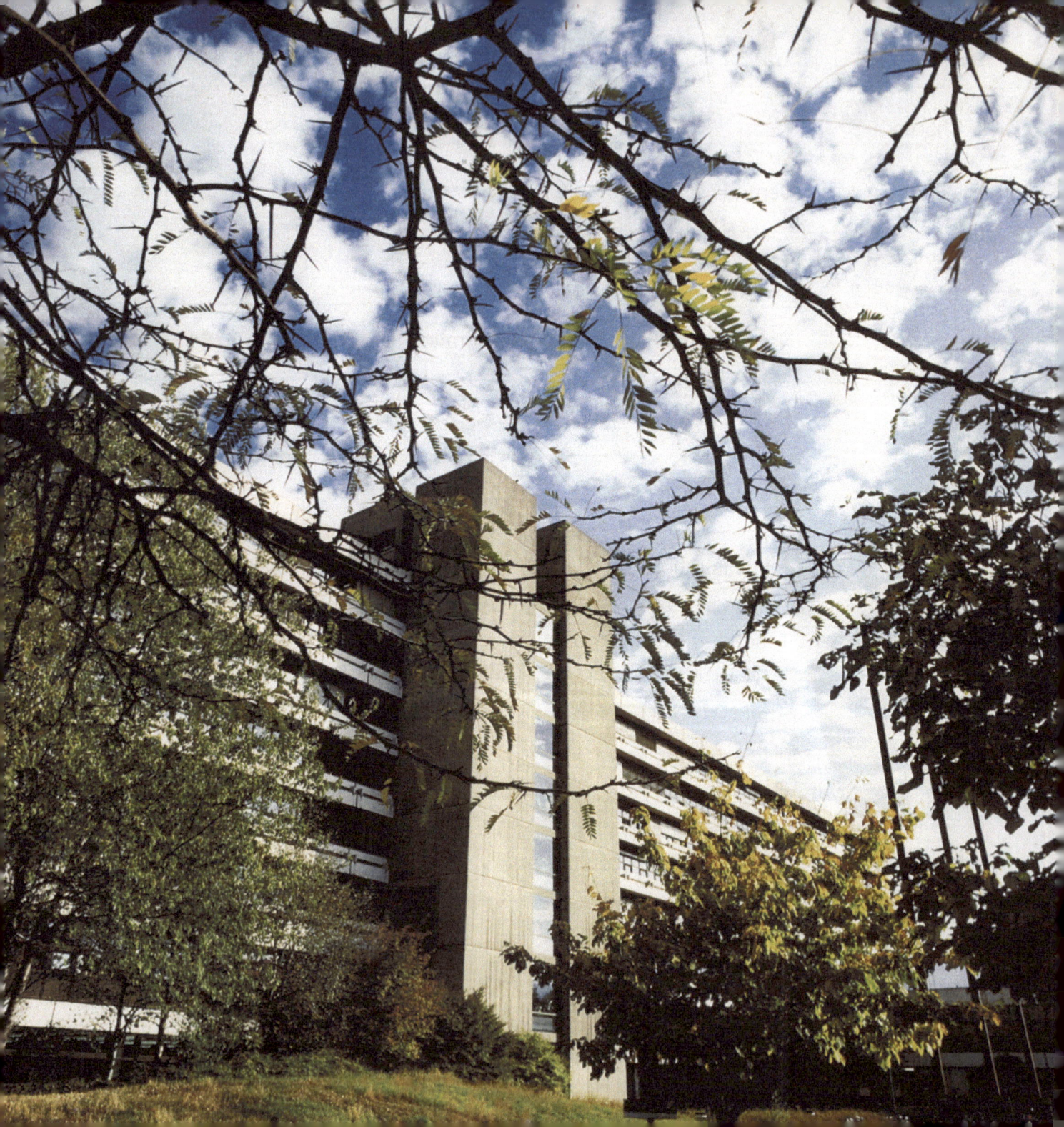

# Deutsches Krebsforschungszentrum Status and Perspectives

by Harald zur Hausen

The past five years have seen particularly significant advances in research on the causes of cancer and in the detection of cancer risk factors. This justifies the hope that cancer prevention, tumor diagnosis and tumor therapy will make rapid progress in the coming years owing to new approaches and new knowledge.

## Advances in Cancer Research

Research on the causes of cancer received a decisive impetus from the discovery of specific genetic structures ("oncogenes") which occur in every normal cell (probably as growth-regulatory and differentiation-specific genes) and which can become "cancer genes" after certain structural or functional changes.

In addition, investigations on carcinogenesis due to viruses, which also led to the discovery of the oncogenes, show how genes introduced into the cell via mechanisms of infection can lead to carcinogenesis. Successful research on the causes of cancer is being carried out today, especially in the combination of molecular biology with tumor biology and immunology.

The detection of risk factors for the genesis of human cancer forms has been remarkably successful. Habits of life (e. g. smoking or tobacco chewing), environmental factors (e. g., ultraviolet radiation from the sun), occupational noxae (e. g. inhalation of asbestos dust) and to an increasing extent viral infections (e. g. hepatitis B virus in primary hepatocellular cancer, papillomaviruses in genital cancer) have proved to be risk factors for a substantial number of human cancers.

The investigation of habits of life by epidemiologists in combination with the work of toxicologists, virologists and pathologists has led to an appreciable increase of our knowledge in recent years.

In the field of cancer prevention, progress has been more gradual. It has been most impressive in the context of the relatively small number of identified occupational noxae in the world of work and in terms of measures for the early diagnosis in cervical and colon cancer. At present, successful strategies leading to the elimination of recognized risk factors resulting from our life style, e. g., smoking, are lacking. However, promising new approaches can be discerned in the prevention of cancer forms associated with viral infections. A dramatic change in the risk developing cancer may result from vaccination in good time. A first attempt in this direction is the vaccination with a vaccine against hepatitis B virus in areas of Central Africa. An infection produced by this virus is regarded as a precursor of liver cancer. The future will show whether the rate of liver cancer is reduced by this vaccination.

Research on improvement of early diagnosis of cancer is concentrated on novel techniques (e. g. computer tomography, nuclear magnetic resonance, positron emission tomography), as well as in the field of development of biochemical-serological "cancer tests". The possibilities opened up by these tests are still unsatisfactory. The development of an increasing number of differentiation-specific and possibly also tumor-specific monoclonal antibodies might lead to a breakthrough in the long run.

Fig. 1
Deutsches Krebsforschungszentrum (German Cancer Research Center), partial view

Fundamentally new concepts from the past five years on the therapeutic influence of tumor growth are hardly discernible. Nevertheless, the further development of radiological therapy, the improvement of chemotherapeutic schemata and the development of new groups of active substances have led to noteworthy progress in the therapy of individual tumor forms. In the long term, we hope that a new generation of treatment approaches will be developed and applied based on DNA recombination technology. This could be achieved by using carriers for specific lethal factors which convey the anticancer agent directly into the genetic information of the cell. Carriers may be e. g., viruses, which have been modified by genetic engineering.

Fig. 2

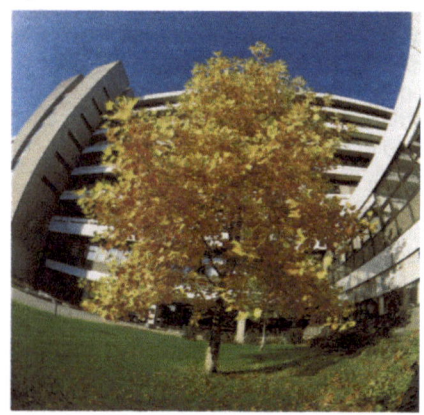

10

## Main Topics of Research in the Deutsches Krebsforschungszentrum

At the Deutsches Krebsforschungszentrum, scientific work in the past years has been increasingly influenced by two factors:

– by new methodological approaches which result from molecular biological and immunological techniques or from their combinations, and
– by an increased attention to the analysis of human tumor systems.

The original conception of the Deutsches Krebsforschungszentrum which was founded 22 years ago foresaw a relatively rigid structure with independent institutes. In the course of time work was concentrated at the level of the departments. The idea that all fields of cancer research could be combined under one roof may have played a role in the initial planning of the early phase, but proved to be unrealistic in practice.

Today, the work of the Deutsches Krebsforschungszentrum is concentrated on four areas:
– Tumor Biology,
– Mechanisms of Carcinogenesis,
– Carcinogenic Factors and Cancer Prevention,
– Research on Diagnosis and Therapy.

Scientific results within these areas are multifarious and are illustrated by a few examples in this edition of "Cancer research today".

Certain scientific groups of the Center hold a leading position which is internationally recognized. This applies in particular to cellular and tumor biology, where investigations on structural components of the cell, the cytoskeleton, have led to new techniques with appli-

cation of monoclonal antibodies in tumor diagnosis. It has become possible to characterize components (proteins) of the cytoskeleton to identify metastases and thus primary tumors of certain cancer forms. Molecular biological investigations on questions of hormone-dependent gene regulation and the processing of genetic information in the cell are widely recognized.

In virology, the identification of certain papillomavirus types in human genital cancer has given rise to a new concept. The carcinogenic role of these viruses is regarded as increasingly more probable. The identification and definition of certain papillomaviruses (e. g., in the smear from the uterine cervix) is gaining increasing importance in the diagnosis of this widespread cancer. In the long run, preventive measures are conceivable, e. g., vaccinations.

Research on metastases and cell surface analysis by means of monoclonal antibodies in the Institute of Immunology and Genetics, for the detection of cancer-promoting and cancer-initiating factors in the Institute of Biochemistry and the Institute of Toxicology and Chemotherapy as well as in the Institute of Experimental Pathology should be mentioned here.

In view of the reactions it called forth, we hope that the Cancer Atlas of the Federal Republic of Germany, which is based on the analysis of death certificates, will motivate the establishment of cancer registries. These cancer registries which collect data on disease incidence are a prerequisite for evaluation of the actual situation in the Federal Republic of Germany.

The close link between diagnostics and treatment techniques based on physical methods practiced by the Institute of Nuclear Medicine together with the Heidelberg University Hospitals is of fundamental importance for the development of new forms of cooperation between physicians and scientists in the preclinical and clinical research in the Heidelberg/Mannheim Tumor Center.

After a phase of orientation which lasted several years, the institution has found its place amongst the international cancer centers and is giving new impulses to cancer research.

## Controlling and Appraisal, New Structures and Planning

For two years, the Deutsches Krebsforschungszentrum has now subjected itself to internal "inspections" of the departments which take place at regular intervals. Besides the promotion of communication and the development of interdisciplinary concepts, this procedure is also intended to enable a redistribution of resources in accordance with productivity. In the last two years, all departments have subjected themselves to a critical evaluation by their colleagues in four to six-hour presentations of program of work, future objectives, working accomodation and personnel. In addition, Institute appraisals are carried out in coordination with the Scientific Committee of the Board of Trustees at five-year intervals. These are carried out exclusively by outside scientists with a large proportion of foreign specialists.

The following new departments were founded within the last two years:
Genome Modifications and carcinogenesis (Institute of Virus Research)
Epidemiology (Institute of Documentation, Information and Statistics)
Applied Immunology (Institute of Nuclear Medicine)
Biochemistry of Tumors (Institute of Nuclear Medicine)

In addition, the preconditions for the establishment of a new working group on classical and molecular cytogenetics was created via the financing by the Verein zur Förderung der Krebsforschung (Heidelberg). The functions of the working group will comprise investigation of the significance of various genes and gene amplifications for carcinogenesis or cancer development. It

has been known for a few years that gene amplifications play a major role in the resistance of the cells to some drugs and noxae. Structural alterations are often found in regions bearing growth genes, potentially oncogenes. These gene regions are evidently responsible for products which regulate growth and development in the normal cell.

In the same period, the departments of Nuclear Medicine and Special Radiotherapy (Institute of Nuclear Medicine), Nuclear Medical Diagnosis (Institute of Nuclear Medicine), RNA Viruses (Institute of Virus Research) were closed in connection with the retirement or departure of the heads of departments or transfer of the department in question to the University of Heidelberg, or the posts were not filled again (RNA Tumor Viruses, appointment of Dr. Thomas Graf to the European Laboratory for Molecular Biology).

In order to give up-and-coming scientists a chance to develop research concepts under their own initiative, the Cancer Research Center has promul-

Fig. 3

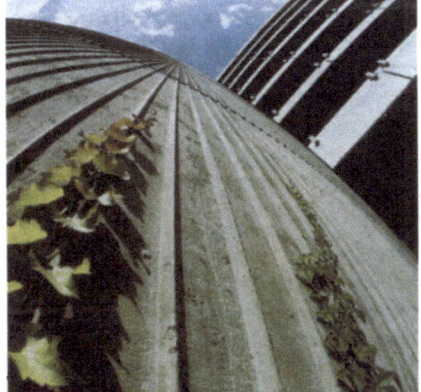

gated a project statute which foresees the establishment of project groups for a specific period of time (five years) besides the organization of research in departments. At the beginning of 1985, four project groups were established which deal with the following topics:
– Molecular Biology of Mitosis
– Cytometry with attached Tumor Bank
– Regulation of Differentiation
– Cancer Encyclopedia.

Internal structural changes such as the transformation of the Central Data Processing into a central service facility of the Cancer Research Center are intended to improve the conditions of scientific work.

The application of molecular biological methods in cancer research has provided entirely new preconditions for understanding carcinogenesis, for the detection of cancer risk factors, for cancer prevention, cancer diagnosis and (as is already apparent) for cancer therapy. This will necessarily be a new focal point for the work of the Deutsches Krebsforschungszentrum without detracting from the importance of the traditional approaches to cancer research, e. g., in the fields of toxicology and pathology. The combination of both approaches in terms of conception and methods will provide a particular chance of successful research. Plans to establish a new research group which is to investigate the molecular biology of aging and the connection between the processes of aging and carcinogenesis are also moving in this direction.

Our scientists have received international recognition for their achievements. This is demonstrated in particular by the number of international scientific congresses and symposia organized or managed by the Deutsches Krebsfor-

schungszentrum (60 from 1983/84 up to the middle of 1985). The increasing number of invitations to accept appointments received by scientists of the center (cf. page 205) and the increase of offers of cooperation from all over the world also document our standing. The cooperation with Israel in the field of cancer research is now in its tenth year. Programs of cooperation with India, Italy, Hungary, the People's Republic of China, Saudi Arabia and the Tanzania Tumor Center are in preparation. Joint

symposia next year will be a visible sign of the deepened German-Japanese and German-American cooperation.
The integration into current national cancer research promotion programs with critical appraisal of research projects is shown by the increased acquisition of funds from other sources, e. g., from the Deutsche Forschungsgemeinschaft. The third-party funding of the Cancer Research Center has risen by 59% from 1983 up to the middle of 1985.

Fig. 4

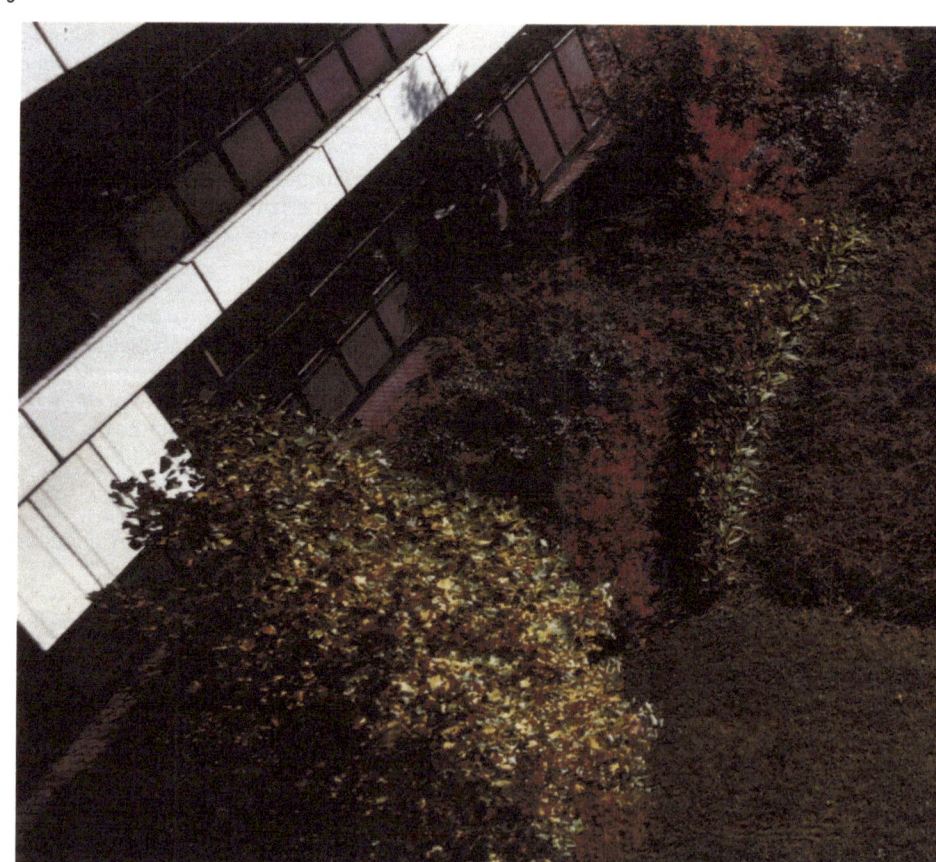

## Perspectives

We require public support for our efforts. It is quite understandable that the individual member of the public would like to see rapid results which help his relatives and friends suffering from cancer. However, he or she must come to understand that insights into basic research which bring us further often require years before they can be practically applied in diagnosis or therapy. A new anticancer drug requires about ten years until it is licensed for the first clinical trial in humans. One must then reckon with at least four years up to its routine application in hospitals.

On the other hand, the development has actually been remarkably rapid. Köhler and Milstein only succeeded in manufacturing the first monoclonal antibodies in 1975. This is an instrument which can be used to identify certain cell structures or cells and also as a potential vehicle of transport in cancer therapy. Monoclonal antibodies open up quite new perspectives in basic research on cancer. First clinical trials on the use of monoclonal antibodies in therapy and diagnosis are in progress at present, e. g., in collaboration of the Deutsches Krebsforschungszentrum with the Dermatology Hospital, University of Heidelberg, and the Heidelberg University Policlinic.

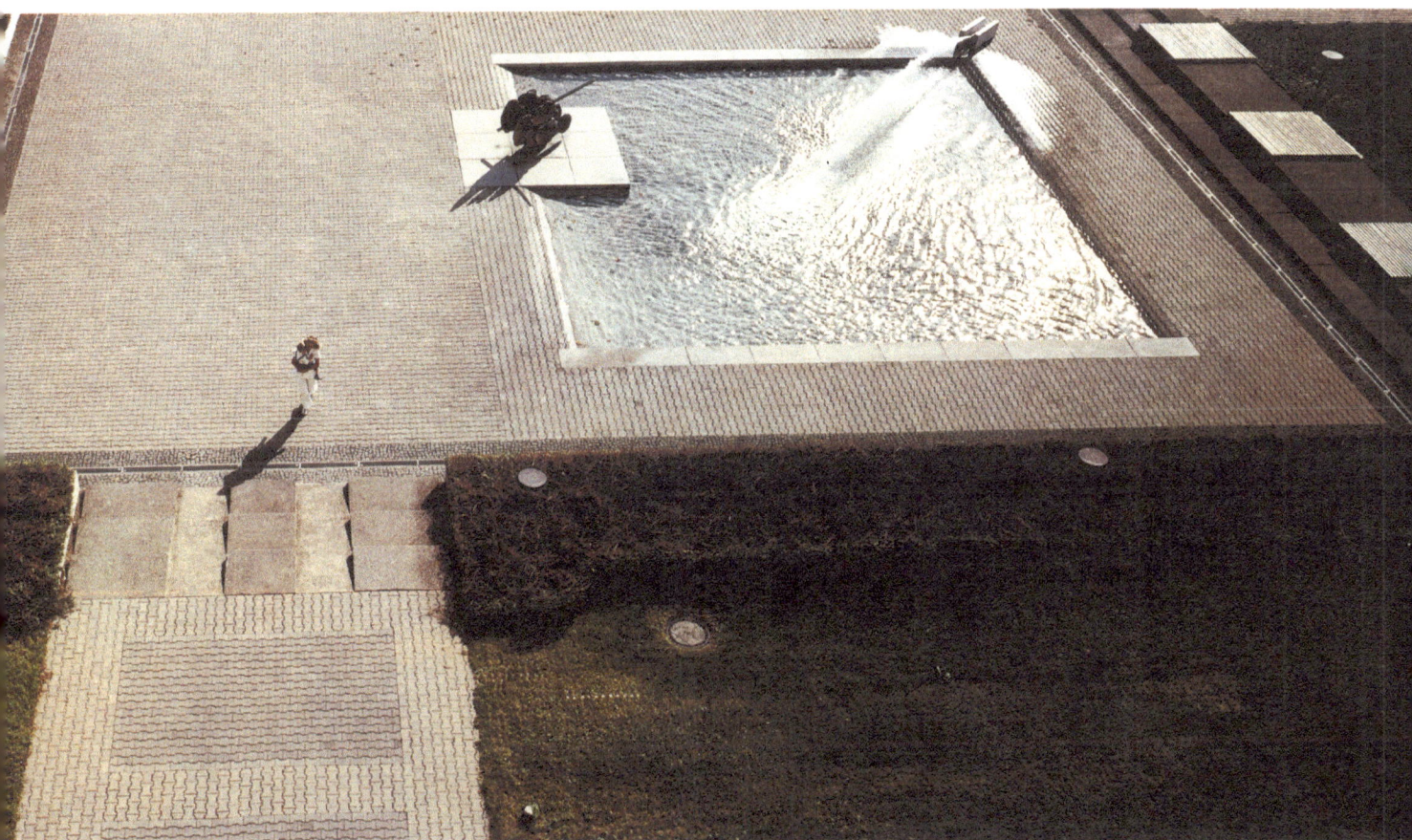

The development is also especially
rapid in other sectors. Autologous substances, interferons, lymphokins, tumor
necrosis factor (TNF), etc. are being increasingly used for specific therapies.
Genetic engineering also opens up very
promising new perspectives for cancer
therapy. We cannot predict whether
gene therapy will ever be applied in humans. However, this is *one* new approach among many which have become possible in the last two to three
years. They all provide a realistic basis
for our hopes that ever more cancer diseases will be successfully treated in the
future and that ever more diseases can
be successfully prevented. However,
not only the efforts of the scientist, but
also the efforts of every citizen in his
lifestyle are required to contribute to the
prevention of cancer.

Prof. Harald zur Hausen
Chairman and Scientific Member of the
Management Board
Deutsches Krebsforschungszentrum

# Scientific Mission and Structure of the Deutsches Krebsforschungszentrum

The Deutsches Krebsforschungszentrum (DKFZ) was founded in 1964 on the initiative of the Heidelberg surgeon Professor K. H. Bauer, who died at the age of 86 in 1978. By decision of the State Government of Baden-Württemberg, the DKFZ was established as a foundation of public law. Since 1975, it has been a national research facility and is being financed by the Federal Government and the State of Baden-Württemberg at a ratio of 90 : 10 on the basis of § 91 b of the German Constitution ("Basic Law"). The Center has consisted of eight institutes since 1976.

According to its statutes, it is the aim of the Center to "pursue cancer research". In view of this general formulation, it is evident that the question will be repeatedly posed in the Center as to whether all research projects entail "cancer research". This term is differently defined from the viewpoint of each specialist discipline. This means that the discussion as to the contents of the research program never ceases in a center with a multidisciplinary structure and that the "equilibrium of forces" must be repeatedly re-established. This process is continuous, not least in view of new discoveries, the significance and weighting of which must be determined in the context of the statutory objectives. It consists in a necessary balance of the interests of scientists who see the problem of cancer in terms of the different methodological approaches and give them different priority in the competition for financial resources. The benefit gained by scientists for the solution of their research problems from discussion and collaboration with a large number of experts from all fields relevant to cancer research in one center is exceedingly great and cannot be provided by any other form of organization.

The battle against cancer is one of the most important tasks of health policy and science in our time. The exceedingly complex problems of cancer research and cancer control touch on many fields of biological sciences, natural sciences and social sciences. They can be approached with prospects of success only by close collaboration of scientists from all these disciplines on a national and international level and by the concentration of available research capacities.

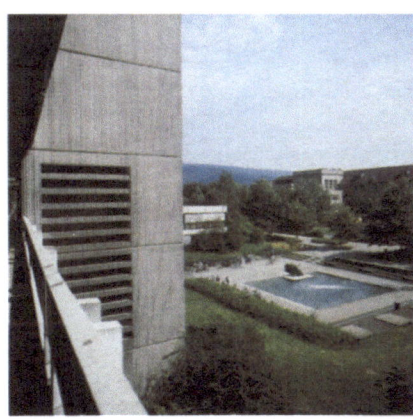

Fig. 5
The German Cancer Research Center is situated directly opposite the Surgery Division of the University Medical School. To the left of the Surgery Hospital is the Max Planck Institute of Medical Research, on the right the Pediatrics Hospital of the University Medical School, and on the other side of the Cancer Research Center are the Institutes for Theoretical Medicine of the University

The objective of the research program of the Deutsches Krebsforschungszentrum is to make major contributions to understanding carcinogenesis and to elaborating scientifically well-founded concepts of therapy. It is today assumed that there are more than 100 different types of cancer in man which can occur in individually different forms.

The program of the Center is concentrated on four multidisciplinary focal points, taking into account the diversity of methods and conceptual approaches in cancer research:

– tumor biology,
– mechanisms of carcinogenesis,
– carcinogenic factors and cancer prevention,
– diagnosis and therapy research.

This problem-oriented research program is worked on in eight scientific institutes which are all accommodated "under one roof".

Research

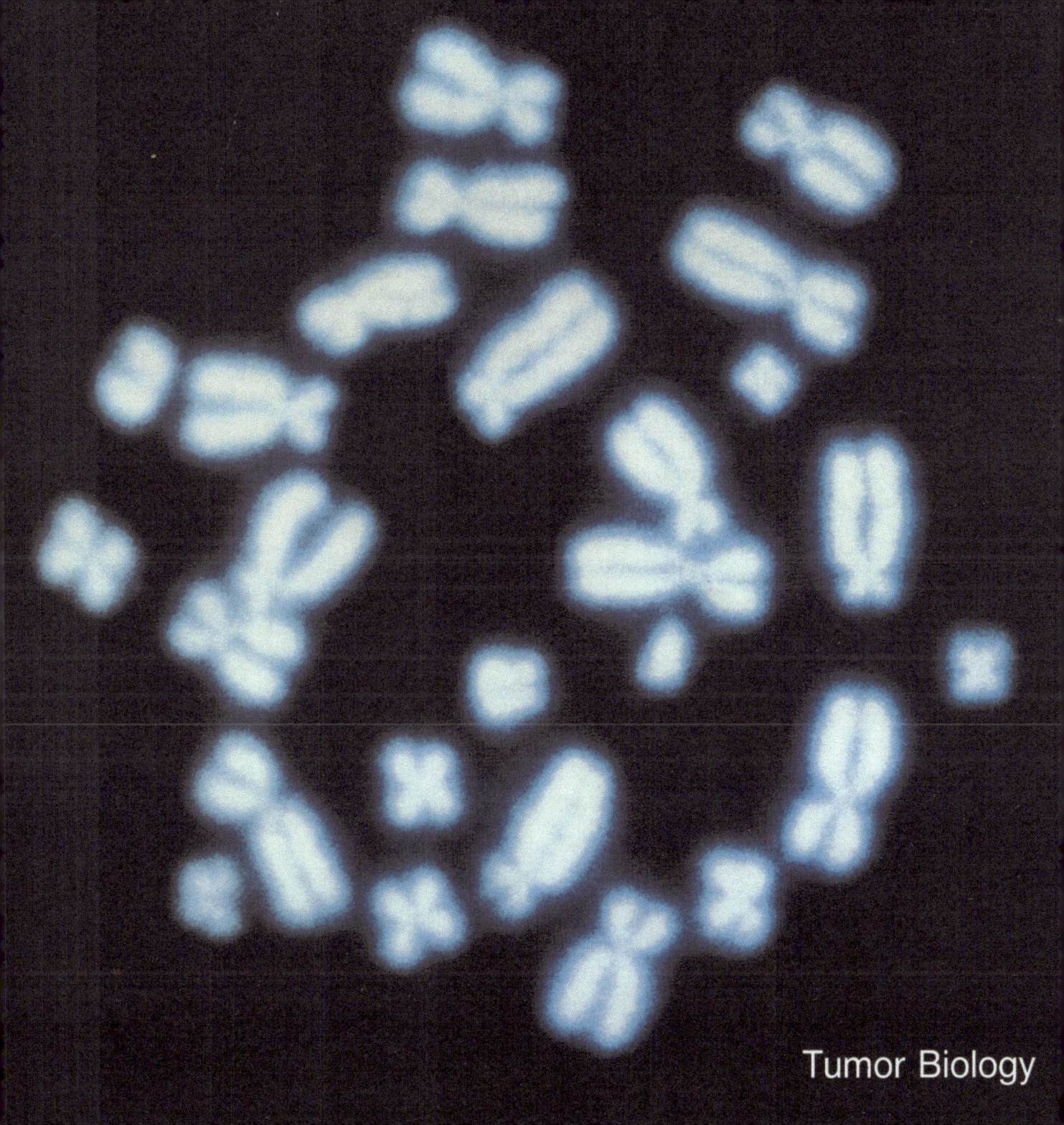

Tumor Biology

# 2

# Tumor Biology

Even if all cancer risk factors in the environment could be identified, it will never be possible to eliminate them completely. Even if the rate can be reduced, there will always be a certain incidence of cancer.

Since cancer will thus not be entirely avoidable despite all precautionary measures, cancer research requires methods which can reliably and specifically inhibit the growth of tumor cells in the body, or therapeutic measures by which these cells can be killed. A major problem is the fact that, apart from their uninhibited growth and their "unresponsiveness" to the control signals of the host body, tumor cells do not differ appreciably from "normal" cells. Crude attacks by chemotherapy and irradiation will (almost) always also affect normal cells. Moreover, tumor cells can evade

the therapeutic attack owing to their astonishing flexibility (development of resistance) and thus gain a lead over normal cells in the competition for survival.

In view of this, cellular and molecular biologists as well as immunologists are challenged to explore and define the existing fine differences between tumor cells and normal cells so that new approaches to diagnosis and therapy can be developed. This line of research entails an option for the future. No one can know today which of the new approaches will permit a fundamental break-through.

Fig. 6a

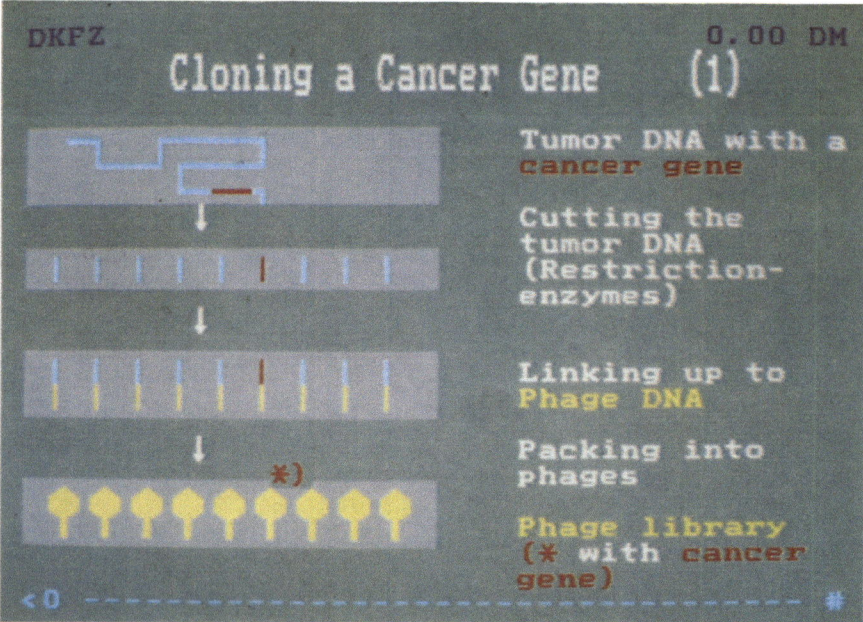

The main activities of scientists in the Deutsches Krebsforschungszentrum concentrated on the field of "tumor biology" can be defined as follows:

## New Insights Into the Structure and Function of Cells

In relation to the complexity of the structures and functions of the cell, we are in the situation of a pupil at an elementary school who wants to grasp the information contained in a huge library. The moral of this analogy is that we must get to know more, i. e., to stick to the metaphor, we must attempt to understand at least some books in the library. In concrete terms, parts of the cell (proteins, nucleic acid molecules, membrane complexes, etc.) must be analysed and their structural and functional significance recognized. To this end, it is sometimes useful to have recourse to simpler systems (unicells, frog eggs, fungi, etc.) in order to explore in the simpler model the principles which are then to be rediscovered in an identical or different form in the human cell. With regard to the problem of cancer, this research is focused on functions and structures which may entail possible differences between normal and transformed cells: organization of genetic information in the cell nucleus, apparatus of cell division, cell surface structures.

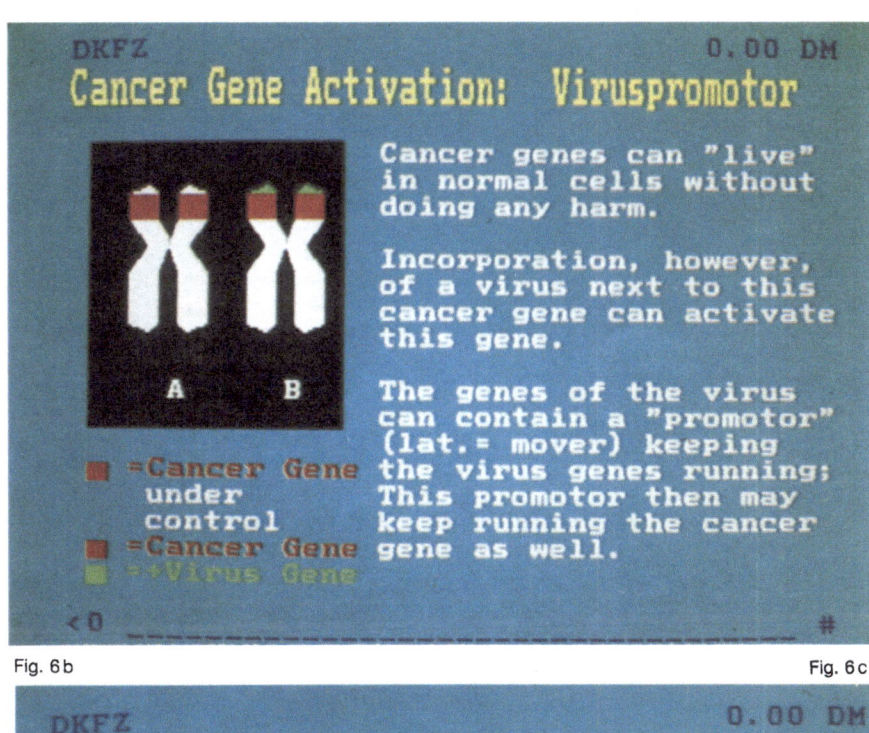

Fig. 6b

Fig. 6c

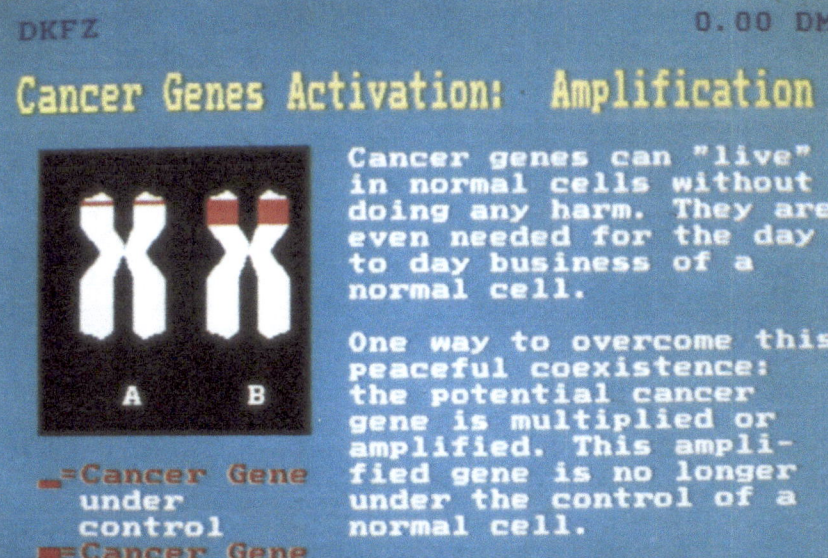

21

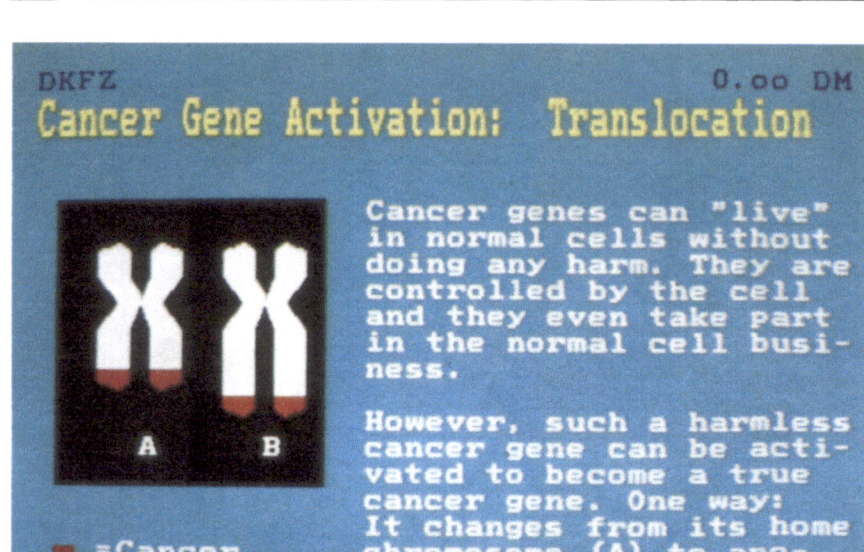

DKFZ                    0.oo DM
**Cancer Gene Activation:  Translocation**

Cancer genes can "live" in normal cells without doing any harm. They are controlled by the cell and they even take part in the normal cell business.

However, such a harmless cancer gene can be activated to become a true cancer gene. One way: It changes from its home chromosome (A) to another one (B). In its new position it is no longer under control.

■ =Cancer Gene

< 0                                    #

Fig. 6 d                                    Fig. 6 e

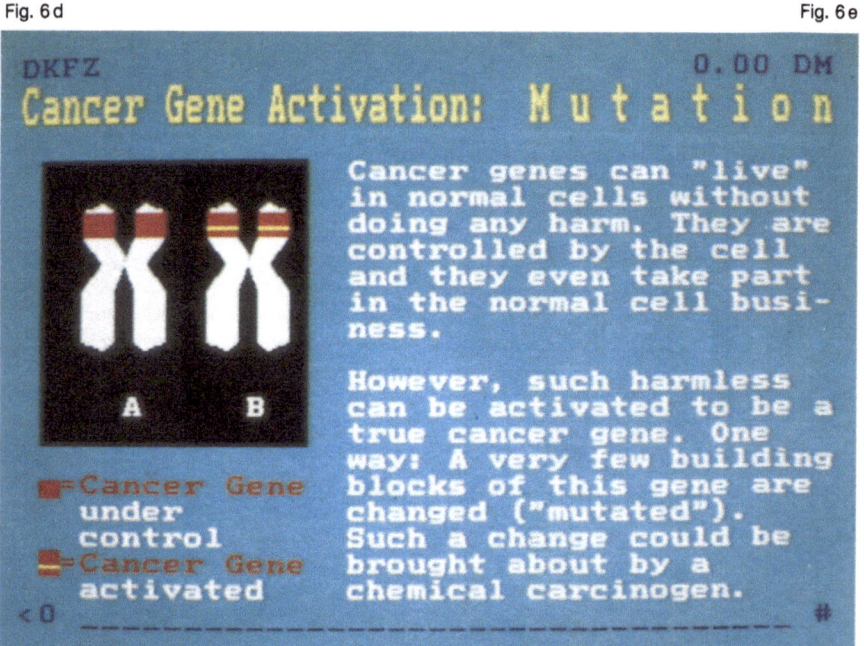

DKFZ                    0.oo DM
**Cancer Gene Activation:  M u t a t i o n**

Cancer genes can "live" in normal cells without doing any harm. They are controlled by the cell and they even take part in the normal cell business.

However, such harmless can be activated to be a true cancer gene. One way: A very few building blocks of this gene are changed ("mutated"). Such a change could be brought about by a chemical carcinogen.

■ =Cancer Gene under control
■ =Cancer Gene activated

< 0                                    #

## Regulation of Gene Expression

Any alteration of the properties of a cell is conditioned by switching a series of genes on or off. Accordingly, the transformation of a normal cell into a degenerated cell must at least be accompanied by or is very probably due to a change in genetic expression, i. e. a different pattern of genes is active in the tumor cell. By means of molecular biological methods, it is possible today to locate altered or activated genes and to investigate their significance in malignant transformation (transformation into cancer). If it should turn out to be the case that such genes (also termed oncogenes) cause the transformation, it is theoretically conceivable that these might be specifically switched off or their expression neutralized. Since every gene is expressed via the insertion of a messenger model (messenger RNA) and molecular biology is familiar with methods of preparing specific anti-messenger RNA, the neutralization of certain messages by anti-messages is not an utopian concept.

## Ultrasensitive Probes

It is possible today to prepare molecules against any given biological substructure (monoclonal antibodies) which can identify and localize the substructure with extreme accuracy of fit. Such probes can already be used to identify certain cells in the human body. Once tumor cells have developed, they can be typed with regard to their tissue origin (as metastases of a tumor which is located in a certain tissue of the human body) by means of such probes and appropriately treated. Monoclonal antibodies against tumor-specific substructures loaded with radioactive material or toxins might in theory transport their deadly freight specifically to the tumor cells in an organism.

## Physiological Growth Regulation

All cells in a body are subject to an extremely complex system of regulation by growth or inhibitory factors. As a consequence of this system, the cells which are destroyed daily by injuries, attrition and other processes of wear and tear are replaced by new cells. This changing of the guard occurs with enormous precision: exactly the same number of cells are always supplied as have been lost by cell death. Cell divisions are only admissible in accordance with an exact timetable. In this concert of regulatory factors, tumor cells are at least partially "unresponsive"; however, there are indications that tumor cells receive quite specific regulatory signals. If it were known how the system of phy-siological growth control functions or what the tumor cell "lacks" in order to receive these signals in their full bandwidth, it is conceivable that such defects could be compensated (e. g., by excessive administration of the factor). There are already indications that the code of physiological (i. e. tissue-specific) regulation can be "cracked".

## Approaches to Immunotherapy

By nature, the tumor cell is part of the respective organism. It is, therefore, not recognized by the latter as fundamentally "foreign" and is accordingly not rejected by the immune system. However, it is conceivable in principle that the tumor cells can be modified in such a way that they are recognized as "foreign" by the immune system. Conversely, it is conceivable that the immune system can be manipulated in such a way that it already reacts to the tiniest differences between tumor cells and normal cells. A great deal of work in fundamental research is required before one of these concepts can be applied in practice.

## Metastatic Growth and Invasion

A tumor cell, which has merely escaped growth control, is not by any means always already potentially fatal. However, tumors always become malignant when they succeed in infiltrating healthy adjacent tissue (invasion) or become established as metastases in tissues far removed from the site of origin (metastatic spread). The analysis of why and how tumor cells migrate might help in developing therapeutic strategies in order to stop this potentially fatal step in the development of a tumor.

Fig. 7

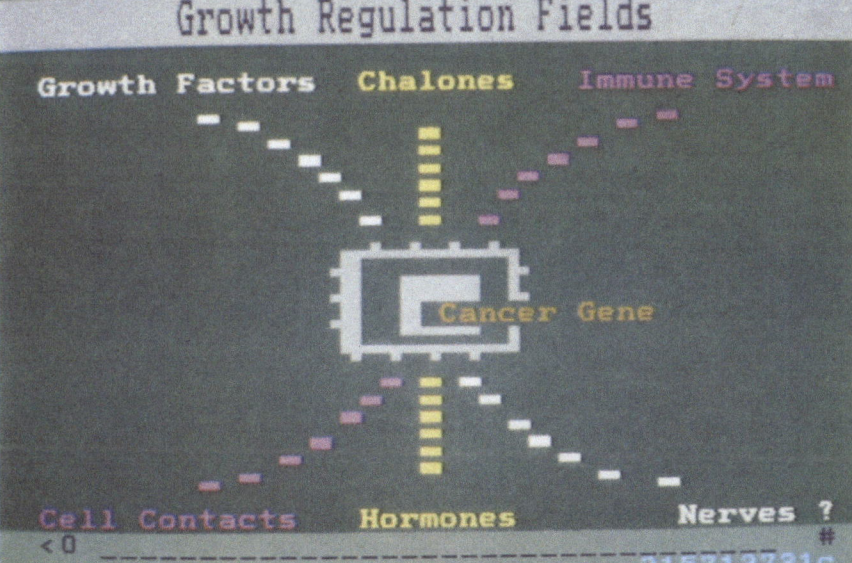

## Research Activities Focused on Tumor Biology

Chromatin structure and gene regulation

Tumor banks

Sessile macrophages with cellular resistance ("instant defense")

Protein kinase and substrate on the surface of human cells

Bioregulation of the catalytic subunit cAMP-dependent protein kinase

Physicochemical and molecular genetic characterization of chromosomes of experimental tumor cells (CATES)

Cellular control mechanisms in cell devision

Model trials on the problems of invasion and metastatic spread

Cytoskeleton and karyoskeleton of normal and transformed cells for tumor diagnostics (basis of tumor diagnosis with antibodies against cell type-specific proteins)

Membranes and redox components of the mammary gland and breast tumors

Structure and function of chromatins: mechanisms of gene activity and regulatory interventions

Characterization of transcription units and transcription products in lampbrush chromosomes

Relatedness, formation and functions of plasma membrane-associated electron transport systems in animal cells

Interaction of proteins of intermediate filaments with other cell constituents

Correlation of DNA sequence and chromatin structure of primary transcription units

Involvement of mitotic $Ca^{++}$-ATPase in intracellular $Ca^{++}$ regulation; application of monoclonal antibodies

Control of gene function by steroid hormones

Development of eukaryotic vectors

Cloning of messenger RNA for preproneurophysins I and II

Structure and expression of chicken lysozyme genes

Expression of the genes for tryptophan oxygenase and tyrosine aminotransferase after transfer into homologous and heterologous cells

In vivo expression of modified lysozyme genes

Regulation of transcription in dictyostelium

Correlation and structure of the dictyostelium genes

Transcription of messenger RNA in vitro and in vivo

Structure and functions of the achromatinized cell nucleus

Genome alterations of mutated tumor cells

Mechanism of mitosis

Localization of the binding sites of cytostatics on tubulin, testing of a photoreactive derivative for possible therapeutic use

Growth and organization behavior of transformed epidermal cells

Regulation of differentiation of keratinocytes in culture

Cytogenetics of skin carcinoma cells

Structure of viral and cellular chromatin

Characterization of immunologically significant membrane antigens (tumor antigens, histocompatibility antigens, differentiation antigens) on malignant tumors

Antitumor immune responses as the basis for antimetastatic immunotherapy

Investigations on the mechanism of metastasis

Cancer cells and basement membrane

The physiological basis of "immunogenicity" in cytostatic reactions

The influence of persistent antigen contact on the T cell repertoire

Biological, biochemical, molecular biological and genetic analysis of the lympho-kins, their receptors and target cells in mice and humans

Tumor growth and histocompatibility antigens

Structure of immune response antigens

Receptors on T lymphocytes

Function of the main histocompatibility antigens

Identification of antigens of the main histocompatibility complex

Development of computer-oriented techniques for application in molecular biology

Mathematical-statistical analysis of cell biology experiments

Elaboration and further development of statistical software (nonstandard software)

## 2.1 Molecular Biological Methods – Motor of Progress in Cancer Research

by Werner Franke

The widespread perplexity of the public and the often distinctly articulated irritation that the great expense has still not led to a "solution of the cancer problem" or to general improvements for cancer patients – despite a profusion of research results and even partial successes in the diagnosis and therapy of cancer – is understandable. However, this disappointed expectation is based on a fundamental misunderstanding between the public and research to which many cancer researchers have themselves contributed. The goal of cancer research is the promotion of knowledge about the normal and degenerated cell, normal and degenerated tissue, healthy subjects and cancer patients, naturally associated with the well-founded hope that knowledge of practical value can be derived for healthy and diseased human beings. However, possible applicability can never be the a priori objective of research – i. e. research of the fundamentally unknown. This also applies to cancer research. Whoever puts pressure on research fields and researchers with an impatient anticipation and speculation, wanting to obtain results of practical significance at all costs is naturally exposed to the same risk as that entailed in the hectic support of alchemists in past centuries. One is easily susceptible to the charlatans who promise to supply useful results and solve practical problems quickly by shortcuts. Whoever wishes to have serious research, must be a patron of science and must himself be able to wait for results.

The patron (i. e. in our case the taxpayer) can and should expect that researchers promoted in this way be prepared to give their best and to submit to a control of their achievements.

First of all, I should like to postulate that, as in many fields of medical research, the present state of the art in cancer research does not allow the formulation of rationally structured "strategic" approaches to the solution of most problems. Neither does it reveal a coherent concept for the prevention and therapy of cancer diseases, apart from certain exceptions of some virus-induced cancer conditions. The reason for this is the still inadequate knowledge about the composition of living matter, in particular human cells and tissues, and the lack of understanding even of simple reactions and their regulation. It is especially problematic that we are not yet even able to estimate the extent of our ignorance. If one reads the research grant applications of cancer researchers from the 1960s (which would doubtless be very instructive, even if sometimes painful), one would have to conclude in many cases that the information available at that time was not only inadequate but frequently quite wrong. Our modern concepts in cancer research, as in biological medical research in general, are still on uncertain grounds, even if our ignorance is at a higher level, so that we ask ourselves questions today which we would not even have been able to conceive 20 years ago.

Secondly, I should like to assert that our knowledge of living matter has changed during the last decade to an extent without parallel in history. The increase in knowledge in the individual specialties is frequently a dribble, slow and sporadic. However, there are periods in which a certain discipline passes through a stormy phase when the increase of knowledge is like an avalanche, giving rise to new research directions and ever new hypotheses, a rather disordered process. We all know examples of such phases from the history of chemistry and physics. Biological knowledge, especially in cellular and molecular biology, is today passing through its "golden age". It is only now gradually becoming possible to describe and to understand life on a scientifically adequate level, i. e. as an interaction of cells and molecules. These abrupt advances in knowledge, as almost always in the history of natural sciences and medicine, are associated with the development of new methods, often not even especially spectacular methods. For example, it is all too easily forgotten that only the development of the light microscopical optics and the selective staining methods almost a century ago, which in retrospect does not seem to be very exciting, has enabled one of the most important advances in medicine, the systematic discovery of the causative agents of bacterial infections.

Let us reflect today on the revolutionary advances in knowledge which have occurred during the last decade. We only discovered in 1977 that the genes of our chromosomes do not have to be continuous, but are in many cases interrupted; that the synthesis of gene products not only requires correct reading of the information of the genetic material (the DNA), but likewise correct "splicing", i. e. the excision of fragments from the product of transcription (RNA) and joining together of the ends. We have learned that genes can alter their position, that certain genes can be selectively amplified, e. g., after induction by certain substances. It is only in this decade that we found the structure in which the genetic material is arranged in our cell nuclei, the nucleosomes. It is only in recent years that we learnt how protein molecules are channeled through membranes and how they are linked with carbohydrate chains. Astonishingly, the most frequent proteins of the cell plasma as well as of the cell nucleus have indeed only been detected in the last five years. More protein molecules have been discovered in the last two decades than in the entire previous history of science. Especially in cancer research, we have only learned in recent years that certain regions of the genetic material, which are commonly termed oncogens, may suffice to effect the change of a cell in the direction of tumorigenesis. On the other hand, it has also been found that even a cell, which has undergone malignant transformation, may be brought back under the control of the body and generates healthy tissue. And it is only in the last decade that two technical advances in methodology have been made which were never planned and not even guessed at. They did not only alter research but will doubtless become of great significance for medicine in future decades.

These are, on the one hand, the possibility of molecular cloning of DNA, i. e. isolating practically any desired piece of genetic information of whatever origin, of reproducing it in bacteria and thus isolating and propagating it with great purity and in whatever quantities desired and indeed re-introducing into other organisms. The other dramatic advance is the development of methods to immortalize cells which produce a certain antibody so that they can make this antibody available once and for all in a constant quality and purity. This unexpectedly rapid increase in knowledge of fundamental facts of life has made it clear to us how limited our earlier knowledge and how inadequate our methods have been. This personal experience of progress, which often leads to excitement among scientists, also gives us an idea of how fragmentary our present-day knowledge of the complexity of life still is. In order to illustrate this by an image, biology and thus in particular medicine is still in the phase of hunters and gatherers; planned agriculture is a phase which is still before us. I have never been able to and still cannot take it seriously when researchers, especially cancer researchers (with and without inverted commas), give rise to the impression in public that we now have sufficient fundamental knowledge to approach medical problems in a planned way, and that these will be solved if only sufficient money for research were available. This is not the case, and society is ill-advised to believe suggestions that a scientific break-through might be bought with money. This, of course, does not mean that cancer research does not need any money, but money is not everything and perhaps not even the most important factor.

I hope that I have made a sober contribution with regard to the "feasibility" and the possibility of planning research results. Nevertheless, I clearly hear two objections. The first is: But our patients are living today! The second: There are also other ways, short-cuts and approaches which are possibly less satisfying intellectually, but which can also achieve practical results. There is the empirical approach, the probing search, the "screening"! Both objections are justified. Cancer research today is a science in a dualistic dilemma. On the one hand, it must of necessity push forward into new fields of fundamental knowledge and apply new fundamental results to problems of cancer research. On the other hand, it must be expected that the cancer researcher will do everything in his power to make the new results of research available for practical application, if possible without delay. This applies to prophylaxis, diagnostics and therapy.

Incidentally, if one asks what is the difference between a cancer researcher and other basic researchers, for example a "pure" molecular biologist, then this exigency for the researcher himself appears to me to be the most important and distinctive feature. This kind of research is indeed something special: on the one hand, it requires fundamental exploration at the frontiers of knowledge, but on the other hand, it also requires personal endeavors to apply the results of research to benefit the health of patients: a double obligation which makes greater demands on the cancer researcher (also in terms of his personal effort) if he takes his function seriously. With regard to the problem of practical application of the results of fundamental research, there have been many changes for the better in recent years, especially in the field of molecular biology. To describe an example from my research field: a class of proteins, which was recognized as cell type-specific in 1978, was already being tested in clinical pathological tumor diagnostic trials in 1979 and 1980 and their use has become routine today in many centers and hospitals in the world. The discovery by the group of Professor zur Hausen that the presence of DNA of a certain virus is correlated at high frequency with the development of certain forms of cancer in the genital tract has likewise been applied diagnostically within a few years. I believe that a crucial process of learning on both sides (by the molecular biologists as well as by clinicians) has indeed taken place and is still doing so (by the way, this is by no means a simple process).

Molecular biologists and clinicians, often separated by different structures of thinking and preferences, have started to apply the results of research without delay for the benefit of patients.

The second objection rightly points out that many advances in medicine have not been achieved by coherent research oriented toward causal interrelationships, but by pure empiricism, by trial and error, by observations (often fortuitous observations) in the environment and at the bedside. For example, most of the cytostatic drugs used today have been found in this way. In order not to be misunderstood, I should like to observe that this empirical approach, "keeping one's eyes open" and "screening", is still justified today and will be in the near future so long as it subjects its findings and assertions to scientific investigation. Whoever cures is right, provided he can prove that he has indeed cured. Unfortunately, this "empirical approach" has also become the field of activity of cancer alchemists, including in the meantime an academically trained "demi-monde". It is an easy and popular step to look for salvation in the extracts from taiga roots collected under the full moon, or in the body rays of Madagascar lemur skins. And it is left to conventional science to prove the contrary.

Although the undirected search for carcinogenic substances on the one hand and therapeutic agents on the other hand is still indispensable at present, it must be observed that it is in principle an intellectually unsatisfactory method developed in the absence of better and more rational approaches. These probing and testing approaches must, therfore, be supplemented as soon as possible by specific strategies based on a better fundamental understanding of tu-

morigenesis and cancer growth, which it is to be hoped will replace them some day. There has thus been a fundamental change in the situation of cancer research in recent years, even if this has not yet yielded many practical results. We know today how a series of central questions as to the role of certain molecules is to be correctly posed and what methods are required to explore and answer these questions in relation to the sequence of events and building blocks. There is indeed some light at the end of a long tunnel. Moreover, this is the only light which we have in order to clarify processes in living matter and to prove them in the final analysis. We will finally be able to give the processes occurring in transformed and normal cells a molecular formulation, and these processes will thus also become accessible to experimental intervention and rational correction. In addition, we can no longer afford to dispense with molecular biological exploitation of living systems, not only in medicine, but also in other central questions of life and survival on this planet. Incidentally, this is an insight and a postulate which is shared by almost all nations engaged in research, irrespective of their political ideology. Molecular biology in cancer research as in other fields does not require any plea for promotion; it has no alternative.

Prof. Werner Franke, Ph.D.
Membrane Biology and Biochemistry,
Institute of Cell an Tumor Biology

## 2.2 The Effect of Organic Lead on the Cytoskeleton

by Hans-Peter Zimmermann

Environmental noxae can damage the genetic material, cause cancer or promote malignant growth. A series of suspected substances also includes triethyl lead, a decomposition product of the organic lead compound tetraethyl lead used as an antiknock agent in petrol. Tetraethyl lead is a relatively harmless substance which in itself is not injurious to cells, but which decomposes under the action of light and heat into the very much more stable, water-soluble cytotoxic triethyl lead.

Tetraethyl lead is also broken down in the body, primarily giving rise to triethyl lead. The main site for biotransformation of tetraethyl lead in the body is the liver. From there, the cytotoxic degradation product triethyl lead is distributed over the body and can also pass the blood/brain barrier. This is shown by investigations of subjects who died of an acute organic lead intoxication. High concentrations of triethyl lead were found in their brains. An explanation for this particular accumulation of triethyl lead in the brain and for nerve damage due to this substance could not be found so far.

We have concentrated our attention on the points of attack of triethyl lead in the cell and their molecular interaction with this organic lead compound. We found that the cytoskeleton (the skeletal structure of the cell consisting of various proteins) of all mammalian cells investigated, and especially that of the nerve cells, is destroyed by low concentrations of triethyl lead. Such damage is also found in the brain of persons who died of acute organic lead intoxication. The results of our experiments thus correspond to the effects of an acute organic lead intoxication in humans.

Fig. 8
Human fibroplasts in cell culture. Staining with fluorescent antibodies gives rise to fluorescence of the microtubules in the cells

Fig. 9
The fibroblasts were treated with small concentrations of triethyl lead and then stained. The microtubules were destroyed by the triethyl lead. Only the degradation products of the microtubules appear as a diffuse fluorescence in the cells

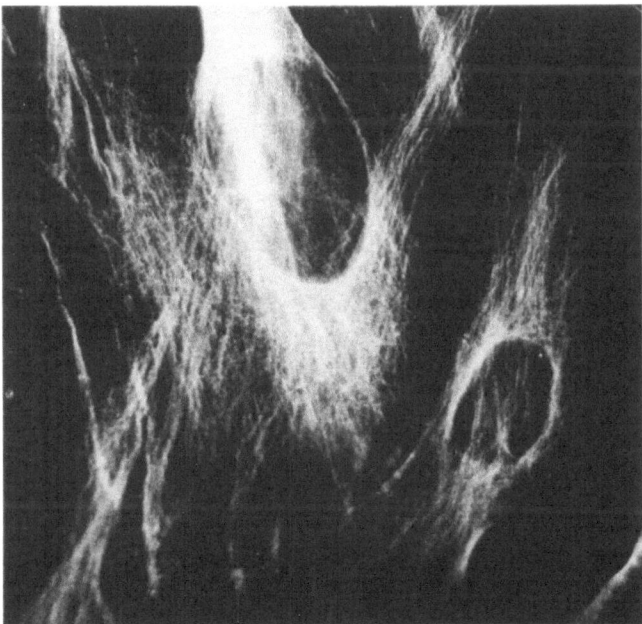

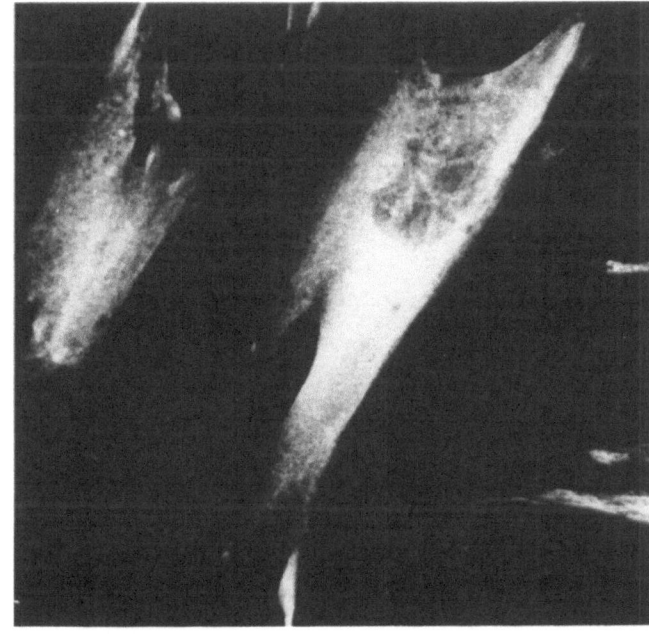

The skeleton of a cell consists of several components. In this structure, the microtubules (tubelike protein structures with an external diameter of about 25 nm (1 nm = 1000 millionth of a meter)) have a superordinate function. These structures are involved in vitally important cellular processes, for example the ordered distribution of genetic material to the daughter cells, intracellular transport mechanisms as well as endocytosis and exocytosis (channeling into and channeling out of substances in the cell). It must be mentioned here that transport processes involving the microtubules also occur in nerve cells. They have especially abundant microtubules.

We have found that triethyl lead acts on the microtubule system to a special extent. The structures are then completely destroyed, so that they can no longer carry out the functions described. Investigations in the test tube with tubulin, the protein which forms the microtubules, do not only show a complete destruction of the microtubules, but also the unrestricted inhibition of their reformation in the presence of triethyl lead. Corresponding findings were later on also made in living mammalian cells in tissue culture. We also clarified the molecular mechanism of the interaction between triethyl lead and the protein tubulin.

We are convinced that the interaction of triethyl lead with the tubulin/microtubule system of the cells is one of the factors responsible for the cytotoxic action of the substance.

New information shows that cell functions above and beyond the function of the microtubules are likewise inhibited by triethyl lead, e. g., the activity of the $Na^+/K^+$ ATPase, a catalytic protein of the cell membrane which is responsible for the vitally important exchange of sodium and potassium ions between the interior of the cell and the extracellular environment.

Fig. 10
The protein tubulin was isolated from porcine brain and reconstituted to microtubules in the test tube. The microtubules are to be seen after negative staining in the electron microscope as bright tubular structures

Fig. 11
Microtubules after short treatment with low concentrations of triethyl lead. Triethyl lead has destroyed the tubular structures. Their breakdown products are to be seen in the electron microscope as bright points which appear to be lined up like a string of beads

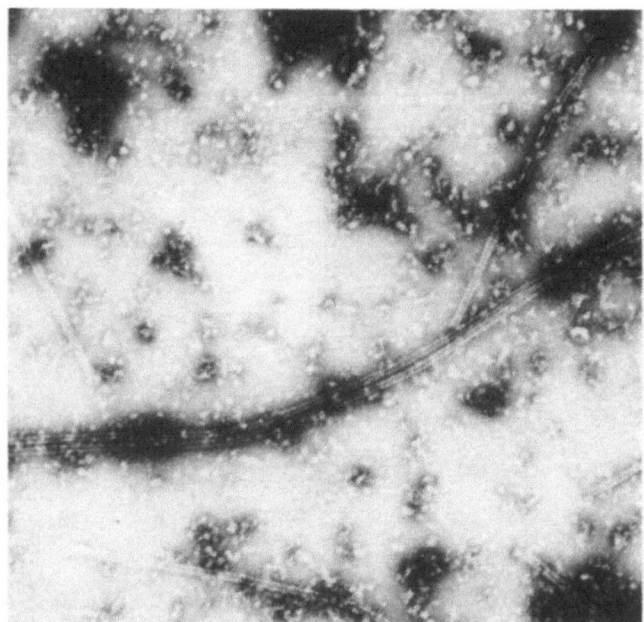
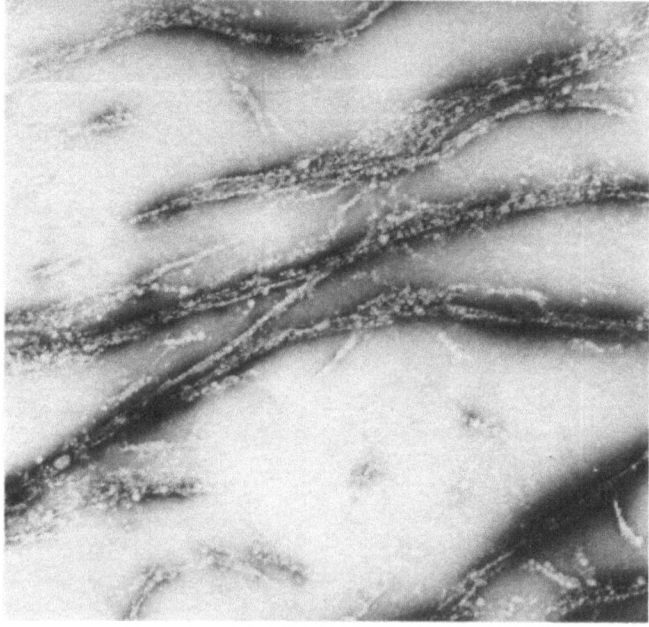

Further investigations are required to clarify unequivocally the extent to which triethyl lead is a carcinogenic or cancer-promoting substance. Recent information suggests this, but the chain of evidence does not yet appear to be complete.

Even on the basis of the available information, the environment should be freed from organic lead as far as possible. As shown here, organic lead compounds in low concentration can cause major damage in mammalian cells. At present, this does not allow any conclusions with regard to possible damage to the entire body. However, the high concentration of triethyl lead in the brains of subjects, who have died from an organic lead intoxication, and knowledge of the cell-damaging effect of this substance in experiments, make it necessary to carry out further investigations in the future which will provide an adequate basis for preventive measures.

Dr. Hans-Peter Zimmermann
Growth and Division of the Cell,
Institute of Cell and Tumor Biology

Participating staff

Joachim Buchholz
Dr. Karl Heinz Doenges
Sabine Mocikat

In collaboration with

Prof. Heinz Faulstich
Dr. Christos Stournaras
Department of Physiology,
Max Planck Institute of Medical Research, Heidelberg

Dr. Gerhard Röderer,
Botanic Institute
University of Hohenheim

Selected publications

Bolanowska, W., Piotrowski, J., Garzcynski, H.: Triethyl lead in the biological material in cases of acute tetraethyl lead poisoning. Arch. Toxicol. 22, 278–282 (1967).

Blumer, W., Reich, Th.: Bleibenzin und Krebsmortalität. Schweiz. med. Wschr. 106, 503–506 (1976).

Zimmermann, H.-P., Röderer, G., Doenges, K. H.: Influence of triethyl lead on the in vitro and in vivo assembly and disassembly of microtubules from mammalian cells. J. Submicrosc. Cytol. 16, 203–205 (1984).

Faulstich, H., Stournaras, C., Doenges, K. H., Zimmermann, H.-P.: The molecular mechanism of interaction of $Et_3Pb^+$ with tubulin. FEBS Lett. 174, 128–131 (1984).

Stournaras, C., Weber, G., Zimmermann, H.-P., Doenges, K. H., Faulstich, H.: High cytotoxicity and membrane permeability of $Et_3Pb^+$ in mammalian and plant cells. Cell Biochemistry and Function 2, 213–216 (1984).

Odenbro, A., Arrhenius, E.: Effects of triethyl lead chloride on hepatic N- and C-oxygenation of N,N-dimethylaniline in rats. Toxic. Appl. Pharmacol. 74, 357–363 (1984).

Grandjean, Ph. (ed.): Biological Effects of Organolead Compounds. CRC Press, Inc. (1984).

Zimmermann, H.-P., Doenges, K. H., Röderer, G.: Interaction of triethyl lead chloride with microtubules in vitro and in mammalian cells. Exp. Cell Res. 156, 140–152 (1985).

## 2.3 Control of Gene Activity by Steroid Hormones – Identification of the Site of Action in the Genetic Information

by Günther Schütz

Steroid hormones are chemical messenger substances which are secreted by endocrine cells, which reach their target cells via the blood circulation and alter the activity of the target cells. The sites of synthesis and action of steroids are thus separate from each other. Steroids play an important role in metabolism, in the differentiation and growth of cells and tissues in the body. Good examples of steroid-controlled complex regulatory processes are the development of secondary sexual characteristics, cyclic buildup and breakdown of the uterine mucosa and the regulation of the electrolyte and water balance, to mention only a few.

The effect of the steroid hormones on these extremely complex processes in the target cell arises in that the expression of genes is specifically switched on and off. The resulting alteration in the protein complement of the target cell constitutes the basis for the altered cell function. There is a double selectivity of the action: firstly, only certain cells are affected by the action of the hormone and, secondly, only a few genes are influenced in these cells.

The effect in the target cell does not occur directly, but is mediated by proteins, the receptors, which bind the steroids with high affinity and specificity. Only

target cells possess such receptor proteins which recognize with very great precision the minor chemical differences between the various steroid hormones. The most important steroid hormones in mammals (glucocorticoids, mineralocorticoids and the sex hormones androgens, gestagens and estrogens) each have a specific receptor which binds the hormone with high affinity. The interaction of the receptor with the hormone probably brings about a change in conformation of the receptor protein. The affinity of the hormone receptor for regulatory binding sites in the deoxyribonucleic acid (DNA) and on the chromatin is thereby increased, regulating the expression of certain genes (Fig. 12).

Fig. 12
Scheme of the mechanism of action of steroid hormones. The hormone (S) enters the cell by diffusion and binds to a receptor protein with high precision. The attachment of the hormone leads to the activated steroid-receptor complex. The complex binds to specific DNA sequences in the control region of hormone-regulated genes. The interaction of the complex with control sequences leads to increased gene expression

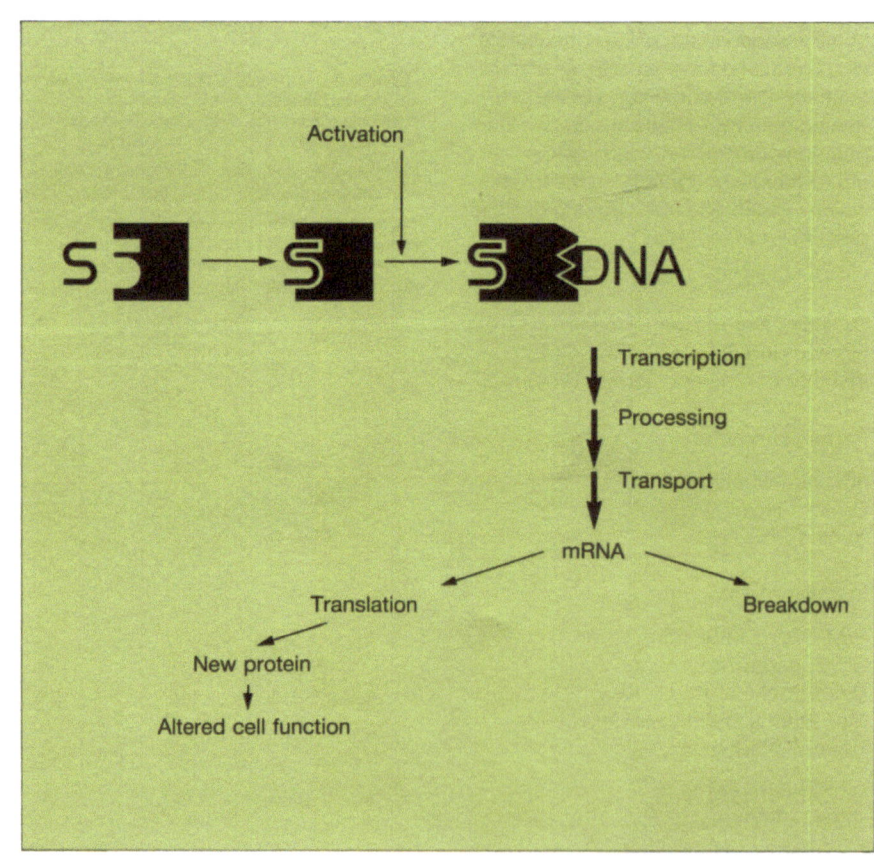

Whereas it has already been assumed for a long time that the binding of the hormone-receptor complex at specific sites in the chromatin regulates gene transcription, it was exceedingly difficult to identify such regulatory sequences and to elucidate their action.

Information on the switching-on and -off of genes is of crucial significance for our understanding of metabolic processes in the normal and transformed cell. The ability to introduce cloned DNA into eukaryotic cells has opened up a way of analyzing the expression of genes and clarifying the mode of action of signal structures, e. g. hormone control sequences. A cloned gene is introduced into animal cells, and the expression of the DNA and its control by steroid hormones is analysed. If hormone-dependent transcription is present, the gene can be specifically altered before transfer and the effect of such alterations on its expression can be investigated. By manipulation of the genes by means of the DNA recombination technique before their introduction into the cell, it is thus possible to identify control sequences which are important for individual steps in gene expression. This will be illustrated by the control of the expression of the chicken lysozyme gene by steroid hormones.

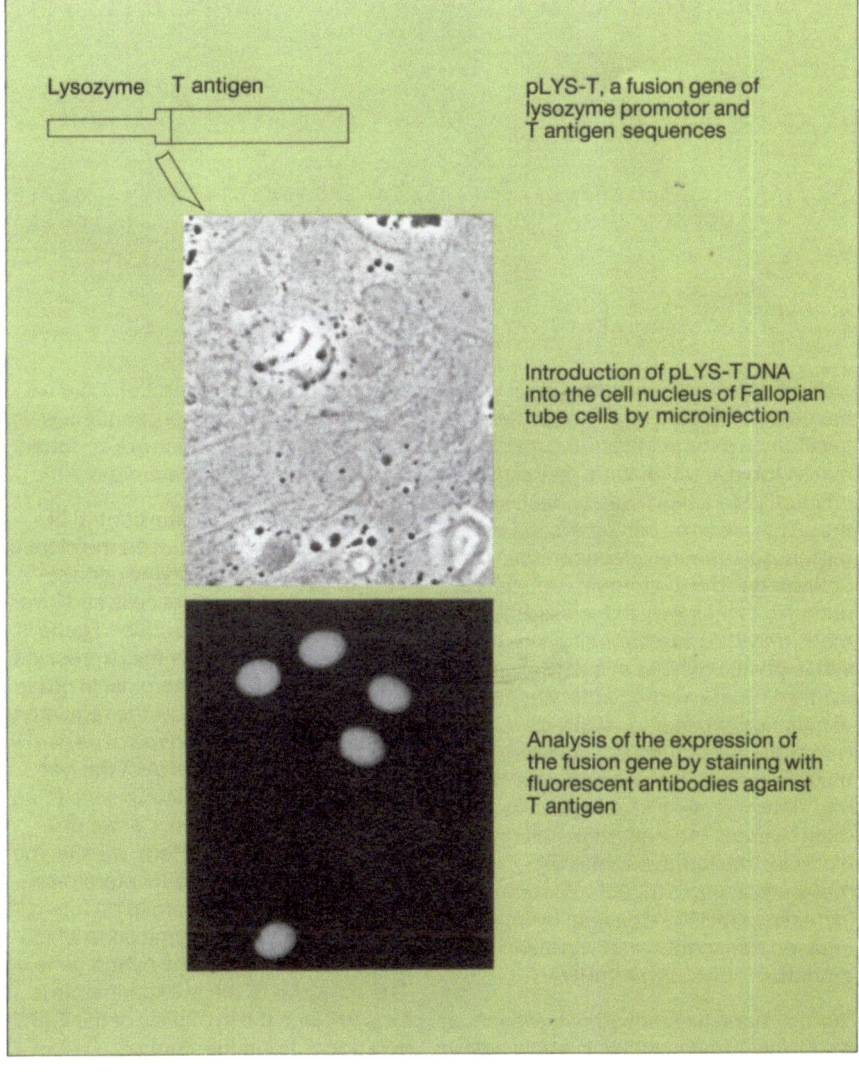

Lysozyme    T antigen

pLYS-T, a fusion gene of lysozyme promotor and T antigen sequences

Introduction of pLYS-T DNA into the cell nucleus of Fallopian tube cells by microinjection

Analysis of the expression of the fusion gene by staining with fluorescent antibodies against T antigen

Fig. 13
Functional test of the control region of the lysozyme gene. A fusion gene with the control sequences of the lysozyme gene before the SV40 T antigen as an indicator gene is introduced into the cell nucleus of primary oviduct cells by microinjection. The expression of the fusion gene is rendered visible by means of fluorescent antibodies against the T antigen. It is a measure for the function of the lysozyme control region

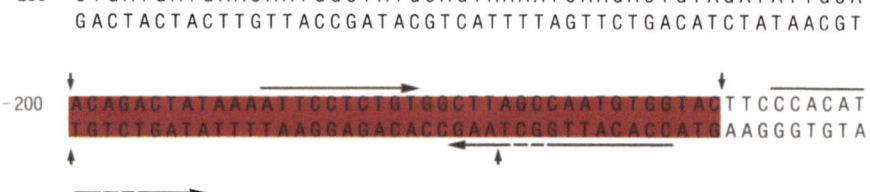

```
-250   CTGATGATGAACAATGGCTATGCAGTAAAATCAAGACTGTAGATATTGCA
       GACTACTACTTGTTACCGATACGTCATTTTAGTTCTGACATCTATAACGT


-200   ACAGACTATAAAATTCCTCTGTGGCTTAGCCAATGTGGTACTTCCCACAT
       TGTCTGATATTTTAAGGAGACACCGAATCGGTTACACCATGAAGGGTGTA


-150   TGTATAAGAAATTTGGCAAGTTTAGAGCAATGTTTGAAGTGTTGGGAAAT
       ACATATTCTTTAAACCGTTCAAATCTCGTTACAAACTTCACAACCCTTTA


-100   TTCTGTATACTCAAGAGGGCGTTTTTGACAACTGTAGAACAGAGGAATCA
       AAGACATATGAGTTCTCCCGCAAAAACTGTTGACATCTTGTCTCCTTAGT


-50    AAAGGGGGTGGGAGGAAGTTAAAAGAAGAGGCAGGTGCAAGAGAGCTTGC
       TTTCCCCCACCCTCCTTCAATTTTCTTCTCCGTCCACGTTCTCTCGAACG


+1     AGTCCCGCTGTGTGT
       TCAGGGCGACACACA
```

Fig. 14
The DNA sequence of the control region of the lysozyme gene is illustrated here. The figures relate to the starting point of transcription at +1, the short arrows mark the binding sites for the progesterone receptor (upper filament) and for the glucocorticoid receptor (lower filament). The long arrows point to repeat sequences, which are important for the function of the control region

Lysozyme is synthesized together with the other important eggwhite proteins (ovalbumin, ovomucoid and conalbumin) in the oviduct of birds. In the differentiated gland cell of the oviduct, synthesis of lysozyme can be elicited by estrogens, gestagens, glucocorticoids and androgens. These steroids each have a receptor of their own in the cell which binds only the corresponding steroid with high affinity. The raised lysozyme synthesis in the oviduct after steroid stimulation is based on a raised level of lysozyme messenger RNA (mRNA) in the oviduct cell. In the uninduced state, 5 to 10 lysozyme mRNA molecules are found per cell. After full stimulation with estradiol, the number of mRNA molecules rises to 30,000. This dramatic increase of mRNA is caused by an increased transcription and reduced degradation of lysozyme mRNA.

We ask ourselves how this elevation of lysozyme mRNA synthesis is achieved after hormone administration? Are we able to identify regulatory sequences in the lysozyme gene which are important for switching – on by steroids?

In order to investigate the control of transcription, we introduced the cloned lysozyme gene or lysozyme gene recombinants into oviduct cells and investigated whether the introduced gene is expressed and whether the expression can be influenced by steroids. In order to be able to easily follow the regulatory sequences of the lysozyme gene, we fused the 5'-flanking DNA of the lysozyme gene with an indicator gene (T antigen of the SV 40 virus), i. e. we produced a hybrid gene. Here, we assume that the control regions for steroid-dependent transcription are to be found in the region of the lysozyme gene which we incorporated into the hybrid gene. The objective of these experiments is thus to place the synthesis of the T antigen under hormone control.

The hybrid gene is introduced into the cell by microinjection, and its activity is determined by T antigen expression. The synthesis of the T antigen can be readily followed in the cell by means of fluorescent antibodies (Fig. 13). The synthesis of the viral protein under the control sequences of the lysozyme gene takes place hormone-dependently. The treatment of the cells with glucocorticoids and gestagens leads to an increased synthesis of T antigen. It is thus possible to identify the region within the lysozyme gene which is important for hormonal control.

Fig. 15
High-resolution sequencer gels serve for the exact determination of the site at which the hormone receptors bind to the DNA

We have altered the DNA in the test tube and investigated what effects these alterations have on hormone-controlled expression. In this way, we were able to determine the minimal region which is important for the effect of the hormone. We were able to show that the first 200 base pairs in the immediate vicinity of the lysozyme gene are sufficient to enable hormone-controlled expression.

In collaboration with the group of Miguel Beato, University of Marburg, we attempted to identify binding sites for the hormone receptor complex in this region. Can binding sites for the steroid receptors be found in the region which we have characterized as the control sequence? Is the region identified in the gene transfer experiments the binding site for the progesterone or glucocorticoid receptor? By analysing the binding of the purified progesterone and glucocorticoid receptor on specific fragments of the lysozyme gene, binding sites could be identified which are selectively recognized by the hormone receptor complex. We find two binding sites in each case. It is surprising that the progesterone receptor complex and the glucocorticoid receptor complex bind to the same DNA regions (Fig. 14).

We can conclude from these results that steroid hormone receptors bind at specific sites of the lysozyme gene and that the interaction with these sequences is of crucial importance for the expression of the gene. If the receptor or the binding site for the hormone-receptor complex is lacking, the lysozyme gene is inactive.

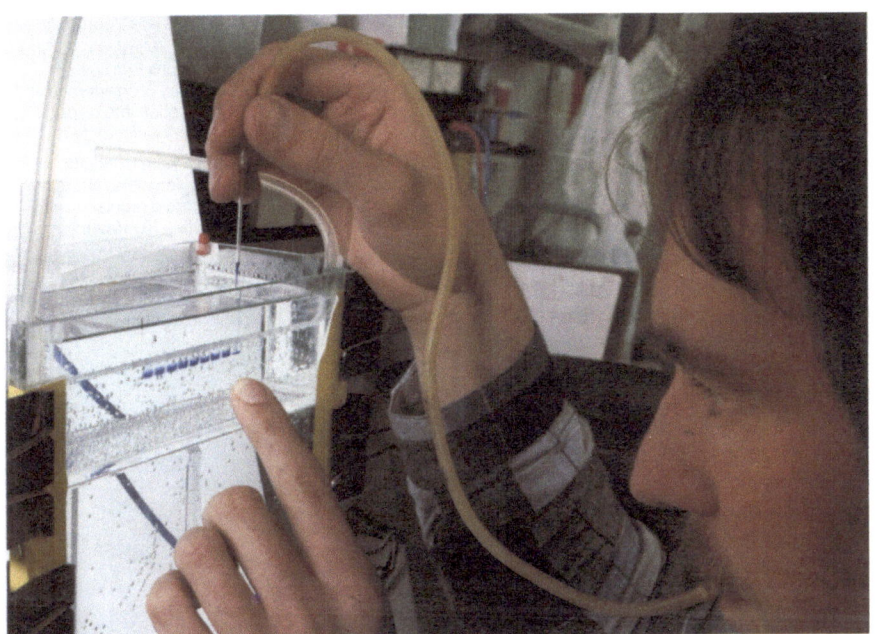

Fig. 16

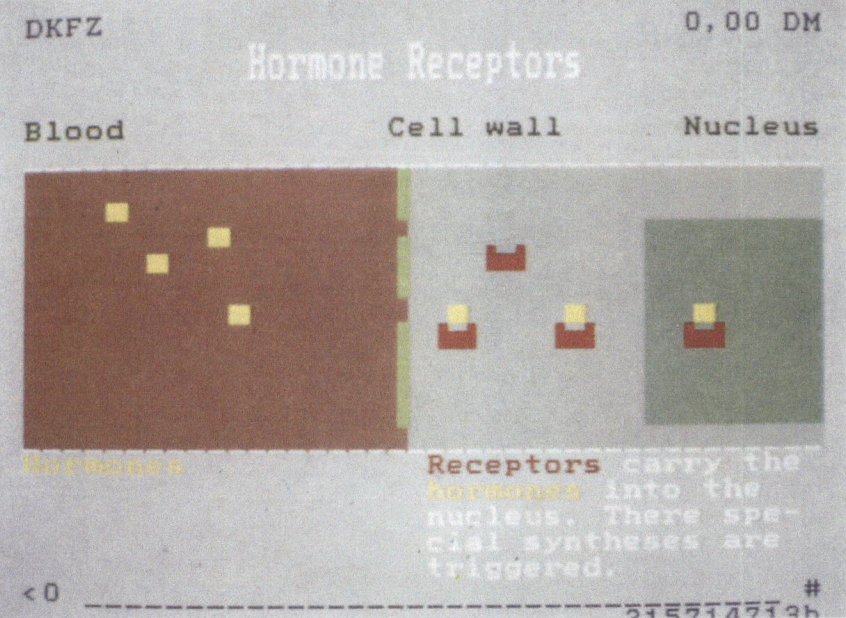

At the moment, we are investigating the mechanism by which the binding of the hormone receptors to these sequences leads to switching on the transcription of the lysozyme gene.

The results of these investigations are significant for our understanding of the molecular basis of the activity of genes and their regulation in the normal and transformed cell. Knowledge of the mechanisms of gene regulation is a necessary precondition for understanding carcinogenesis on the molecular level. Analysis of the mode of action of hormones shows how important functions of the target cell (e. g., cell division, cell differentiation) can be altered by the regulation of gene expression.

Prof. Günther Schütz
Molecular Biology of the Cell,
Institute of Cell and Tumor Biology

Participating staff

Dr. Waltraud Albert
Bruno Luckow
Dr. Richard Miksicek
Dr. Reiner Renkawitz

In collaboration with

Dietmar von der Ahe
Dr. Miguel Beato
Institute for Physiological Chemistry,
University of Marburg

Selected publications

Renkawitz, R., Beug, H., Graf, T., Matthias, P., Grez, M., Schütz, G.: Expression of a chicken lysozyme recombinant gene is regulated by progesterone and dexamethasone after microinjection into oviduct cells. Cell 31, 167–176 (1982).

Renkawitz, R., Schütz, G., v. d. Ahe, D., Beato, M.: Sequences in the promoter region of the chicken lysozyme gene required for steroid regulation and receptor binding. Cell 37, 503–510 (1984).

v. d. Ahe, D., Janich, S., Scheidereit, C., Renkawitz, R., Schütz, G., Beato, M.: Glucocorticoid and progesterone receptors bind to the same sites in two hormonally-regulated promoters. Nature 313, 706–709 (1985).

## 2.4 Chromatin, its Structure and its Function

By Ulrich Scheer

The genetic information, which is laid down as a linear sequence (DNA) of the cell nucleus, is essentially identical in all cells of an organism. Nevertheless, the expression of the genetic information of the individual cell types may be very different. Cell differentiation is lastly based on the activity of different genes in different cell types. Only little is known so far about the fundamental mechanisms regulating such genetic programs. However, it is known that the type of packing of DNA with histones and nonhistone proteins to form chromatin plays a major role in gene expression and that the sequence-specific attachment of proteins as regulatory factors to the DNA specifically modulates the activity of the genes. The investigations described here have the objective of demonstrating the role of chromatin in the regulation of gene expression in the course of cell differentiation in order to render dysregulated differentiation processes, which lead to transformation of normal cells into cancer cells, understandable.

Chromatin is a collective term which comprises the various forms of material in the chromosomes. In molecular biology, in the strict sense, chromatin is the term used to designate the genetic material of the cells, the deoxyribonucleic acid, in its biochemically and structurally well-defined nuclear protein packing complexes which come into being by the attachment of specific nuclear proteins, above all histones.

On the chromatin, the complex chain of action of gene expression begins with the transcription of functional DNA regions or genes into ribonucleic acid (RNA) molecules. The fundamental sequence of gene expression, which comprises all processes from reading the genetic information to the synthesis of the protein products of the genes, is the same in all eukariotic cells.

The transcription of the DNA located in the cell nucleus into precursors of messenger RNA (mRNA) is brought about by specific enzymes, the RNA polymerases. During or after its synthesis, this RNA is processed; thus, for example, the ends of the molecule are modified, sequences are cut out, and the ends are joined up again; certain proteins are attached and thus form compact RNA-protein complexes. After being locked out through the pores of the nuclear membrane, the messenger RNA molecules attach to ribosomes of the cytoplasm and thus transfer to the cellular apparatus for protein synthesis a copy of the genetic information which directs the synthesis of specific proteins (translation).

Other genes in turn code for RNA molecules which are never translated

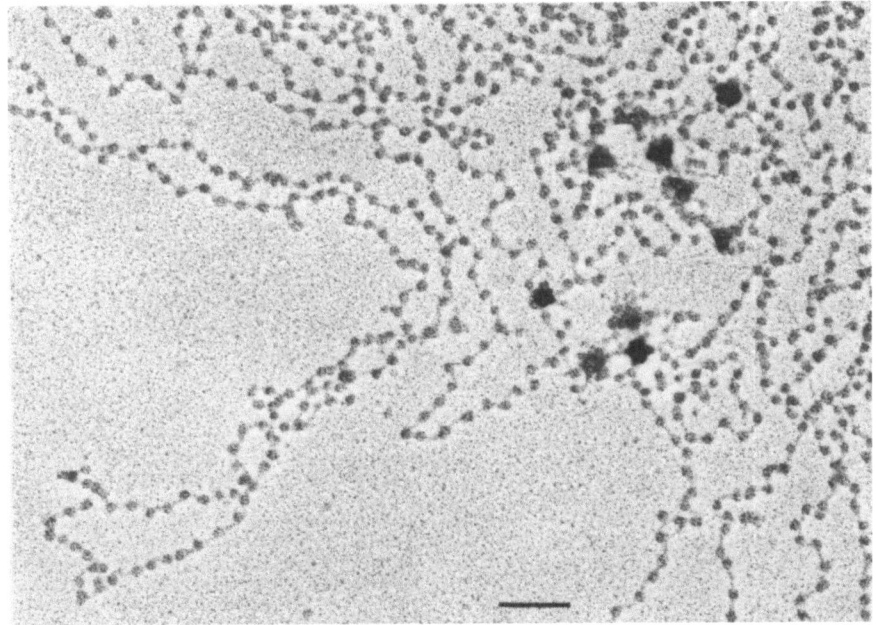

Fig. 17
Human cell (HeLa) with transcriptionally inactive chromatin which is arranged in nucleosomal "string of beads" structures. At some sites, local condensations of the chromatin filaments are seen. Scale calibration = 0.1 μm

into proteins, but which have other functions: examples are the transfer RNAs and ribosomal RNAs. The latter class of RNA is a structural and functional element of the ribosomes.

Chromatin can be demonstrated in the electron microscope by a "spreading technique" introduced by the American cell biologist Oscar Miller. The particular significance of this method is that the transcription of genes can be directly visualized. One thus obtains fundamentally important information on the size of genes or transcription units (from which the size of the primary RNA transcription products can be derived), their arrangement in the genome, the structure of active and inactive chromatin regions and the specific transcriptional status of genes.

The objective of the studies described here is, on the one hand, to define the genetic content of transcription units (e. g., by "in situ hybridization") and, on the other hand, to investigate the biochemical composition of active genes (e. g., by localization with antibodies against certain proteins). The discovery of differences of a biochemical and structural nature between genetically active and inactive chromatin regions provides us with indications about fundamental regulation principles which play a role in the selective transcription of the genome and thus finally regulate cell differentiation and cell transformation, i. e. the transformation of a cell into a tumor cell.

## Inactive Chromatin

In the electron microscope, the major proportion of the chromatin appears as linear chains of globular or discoid subunits, the nucleosomes. This is the case irrespective of whether the chromatin has been isolated from human, animal or plant cell nuclei. The nucleosomes consist of defined DNA-histone complexes and constitute the elementary packing unit of DNA in the chromatin. In the living cell, the nucleosome chains are further condensed to the chromosomes which can already be recognized under the light microscope and which can be observed, e. g., in dividing cells.

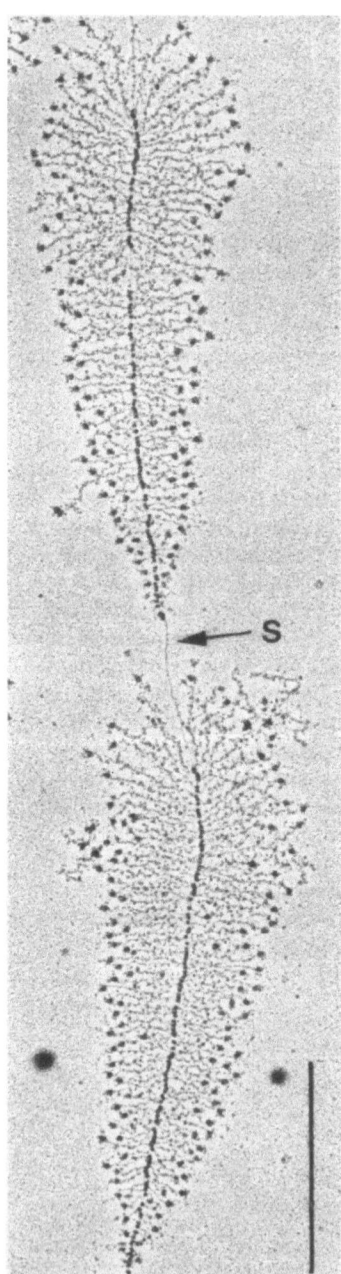

Fig. 18
Transcriptionally active ribosomal RNA genes of a salamander. Each "christmas tree" structure constitutes an active gene which is read simultaneously by numerous densely packed RNA polymerases. The lateral fibrils contain the growing RNA chains. The genes are separated by spacer (S) chromatin which has a smooth, non-nucleosomal organization. Scale calibration = 1 µm

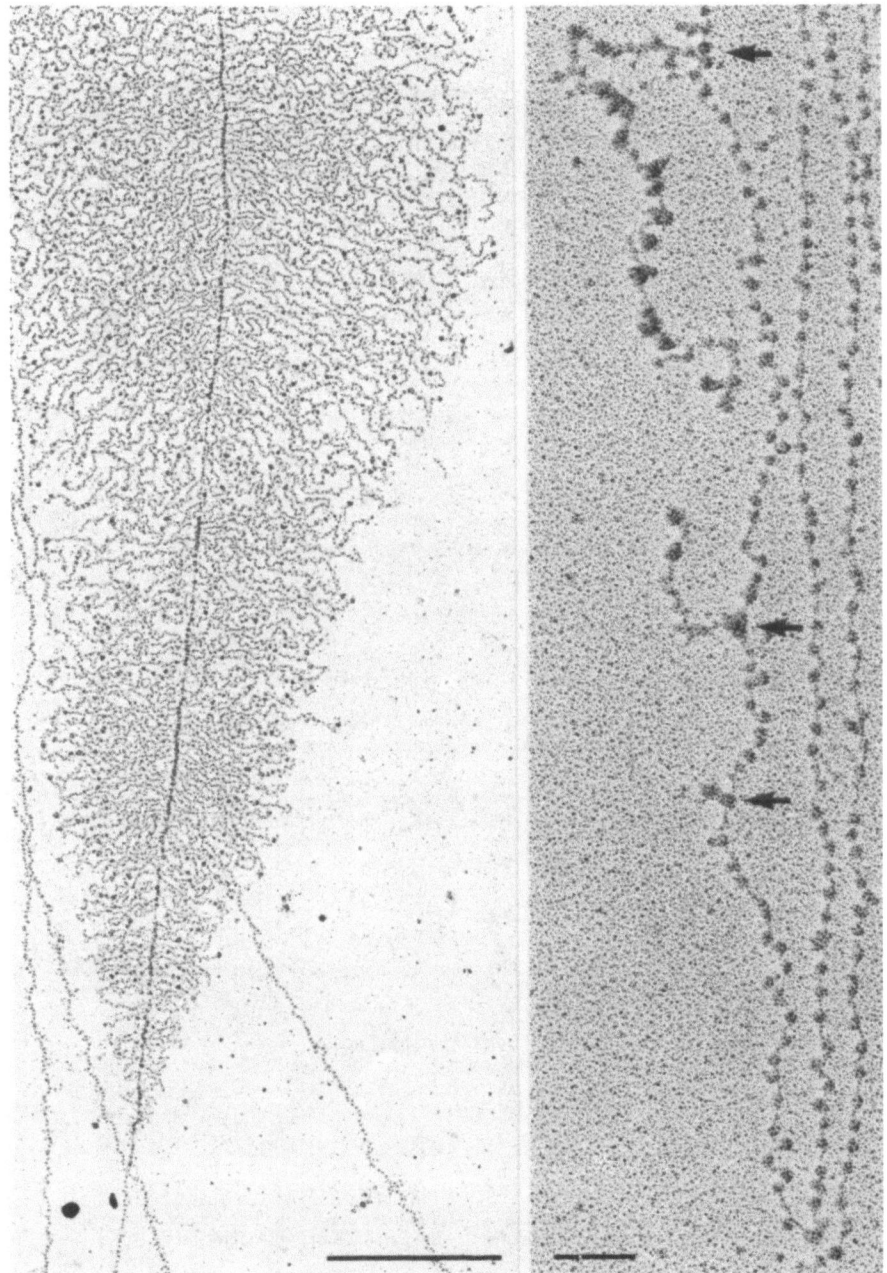

## Active Chromatin

Since the actual process of transcription can be visualized directly in the electron microscope, one can refer unequivocally to active chromatin regions. An active RNA polymerase molecule appears as a globular particle with a diameter of about 15 nm (1 nm = 1000 millionth of a meter), which is located on the chromatin axis and bears a fibril extending laterally to varying lengths. Such a lateral fibril contains the growing RNA chain and RNA-binding proteins. Depending on the state of activity of the specific gene, one recognizes only one or several or (as in the case of the highly active genes for ribosomal RNA (rRNA) in many cells), numerous lateral fibrils following each other in a close sequence. In such cases, the direction of reading the RNA polymerases is indicated by the increase in length of the lateral fibrils. The sites of initiation and termination of the polymerases can be unequivocally located at the beginning and end of a "Christmas tree" structure.

Fig. 19
Protein genes in various activity states. The picture on the left shows the initial region of a highly active gene from a lampbrush chromosome of a salamander. The picture on the right shows an only moderately active gene (three transcription complexes are indicated by arrows) from a cultured cell of Xenopus laevis with a distinct nucleosomal string of beads pattern. Scale calibration = 1 μm (left picture) and 0.1 μm (right picture)

Active rRNA genes, which usually occur in a few hundred copies in the nucleoli (nuclear bodies) of each cell nucleus and which can be easily recognized due to their tandem arrangement and their high transcription activity, are present in a non-nucleosomal packing state: their chromatin axis has a distinctly different arrangement from the string-of-beads structure of inactive chromatin. This also applies to the regions situated between the genes which are mostly not transcribed (spacers). Our investigations have shown that the transition to this non-nucleosomal and largely unfolded chromatin arrangement is the first recognizable structural alteration in the course of the activation of rRNA genes and precedes the actual transcription.

Transcription units of protein genes vary greatly in length; the heterogenous size distribution of their primary products, i. e. the molecules for the precursors of messenger RNAs, the "heterogenous nuclear RNAs", follows from this. As a rule, they only occur singly and without a discernible spatial pattern and with variable polarity along a chromatin strand. Whereas these genes only contain a moderate density of lateral fibrils in most cases, there are a few noteworthy exceptions such as the puffs of the "giant chromosomes" from the salivary glands of some insects and the lateral loops of the "lampbrush chromosomes" of certain plants and animals. Here, protein genes likewise display an almost maximal packing density with RNA polymerases. In such highly active states, the chromatin is once more in a largely unfolded, non-nucleosomal state. In states of reduced transcription activity, however, in contrast to the situation in rRNA genes, a transient folding back of the gene chromatin into the nucleosom-

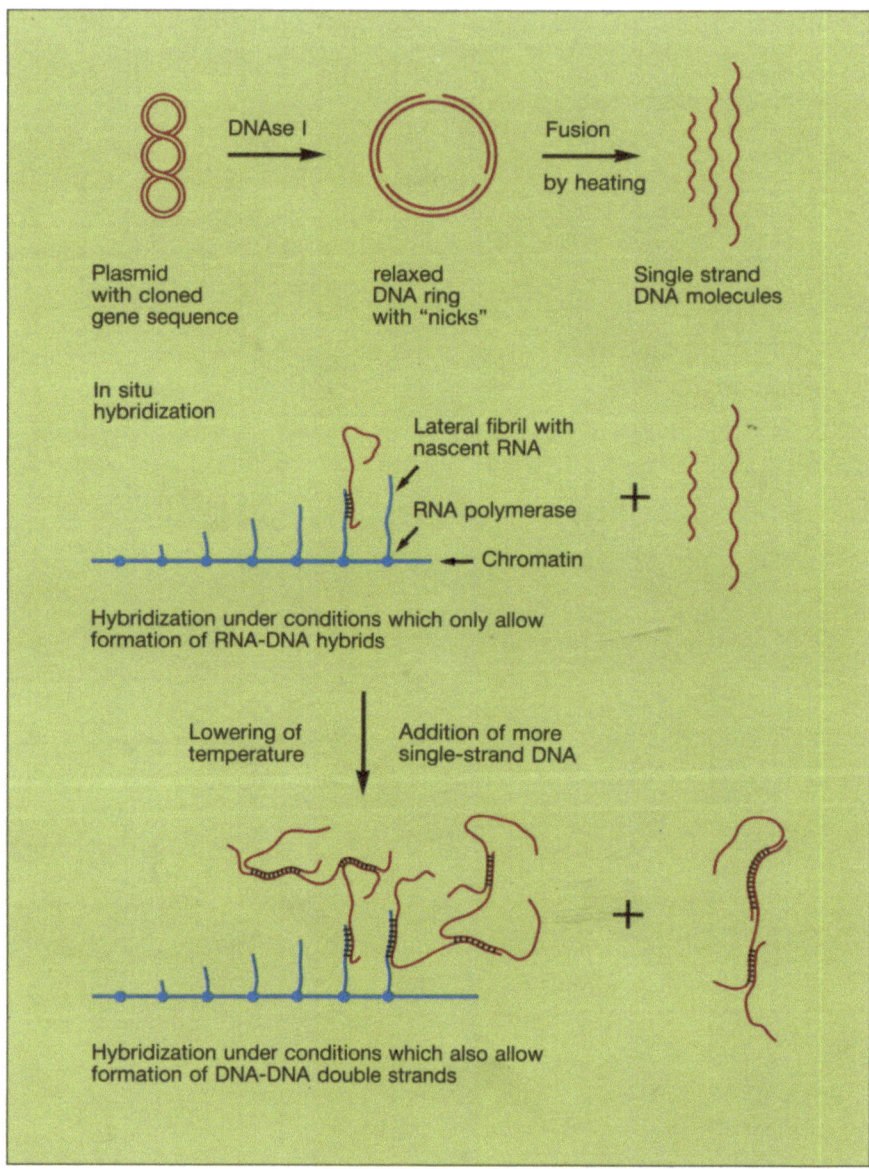

Fig. 20
Schematic representation of an "in situ hybridization" on electron microscopic squash preparations.

The method described here has the advantage that the DNA sample is rendered directly visible due to the formation of large aggregate tufts

al form may occur between two subsequent transcription processes. In the electron microscopic representation, a scattered arrangement of lateral fibrils is discerned; their sites of attachment are separated by regions of the chromatin axis with the characteristic string-of-beads structure.

Fig. 21
Example of an "in situ hybridization" for the identification of active genes under the electron microscope. The specific hybridization of cloned rDNA (arrows) on the lateral fibrils of an rRNA gene is shown here. Scale calibration = 0.5 µm

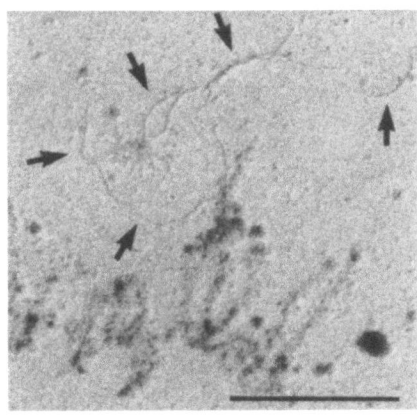

## Identification of Active Genes

The use of methods from genetic engineering allows the production of gene-specific DNA or RNA molecules which can be used to track down the corresponding genes or gene products.

In order to be able to identify active genes (i. e. transcription units) unequivocally, we employ the method of "in situ hybridization" on spread chromatin preparations. By using rRNA genes, we are able to show that cloned DNA molecules containing ribosomal sequences bind specifically to the lateral fibrils of the rRNA genes and form DNA-RNA hybrids (Fig. 21; for a graphic representation, see the scheme of Fig. 20). By use of these methods, we expect that we will be able to identify transcription units of specific genes and visualize them directly in the near future.

## Proteins of Active Chromatin Regions

The biochemical composition of chromatin in various functional states can be investigated by means of electron microscopic immunolocalization, using specific antibodies. For the visualization of antibodies in the electron microscope, they are bound to colloidal gold particles with a diameter of 5 to 20 nm; these appear in the electron microscope as small black granules. The highly active "lampbrush chromosomes" of amphibian oocytes, which have been mentioned, offer an especially favorable model object. For example, antibodies against histone proteins allow these proteins to be demonstrated on transcriptionally active chromatin regions, although these regions are normally not folded into nucleosomal particles. Antibodies against specific RNA

packing proteins in turn show that the pre-mRNA chains being formed are folded into linearly arranged globular RNA-protein complexes immediately after their synthesis, i. e. in the direct vicinity of the RNA polymerase. This method now opens up the possibility of investigating the biochemical composition of transcriptionally active genes at a high level of resolution by use of a variety of antibodies. For example, in this way we were able to demonstrate on nascent lateral fibrils the existence of certain ribonucleoprotein particles (snRNPs), which play an important role in the splicing of precursor mRNA molecules.

Quite a different experimental approach to elucidating the function of certain chromatin constituents is the microinjection of antibodies against chromatin proteins directly into the cell nucleus of living cells. We investigated whether antibodies introduced "on site" inhibit or modify the process of gene expression by specific binding to these proteins.

This is indeed the case: antibodies against histone H2B, certain non-histone proteins (HMG-1, HMG-14/17) and RNA polymerase II inhibit the transcription of protein genes in the living cell, an indication that these proteins are functionally linked with active chromatin regions.

Moreover, by means of the microinjection technique, we were able to show for the first time that a widespread protein present in a high concentration in the cell nucleus, actin, likewise plays a role in processes of transcription in the living cell.

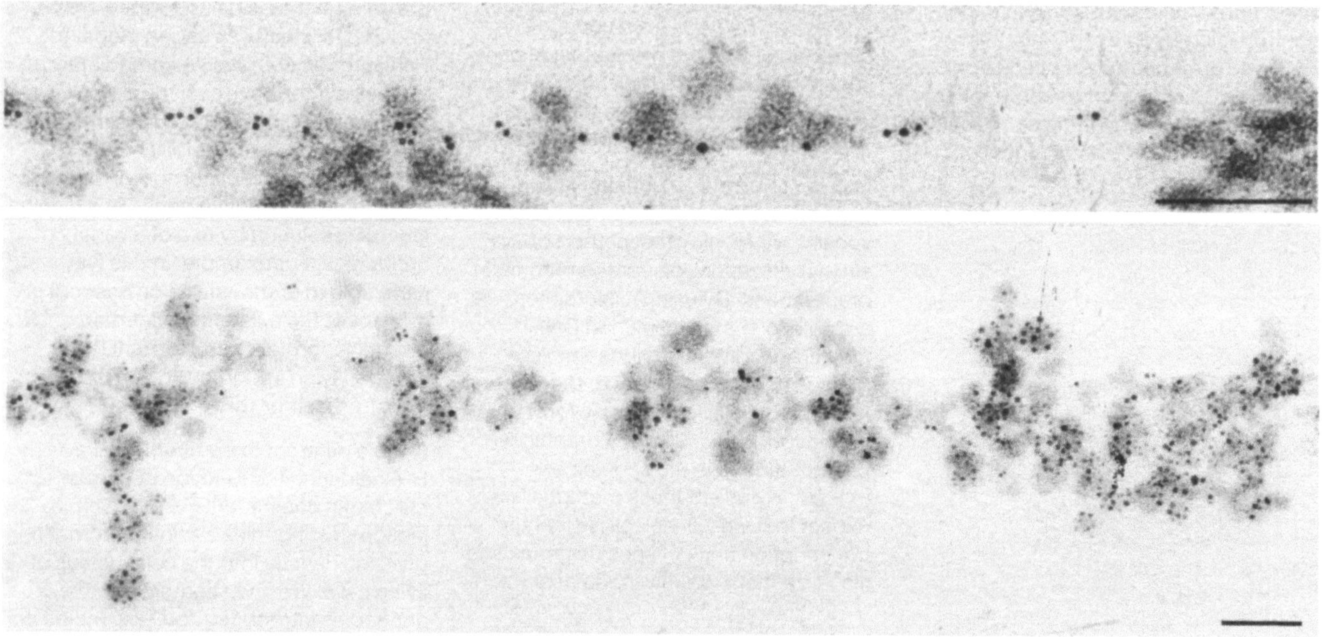

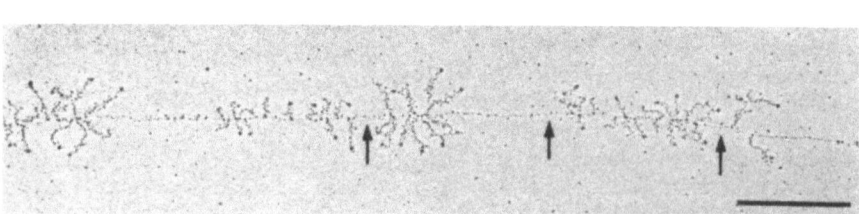

## Molecular Action of Cytostatics

A series of drugs of clinical importance as cytostatics inhibit transcription by intercalation into the DNA molecule. Their action can be directly followed in the electron microscope: shortly after addition of drugs such as actinomycin D or adriamycin to cells, there is a dramatic decrease of the number of lateral fibrils per gene.

Depending on the drug concentration and the duration of its action, transcrip-

tion finally comes to a complete standstill: all lateral fibrils are now shed and the gene chromatin now displays the typical nucleosomal organization of inactive chromatin.

It can often only be inferred with difficulty from biochemical data whether a drug influences transcriptional or subsequent post-transcriptional processes. Electron microscopic analysis of spread chromatin allows a definite decision to be made in this regard.

Fig. 22
Electron microscopic immunolocalization of chromatin proteins. Both pictures show transcribed chromatin regions of lampbrush chromosomes after incubation with antibodies against histone H2B (upper picture) and RNA packing proteins (lower picture). The antibodies have been rendered visible by conjugation to colloidal gold particles (5 nm diameter) (black dots). Histones are located exclusively on the chromatin axis (upper picture), and the RNA packing proteins only on the developing RNP transcripts (lower picture). Scale calibrations = 0.1 μm

Fig. 23
Inactivation of rRNA genes by addition of the cytostatic actinomycin D to the cells: the number of lateral fibrils is already greatly reduced. Some resulting gene gaps are marked by arrows. Scale calibration = 1 μm

## Principles of Order in the Cell Nucleus?

By using the rRNA genes as a model system we have studied the question as to whether functionally active genes occur in a defined topological arrangement within the cell nucleus.

Since this class of genes (and only this class) is read by type I RNA polymerase, antibodies against this polymerase provide a highly specific means of localizing transcriptionally active rRNA genes.

By means of immunofluorescence microscopy and immune electron microscopy, we were able to show that the rRNA genes are located closely together in certain structural components (the "fibrillar centers") of the nucleoli. However, this typical spatial arrangement of the rRNA genes is abolished after experimental interference with maturation processes of the pre-rRNA. An addition of the inhibitory drug DRB (5,6-dichloro-1-β-D-ribofuranosylbenzimidazole), an analogue of the natural nucleic acid building block adenosine, does not interfere with transcription of the rRNA genes but leads, within a few hours, to an unfolding of the nucleoli with a dramatic spatial redistribution of the rRNA genes which now fill almost the entire interior of the nucleus. This effect can be completely reversed after re-

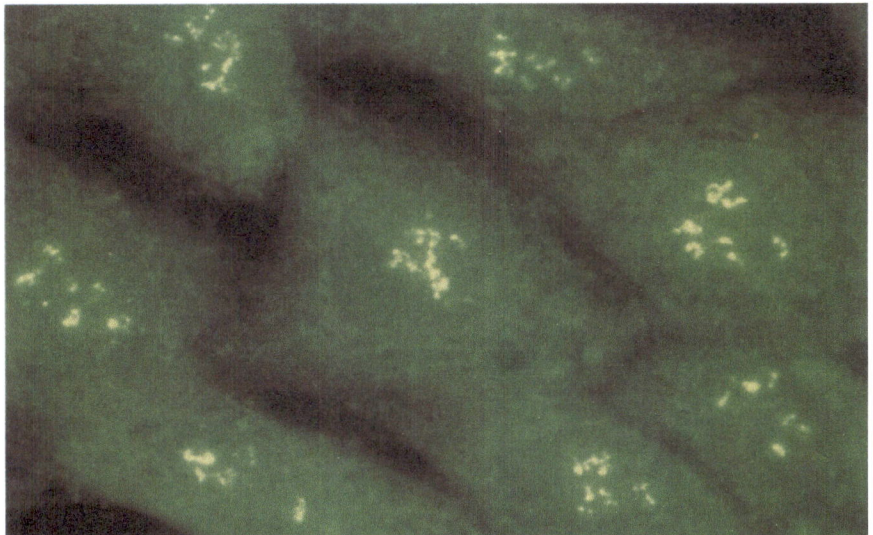

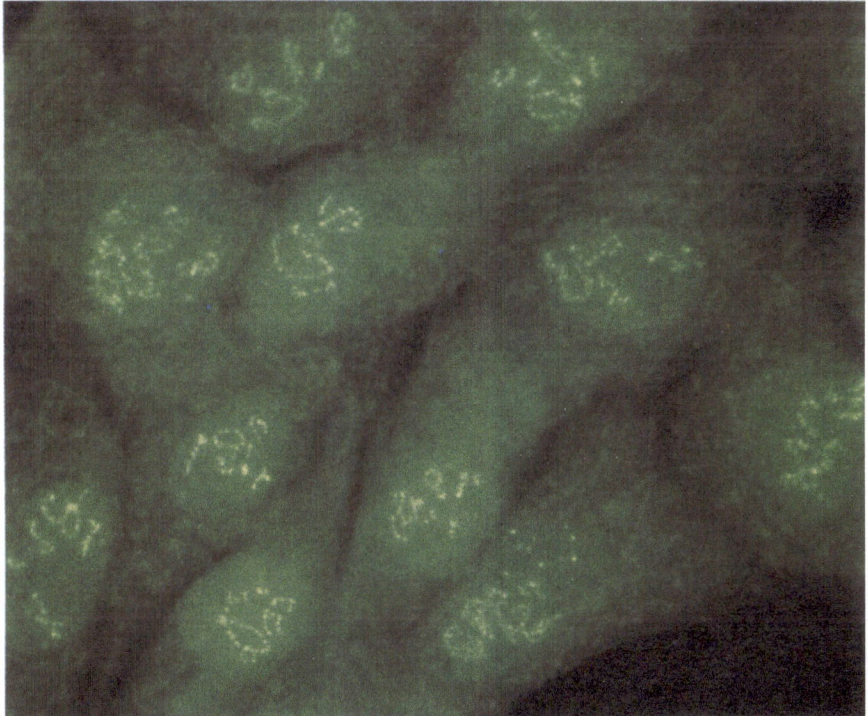

Fig. 24
Localization of active ribosomal RNA genes in cultivated rat cells by immunofluorescence microscopy. Antibodies against RNA polymerase I were used.
Upper picture: in the normal state, the ribosomal RNA genes are densely packed together in the nucleoli.
Lower picture: six hours after addition of the adenosine analog DRB, there has been a great reduction of the density of the nucleoli and the ribosomal RNA genes now traverse the entire inner nucleus in the form of string of beads structures

moval of the drug. It illustrates that the processes of gene expression taking place in the nucleus require a certain topological arrangement of the components involved, here in the nucleoli.

The cell nucleus is thus not (as had been considered for a long time) a kind of bag in which the various constituents are contained in a disordered manner. On the contrary, it is a highly differentiated system with exact topological order in which certain functions are associated with certain structures. In the future, knowledge of these principles of order should enable us to observe disturbances in cellular processes such as they occur, for example, in carcinogenesis.

Priv. Doz. Dr. Ulrich Scheer
Membrane Biology and Biochemistry,
Institute of Cell and Tumor Biology

Scientists participating

Prof. Werner W. Franke

In collaboration with

Dr. Hanswalter Zentgraf
Electron Microscopy Working Group,
Institute of Virus Research

Prof. Ekkehard Bautz
Faculty of Biology,
Department of Molecular Genetics,
University of Heidelberg

Dr. Michael Bustin
National Institute of Health,
Bethesda, USA

Dr. Terence Martin
University of Chicago, USA

Dr. Kathleen Rose
University of Texas,
Houston, USA

Dr. John Sommerville
University of St. Andrews, Scotland

Selected publications

Scheer, U.: Changes of nucleosome frequency in nucleolar and non-nucleolar chromatin as a function of transcription: an electron microscopic study. Cell 13, 535–549 (1978).

Scheer, U., Sommerville, J., Bustin, M.: Injected histone antibodies interfere with transcription of lampbrush chromosome loops in oocytes of Pleurodeles. J. Cell Sci. 40, 1–20 (1979).

Gall, J. G., Stephenson, E. C., Erba, H. P., Diaz, M. O., Barsacchi-Pilone, G.: Histone genes are located at the sphere loci of new lampbrush chromosomes. Chromosoma 84, 159–171 (1981).

Bona, M., Scheer, U., Bautz, E. K. F.: Antibodies to RNA Polymerase II (B) inhibit transcription in lampbrush chromosomes after microinjection into living amphibian oocytes. J. Mol. Biol. 151, 81–99 (1981).

Igo-Kemenes, T., Hörz, W., Zachau, H. G.: Chromatin. Ann. Rev. Biochem. 51, 89–121 (1982).

Scheer, U., Zentgraf, H.: Morphology of nucleolar chromatin in electron microscopic spread preparations. In: The Cell Nucleus, Vol. 11. H. Busch and L. Rothblum, eds., 143–176. Academic Press, New York (1982).

Scheer, U., Rose, K. M.: Localization of RNA polymerase I in interphase cells and mitotic chromosomes by light and electron microscopic immunocytochemistry. Proc. Natl. Acad. Sci. USA 81, 1431–1435 (1984).

Scheer, U., Hügle, B., Hazan, R., Rose, K. M.: Drug-induced dispersal of transcribed rRNA genes and transcriptional products: Immunolocalization and silver staining of different nucleolar components in rat cells treated with 5,6-dichloro-β-D-ribofuranosylbenzimidazole. J. Cell Biol. 99, 672–679 (1984).

Scheer, U., Hinssen, H., Franke, W. W., Jockusch, B. M.: Microinjection of actin-binding proteins and actin antibodies demonstrates involvement of nuclear actin in transcription of lampbrush chromosomes. Cell 39, 111–122 (1984).

Fig. 25

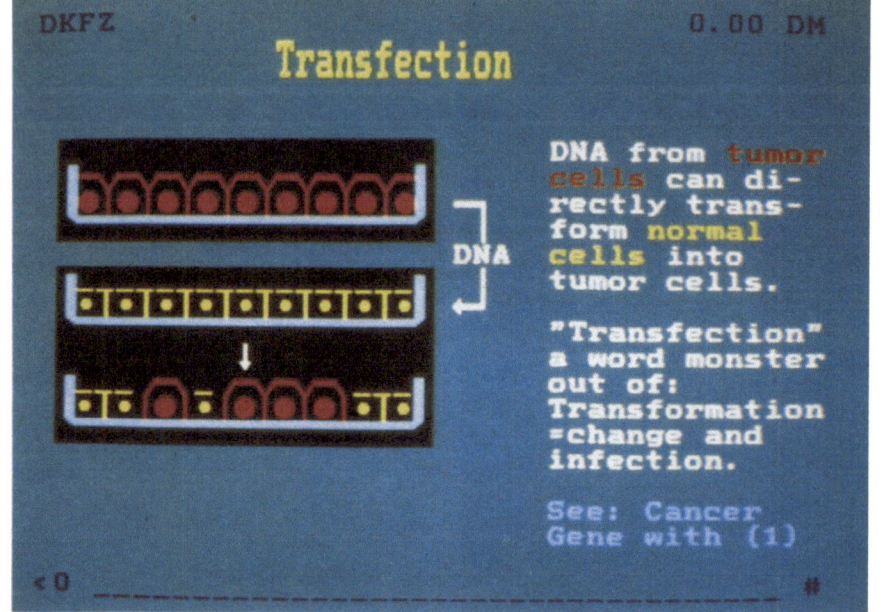

## 2.5 Generation of Metastatic Tumor Cells by Hybridization with Host Cells

by Volker Schirrmacher

The genetic mechanisms leading to the development of malignant tumor cells, which can form metastases, are still largely unknown. Many tumors do not present a uniform appearance. It has already been known for a long time that individual tumor cells of a single tumor can differ in properties such as growth rate, cell surface characteristics (antigenicity), sensitivity to drugs, etc. We have only known for a short time that individual cell groups of a given tumor are also different with regard to their capacity to form metastases. Only certain (especially malignant) subgroups of cells appear to be able to form metastases after transplantation into a suitable animal.

The genetic processes, which lead to the generation of such metastatic tumor cells or tumor cell variants, are still largely unknown. An important factor in the development of various properties and abilities of tumors appears to be the genetic instability of neoplastic cells. Indeed, this instability appears to increase with the progressive development of the tumor. It could thus be shown that metastatic tumor cells are more unstable than nonmetastatic tumor cells and possess a higher rate of mutation.

Metastatic clones (clone = homogenous cell line derived by division from a single initial cell) could, for example, develop drug-resistant variants at a higher rate than nonmetastatic clones. According to the most recent insights of George Poste, interactions between the tumor cell clones themselves may have a stabilizing effect. Such interactions are also of significance for the development of variants.

In view of the diversity of tumors and continuous, complex interactions between the tumor and the host body, it can be assumed that different mechanisms can lead to the development of metastatic variants. A possible mechanism of variant development, which will be specifically discussed here, consists in somatic cell hybridization.

### Somatic Cell Hybridization

The method of hybridization of normal cells (somatic cells) and tumor cells is frequently employed to study chromosomes or genes which are involved in the expression or suppression of properties of the cell and enable transformation of a normal cell into a malignant cell. The results show that in such hybrids the capacity for tumor growth is mostly suppressed, unless certain "suppressor chromosomes" in the normal cell are lost in the hybrid cells (by segregation). The same method can also be used in order to investigate chromosomes or genes which are of potential significance for other tumor properties, e. g., invasive growth and metastatic spreading. They hence open up a possibility for studying genetic control of properties which determine the malignancy of the tumor cell and are, therefore, of particular clinical significance. At the same time, somatic cell hybridization of tumors may also be a process which occurs in nature and which can lead to the generation of metastatic variants.

### Metastatic Spreading Requires Special Properties of the Tumor Cell

One of the objectives of experimental metastasis research is to define the specific properties of highly metastatic tumor cell variants, if possible down to the molecular level. The definition might be the basis for new approaches to the diagnosis and therapy of metastases. Certain cell surface properties as well as functional properties are regarded as especially important, e. g., the invasion capacity, the circulation behavior, the organ colonization capacity or the resistance to immune response mechanisms.

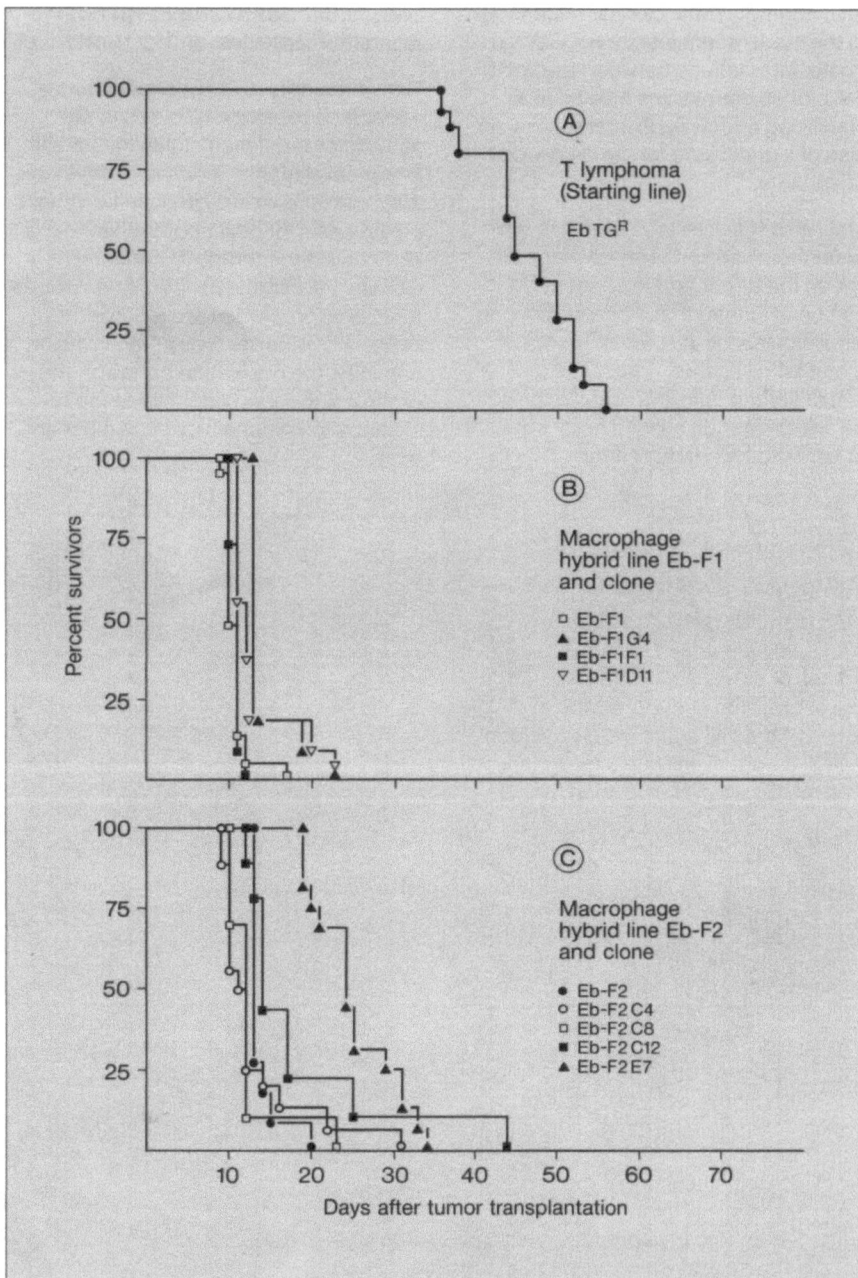

## By Hybridization with a Normal Cell, new Properties can be Transferred to Tumor Cells

By fusion of a tumor cell with an autologous host cell new properties can be transferred to the tumor cell. An impressive example for the transfer of new properties to tumor cells by cell fusion is provided by the hybridoma technique for the production of monoclonal antibodies. By fusion of an antibody-producing B cell, the tumor cell takes over its program for continuous biosynthesis of this one specific antibody. In the hybridoma cell, properties of both fusion partners, e. g., unlimited growth (of the tumor cell) and production of antibodies (of the normal cell), are combined. This process of hybridoma formation sounds simple and plausible, but is highly complicated in practice. After all, the cell must combine two complete chromosome sets and develop hybrids capable of division. This necessitates longer or shorter phases of stabilization.

Fig. 26
Survival curves of mice which have been subcutaneously inoculated either with the non-metastatic initial tumor (EbTGR) or with EbTGR-macrophage hybrid lines (Eb-F1 or Eb-F2). The raised malignancy of the hybrid lines is clearly demonstrated by the drastically shortened survival time of the animals. These animals die above all of metastases in the liver, whereas the animals with the initial tumor died of the primary tumor

## Instability of Cell Hybrids and Chromosome Loss (Segregation)

As already mentioned, investigations into the method of somatic cell hybridization have shown that in hybrids of a tumor cell and a normal cell the tumorigenicity is generally suppressed. The capacity of the tumor cell to undergo unlimited cell division (immortality) is also mostly recessive in such cell hybrids. However, immortality and tumorigenicity might reappear after loss (segregation) of certain chromosomes. Hybrid cells are usually especially labile genetically. Processes such as chromosome segregation are, hence, frequently observed.

## Generation of Metastatic Variants by Cell Hybridization and Segregation

A few years ago, Patrick De Baetselier and co-workers reported for the first time that a nonmetastatic tumor cell (a plasmacytoma) developed metastatic competence after in vitro hybridization with a normal cell of the reticuloendothelial system. The cell hybrids generated formed metastases with a defined organ specificity, i. e. metastases were only formed in certain organs. The results were interpreted in terms of the adoption of new properties by the hybrid cells from the normal lymphocyte fusion partner, e. g., capacity for penetration of blood capillaries, circulation in the blood and "homing" in certain organs. This interpretation might also explain why tumor cell fusions with fibroblasts performed previously have not led to similar results, since fibroblasts are adherent, not circulating cells.

These results obtained by in vitro fusion gave rise to the question as to whether metastatic tumor cell variants might not also arise in vivo under certain conditions from the fusion of a tumor cell with a normal host cell. Tumor-host cell fusions indeed appear to occur occasionally. The literature on such findings goes back to the beginning of the 1970s.

It was only recently observed that metastatic variants can also be formed in vivo by tumor-host cell fusion. In the tumor system of Robert Kerbel and coworkers, highly metastatic variants were repeatedly developed by fusion of a nonmetastatic tumor cell with a cell from the bone marrow. In the tumor system of De Baetselier, the in vivo fusion of a nonmetastatic tumor with a T lymphocyte led to the generation of a highly metastatic cell line.

We also obtained evidence for an important role of somatic cell hybridization in the generation of metastatic variants in the Eb/ESb tumor model. The Eb tumor is a chemically induced T lymphoma of the mouse. From this locally growing tumor line, a highly metastatic variant designated as ESb arose spontaneously in 1968. This variant probably arose from fusion of the T lymphoma Eb with a host macrophage.

We established that the ESb cell expresses surface antigens both of T lymphocytes and of macrophages, whereas the original line Eb only contains markers characteristic for T lymphocytes. Furthermore, we were able to obtain highly metastatic tumor cell variants which were similar in many respects to ESb cells by in vitro hybridization of the Eb lymphoma with a macrophage from the bone marrow.

The reasons for the increased malignancy in the T lymphoma-macrophage hybrids are largely unknown. However, in vitro investigations possibly revealed some important facts:

The hybrids showed a greatly raised enzyme (plasminogen activator) activity, a greatly increased invasive activity in organ cultures and improved adherence properties compared to the original cell line. Furthermore, the expression of new surface glycoproteins, namely the Mac-1 antigen, histocompatibility antigens of class II (I-A, I-E and invariant chain Ii) as well as enhanced expression of a receptor for immunoglobulin ($F_cR$) were noteworthy.

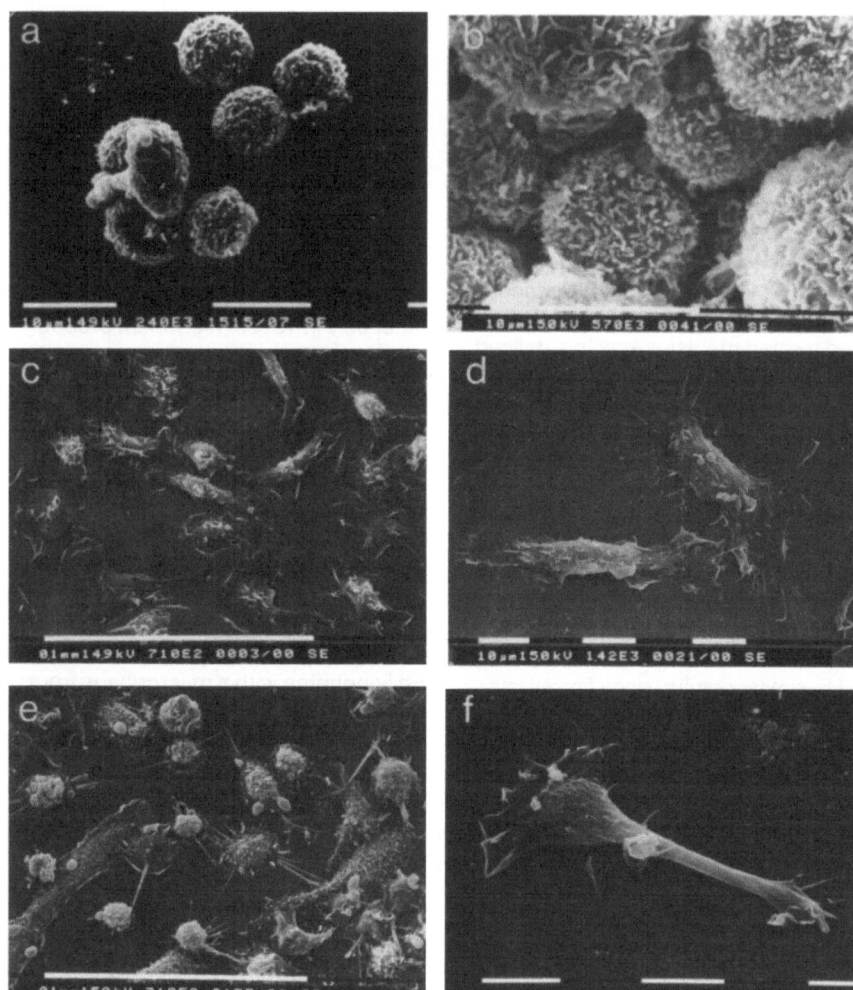

Fig. 27
Tumor line EbTGR, non-metastatic (upper pictures);
below them, host macrophages and at the bottom
the tumor cell variant which gives rise to metastases
and which has arisen by hybridization of the other
two tumor lines

## Significance of Somatic Cell Fusion for the Formation of Metastatic Variants

The question as to the significance of somatic cell fusion for the generation of metastatic variants cannot yet be answered at present. It is not known whether such processes also occur in human tumors. Even in animal tumors, the number of investigations is quite insufficient to enable a rough appraisal of how frequently such fusions occur and what percentage of metastatic variants arises from such fusions.

However, there are nevertheless some observations on human tumors which are possibly to be seen in a fresh light in view of the new results described.

It was recently reported that small cell lung carcinomas, which are very malignant tumors, express a macrophage antigen. Highly malignant tumors frequently display higher chromosome counts and more pronounced heteroploidy than their less malignant precursors. Furthermore, malignant tumor cell lines mostly display an increased number of structurally altered chromosomes (marker chromosomes) and a tendency to gene amplification which are manifested cytologically as HSR (homogeneously staining regions), DM (double minutes), or ABR (abnormally banded regions).

Raised chromosome counts in tumor cells may also be caused by disturbances in the control of chromosome replication and/or chromosome distribution. Such processes leading to hyperploidy or polyploidy are observed both in autochthonous (growing from the body itself, not transplanted) and in transplantation tumors. The common denominator of all these processes appears to consist in the generation of high ploidy cells. By chromosome segregation, new tumor cell variants can arise from them which would lead to an increase in the heterogeneity of the tumor. In addition, chromosome breaks and chromosome rearrangements may occur in high ploidy cells; these may lead to the formation of tumor cell variants which differ from the original tumor both cytogenetically and in their properties. Extensive or even only submicroscopic chromosome alterations can lead in addition to an activation of genes, e. g., of oncogenes. From such a heterogenous tumor cell population, those cells can be selected which are best adapted to the respective microenvironment in which the tumor is situated. Thus, the combination of polyploidization, chromosome segregation and host selection becomes a dangerous cycle of diversification and selection which can lead to the formation of malignant tumor cell variants with the ability to form metastases.

Spontaneous somatic cell fusion can occur both between tumor and host cells (heterokaryotic fusion) and between neighboring tumor cells (homokaryotic fusion). Little is known so far about the mechanisms leading to fusion. It is possible that viruses are involved whose fusion proteins are activated by proteases. It is also conceivable that an incomplete host defense reaction against the tumor by T lymphocytes or macrophages may lead to a fusion of the cells involved.

Naturally, such a process must not always lead to the development of malignant tumor cell variants as described above. It is likewise conceivable that nonviable hybrids may be formed by such fusions. However, the most recent results and theoretical considerations indicate that somatic cell hybridization has a particular significance for the generation of metastatic variants.

Prof. Volker Schirrmacher
Cellular Immunology,
Institute of Immunology and Genetics

Scientists participating

Dr. Peter Altevogt
Eckhard Pflüger
Eberhard Rußmann
Dr. Lynn Graf
(at present Department of Medical Oncology, Fred Hutchinson Cancer Research Center, Seattle, USA)

In collaboration with

Dr. Lidia Larizza
Istituto di Biologia Generale,
Universita Studi di Milano, Italy

Dr. Norbert Koch
Department of Somatic Genetics,
Institute of Immunology and Genetics

Prof. Dymitr Komitowski
Department of Histodiagnostics and Pathomorphological Documentation,
Institute of Experimental Pathology

Dr. Rule Petrusevska
Department of Differentiation and Carcinogenesis in vitro,
Institute of Biochemistry

Dr. Michael Stöhr
Project Group Cytometry and Chromosome Sorting, Tumor Bank,
Institute of Experimental Pathology

Fig. 28

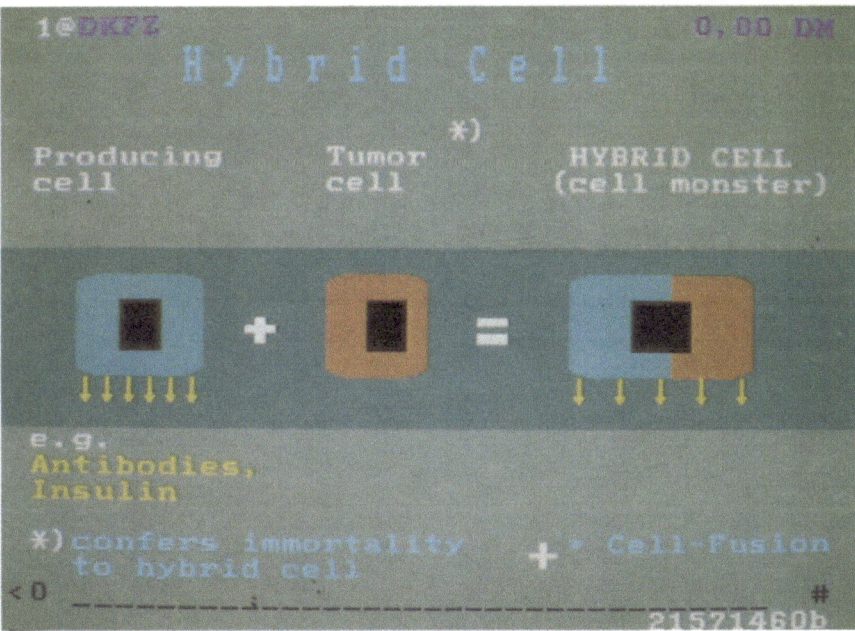

Dr. Hans-Peter Zimmermann
Department of Growth and Division of
the Cell,
Institute of Cellular and Tumor Biology

Dr. Mathias Peres-Martinez
Ciudad Sanitaria "Virgen de Las
Nieves", Granada, Spain

Dr. Israel Vlodavsky
Hadassah Medical Center Kiryat Hadassah, Jerusalem, Israel

Selected publications

Schirrmacher, V., Fogel, M., Rußmann, E., Bosslet, K., Altevogt, P., Beck, L.: Antigenic variation in cancer metastasis. Immune escape versus immune control. Cancer Met. Rev. 1, 241–274 (1982).

Schirrmacher, V., Altevogt, P., Fogel, M., Dennis, J., Waller, C. A., Barz, D., Schwartz, R., Cheingsong-Popov, R., Springer, G., Robinson, P. J., Nebe, T., Brossmer, W., Vlodavsky, I., Paweletz, N., Zimmermann, H.-P., Uhlenbruck, G.: Importance of cell surface carbohydrates in cancer cell adhesion, invasion and metastasis. Does sialic acid direct metastatic behavior? Invasion and Metastasis 2, 313–360 (1982).

Kerbel, R. S., Lagarde, E. A., Dennis, J. W., Donaghue, T. P.: Spontaneous fusion between normal host and tumor cells: possible contribution to tumor progression and metastasis studied with a lectin resistant mutant tumor. Mol. Cell. Biol. 3, 523–538 (1983).

Schirrmacher, V., Vlodavsky, I.: Interaction of metastatic and non-metastatic tumor lines with aortic endothelial cell monolayer and their underlying basal lamina. In: Hormonally Defined Media. A Tool in Cell Biology (Fischer, Wieser, eds) Springer Verlag, Heidelberg, pp. 151–161 (1983).

Larizza, L., Schirrmacher, V., Graf, L., Pflüger, E., Peres-Martinez, M., Stöhr, M.: Suggestive evidence that the highly metastatic variant ESb of the T cell lymphoma Eb is derived from a spontaneous fusion with a host macrophage. Int. J. Cancer 34, 699–707 (1984).

## 2.6 Gene Transfer – Alteration of Tumor Growth and Metastatic Spreading

by Günter Joachim Hämmerling

The most natural kind of tumor defense is mediated by the body's own immune system. In recent years, a great deal has been learned about cellular interactions in the immune system and the molecules involved. The histocompatibility antigens hold key position. In humans, these are termed HLA, and in the mouse H-2 antigens. We are only beginning to understand their biological function. It has become apparent that histocompatibility antigens are guidance structures for the recognition of foreign antigens by "killer cells". Killer cells can recognize, e. g., viruses or their determinants only together with the histocompatibility antigens on the virus-infected cell and can then kill them. If virus-infected cells do not display any histocompatibility antigens, they cannot be eliminated by autologous resistance.

We have posed the question as to whether similar preconditions also apply to the rejection of tumors. This reflection was occasioned by our observation that a considerable percentage of tumors in the mouse displays a defect in the expression of histocompatibility antigens. This applies both to the tumor lines, which have been established for a long time in the laboratory, and to new tumors produced in the mouse with the cancer-inducing substance methylcholanthrene A. In quite a few tumors, one of the two different histocompatibility antigens of the mouse (K and D) was absent. On the other hand, normal cells always have both histocompatibility antigens. The genetic defect, which leads to defective expression of the histocompatibility antigens, is not yet known, and we are investigating it at present. The question arises as to whether the defect in H-2 expression has something to do with the growth and the metastatic behavior of the tumors. Put in another way: how would the tumors grow in animals if they were to express their complete set of histocompatibility antigens like a normal cell?

The modern methods of molecular genetics open up an experimental approach to this question. From normal cells, the genes for the histocompatibility molecules, which were not switched on in the tumor cells, were isolated by cloning. Their nucleotide sequence was determined by Dr. Bernd Arnold from our Institute of Immunology and Genetics. These cloned H-2 genes were introduced into the defective tumor cells by appropriate transfection methods. Such externally supplied genes are incorporated into the genome of the host cell and frequently also become active. Investigations of the manipulated tumor cells with monoclonal antibodies reveal that the externally supplied H-2 genes in the tumor cells were switched on and led to an expression of the corresponding histocompatibility molecules on the cell surface. The defect in the H-2 expression of the tumor cells had thus been successfully repaired by gene manipulation.

In the following experiments, the manipulated tumors were injected into mice and their growth and metastasis behavior was determined. The results will be illustrated by two examples.

Case 1: Methylcholanthrene A-induced fibrosarcoma IC 9 of the (CBH × C 57 B 1/6)F$_1$ mouse carries only the D but no longer the K histocompatibility molecule. This tumor grows exceedingly aggressively but does not metastazise in the mouse. By gene manipulation, IC 9 cells, which again carry the K molecule, were produced in vitro. The presence of the K molecule dramatically altered the

Fig. 29
Repair of an H-2-K-defective tumor cell by gene transfer

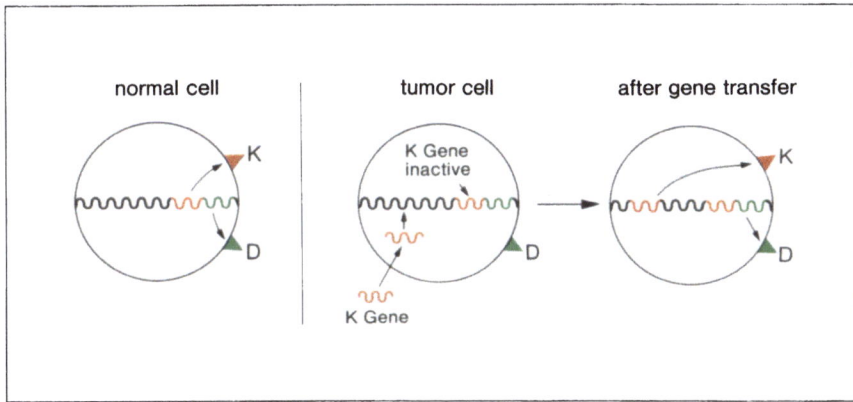

normal cell    tumor cell    after gene transfer

K Gene inactive

K Gene

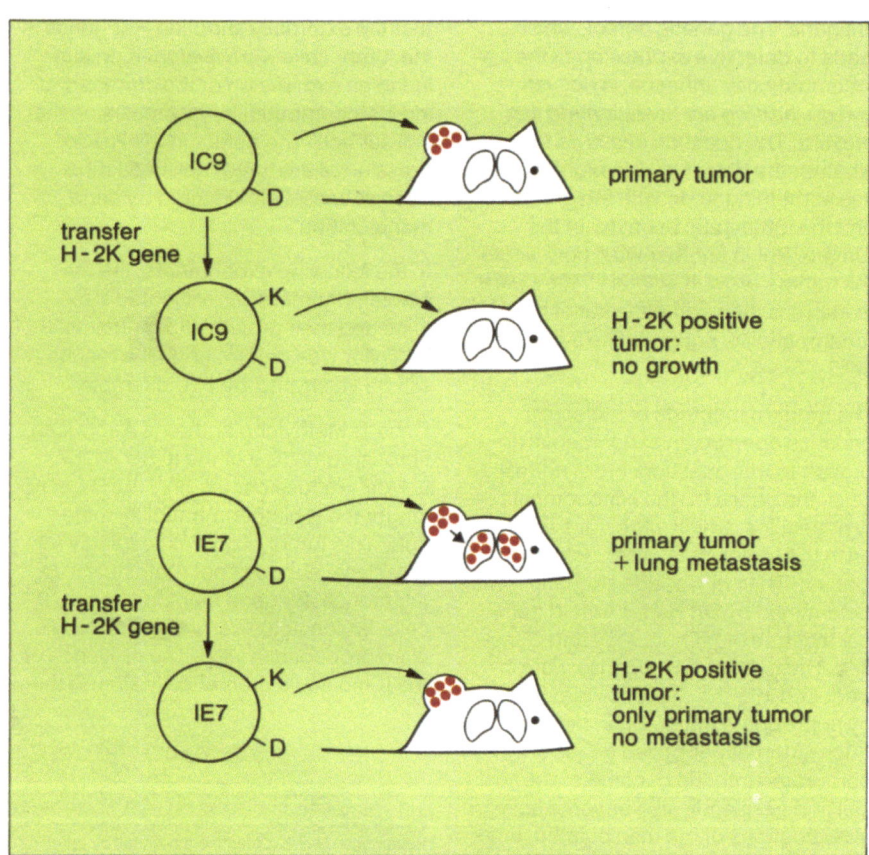

Fig. 30
Alteration of tumor growth and metastatic spreading due to gene transfer

situation: the implantation of K-positive cells into genetically identical $F_1$ mice no longer led to formation of a tumor. The tumor cells were eliminated from the mouse.

Case 2: The fibrosarcoma IE 7 likewise carries only the D but not the K antigens. This tumor also grows very aggressively and forms metastases in the lungs. K-positive tumors, which have arisen by K gene transfection, still grew at the subcutaneous injection site as a primary tumor but could no longer form metastases (Fig. 30).

Further experiments revealed that in both cases the mice formed killer cells against the K-positive transfected tumors, whereas there was no immune reaction against the unmanipulated parent tumors. In the first case, the immune resistance was so strong that it completely suppressed tumor growth, whereas in the second case the resistance was "only" able to prevent the formation of metastases, but not the growth of the primary tumor.

These experiments show that histocompatibility antigens on tumor cells are ex-

ceedingly important for a successful tumor defense by the autologous immune system. Tumor cells, which no longer bear certain histocompatibility antigens, are consequently not rejected and can grow without impediment. These results explain why many mouse tumors display a defect in the expression of histocompatibility molecules.

The following hypothesis can be postulated to explain tumor progression: A tumor cell arises in several transformation steps from a normal cell. Alterations of the cell surface may also occur in this process. The tumor cell divides and can form a primary tumor. If these tumor cells activate the immune system, which is not always the case, they are attacked and killed. For reasons, which have not been clarified so far, some daughter cells, which no longer express the histocompatibility antigens, may be formed during the division of the tumor cells. These daughter cells escape the attack of the immune system and survive, since they no longer expose the histocompatibility guidance structures that are necessary for recognition by the immune system.

In future studies, we wish to investigate whether expression of the histocompatibility antigens can be induced in the K-negative tumors, e. g., by interferon, and whether these tumors are thereby rendered immunogenic, i. e. are rejected by the immune system. It is also important to investigate whether immunization with gene-manipulated tumors protects the animals against the effect of a subsequent implantation of negative parent cells.

Tumor growth and metastatic spread are doubtless not controlled by histocompatibility antigens in every case. Many tumors carry the normal set of histocompatibility antigens and can nevertheless grow and metastasize without impediment. The question is whether the findings in the mouse can be transferred to humans. Preliminary investigations by Dr. Frank Momburg in our laboratory and by other laboratories have revealed that several human

tumors also display a defect in the expression of histocompatibility antigens. Since immune reactions occur according to the same principles in humans as in the mouse, it is consequently very probable that the histocompatibility antigens also play an important role in tumor rejection in humans.

Part of the studies described above was carried out in the context of the German-Israeli Cooperation on Cancer Research promoted in the German Cancer Research Center.

Fig. 31

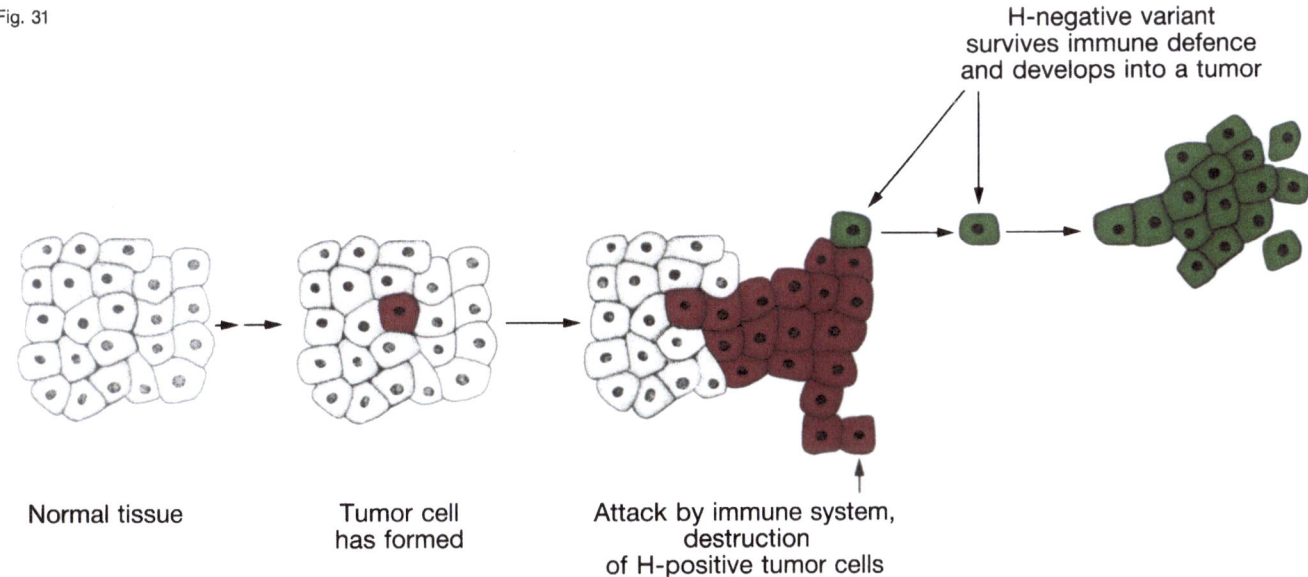

H-negative variant survives immune defence and develops into a tumor

Normal tissue

Tumor cell has formed

Attack by immune system, destruction of H-positive tumor cells

Fig. 32
A classical experiment which proves that autologous defence can be developed against tumor cells. Whereas the inoculated tumor A "takes", defence cells are produced against this tumor. If one attempts to transfer the tumor for a second time to (operated) animals, the defence reaction prevents "taking" of the tumor. However, defence is restricted to this one tumor; another tumor B "takes"

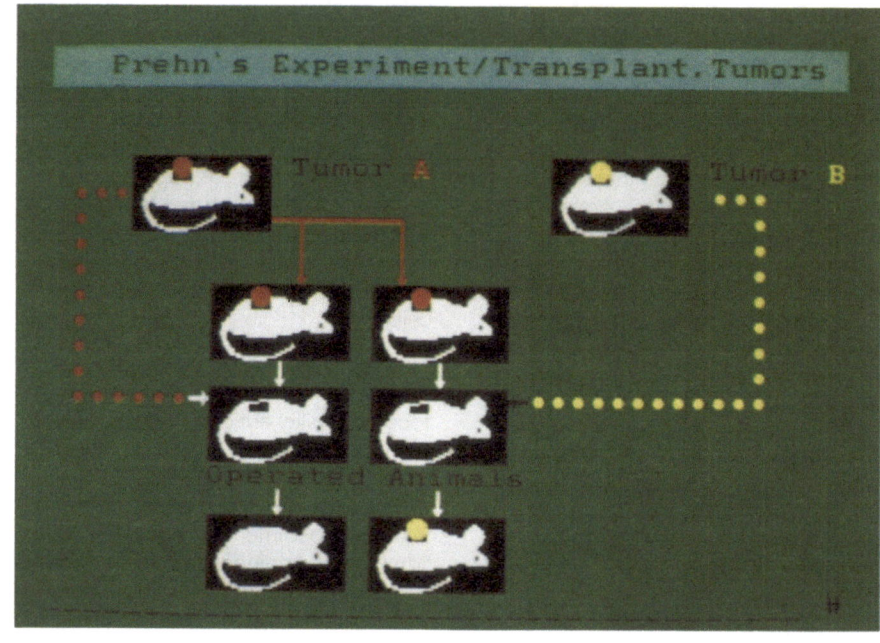

Prof. Günter Joachim Hämmerling
Somatic Genetics,
Institute of Immunology and Genetics

Staff participating

Nadja Bulbuc
Angelika Hemmerling
Daniela Klar
Dr. Reiner Wallich

In collaboration with

Prof. Michael Feldman and
Shulamit Katzav
Department of Cell Biology,
Weizmann Institute of Science
Rehovot, Israel

Prof. Shraga Segal
Ben-Gurion University,
Department of Immunology,
Beer-Sheva, Israel

Selected publications

Momburg, F., Degener, T., Bacchus, E., Moldenhauer, G., Hämmerling, G. J., and Möller, P.: Loss of HLA-A, B, C and de novo expression of HLA-D in colorectal cancer. Intl. J. Cancer, in press.

Wallich, R., Bulbuc, N., Hämmerling, G. J., Katzav, S., Segal, S., Feldman, M.: Abrogation of metastatic properties of tumor cells by de novo expression of H-2 K antigens following H-2 gene transfection. Nature 6017, 301–305 (1985).

## 2.7 High-Resolution Electronic Chromosome Sorting

by Michael Stöhr and Karl-Josef Hutter

Molecular genetic investigations and theories increasingly predominate in fundamental research on carcinogenesis. Cytogenetic aspects play an important role. These are investigated with the methods of classical genetics on the one hand, but to an increasing extent with the techniques of modern molecular biology on the other hand. Besides other theories, the concept that alterations in the genetic material of cells may lead to malignant cell growth by interruption of corresponding control mechanisms is being explored.

In these terms, studies on chromosomes attain a new significance. A close link between classical and modern molecular cytogenetics is aimed at. One of the most important connecting links is high-resolution electronic chromosome sorting. The chromosomes of a cell become clearly visible at a particular time in cell division (mitosis); they assume a typical rod form.

In this state, they are labelled with a specific dye (fluorochrome) which shows bluish fluorescence under irradiation with ultraviolet light (Fig. 33). The intensity of this blue radiation is characteristic for each chromosome type: small chromosomes fluoresce more faintly than large chromosomes.

The method now consists in artificially converting many cells into the mitotic stage. The chromosomes of these cells can be isolated and are available in an aqueous solution at the end of the procedure, suspended singly and stained at the same time. A sophisticated pressure system now ensures that this chromosome solution is pressed out in the form of a fine filament of fluid from a small jet (60 μm diameter). At right angles to this, a laser beam is focused on this filament so that all chromosomes (like beads on a string) are consecutively irradiated for a short time (5 μsec) so that they give off their characteristic intensity of fluorescence. Light receivers register these impulses, and digital signal processing sorts them according to their intensity. At the end of each flow cytometric measurement, there is a frequency diagram of the registered fluorescence intensities of all chromosomes which provides information on the cytogenetic characteristics of the cells investigated. In a routine run of a few minutes, about 100,000 chromosomes are analyzed.

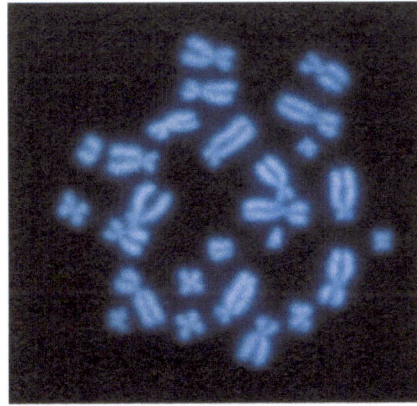

Fig. 33
Chromosomes in cell division. Cell line of the Chinese hamster stained with a dye which gives blue fluorescence under ultraviolet light. The Chinese hamster possesses 21 chromosomes of varying length and shape.

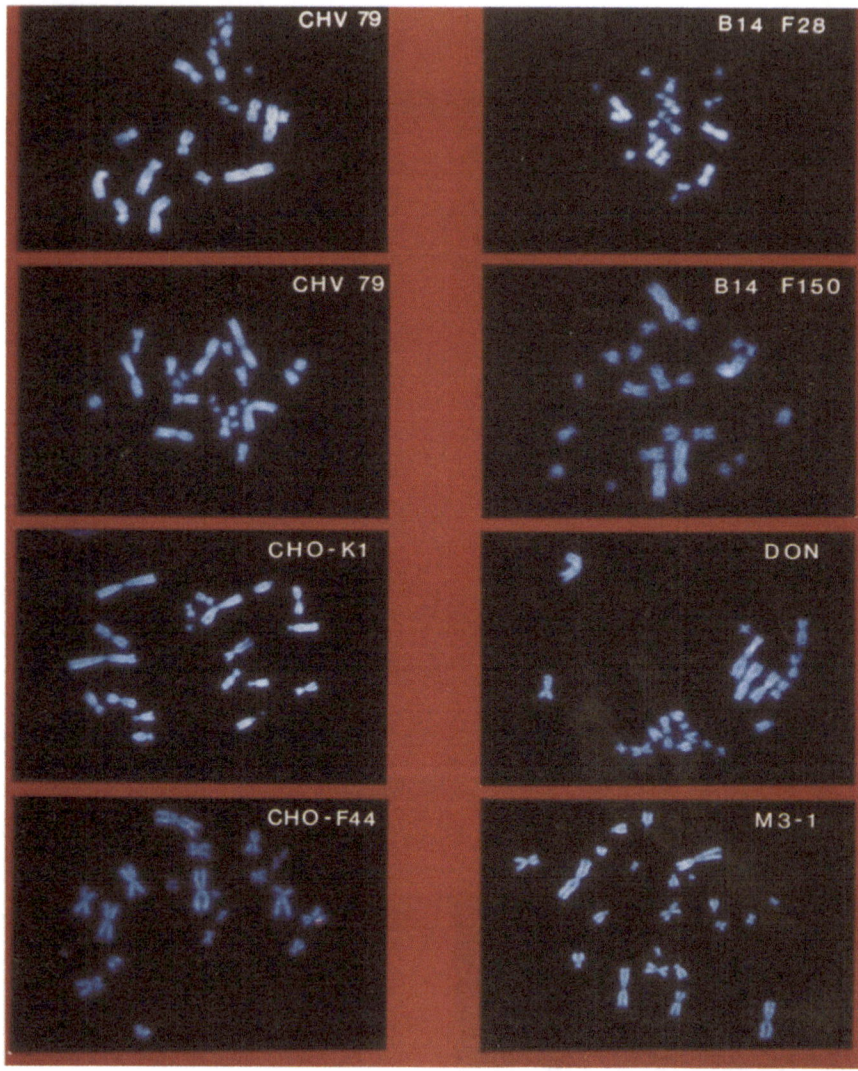

CHV 79

CHV 79

CHO-K1

CHO-F44

B14 F28

B14 F150

DON

M3-1

**Fig. 34**
Chromosomes in cell division from eight different cell lines of the Chinese hamster which differ from each other to a greater or lesser extent in terms of the number and shape of their chromosomes due to the artificial cultural conditions

Fig. 34 and 35 serve to illustrate how informative such distribution diagrams may be. Here, eight cytogenetically different cell lines of the Chinese hamster were investigated both in the classical mitotic preparation (Fig. 34), and with measurement techniques (Fig. 35). In the classical preparation, the variations among the mitoses can only be discerned after lengthy examination (the number of chromosomes and their shape vary). In addition, only a few mitoses of each line can be evaluated, which is why it is very difficult to appraise the cytogenetic variance. The situation is completely different in the diagrams in Fig. 35. It can already be discerned at first glance that all cell lines differ from each other. The position (chromosome class) and height (number of chromosomes per class) of the peaks display a specific pattern for each cell line, enabling them to be readily identified and excellently distinguished from the rest.

After the methodological basis for the cytometric flow measurement of chromosomes could be refined on the cell lines of the Chinese hamster, the way was clear to switching to tumor lines of which the cytogenetics is by no means so clearcut as that of the hamster. As a rule, malignant tumors display an especially striking and mostly very large chromosome (marker) which is absent in healthy cells. Until today, it is still unclear whether such marker chromosomes play a causal role in carcinogenesis or are only an unsignificant concomitant manifestation. Application of modern molecular biology techniques might provide further information for the clarification of this question.

For this purpose, however, it is necessary to obtain a pure fraction of marker chromosomes so that the results are not masked by the presence of the remaining chromosomes. The technique of specific staining and measurement in the liquid stream would be suitable to sort out pure preparations of marker chromosomes.

This is achieved in cytometric flow measurement by means of a very ingenious technique. After formation of the liquid filament, a vibration system (oscillating quartz) ensures that the filament breaks down after a few millimeters (about 5 mm) into small droplets of uniform size (about 60 µm diameter). If these include corresponding chromosomes, they can be given electrical charges which undergo a deflection in a subsequent electrical field of high voltage (6,000 volts/cm). They are thus physically separated from the rest of the stream of drops, which contains the undesired chromosomes, and can be collected in small containers placed in readiness.

First experiments were carried out with an experimental tumor which is a very frequently used experimental model in the rat (Walker 256, a carcinosarcoma). Fig. 36 shows a typical mitotic figure of this tumor and the cytometric flow diagram. The marker chromosome is designated with an arrow. Its position in the distribution curve is on the extreme right. So far, several million marker chromosomes have been sorted out in flow-through technique. The purity was 85%. At present, the chromosome material is being processed molecular-biologically and subjected to a more precise characterization of its genetic composition.

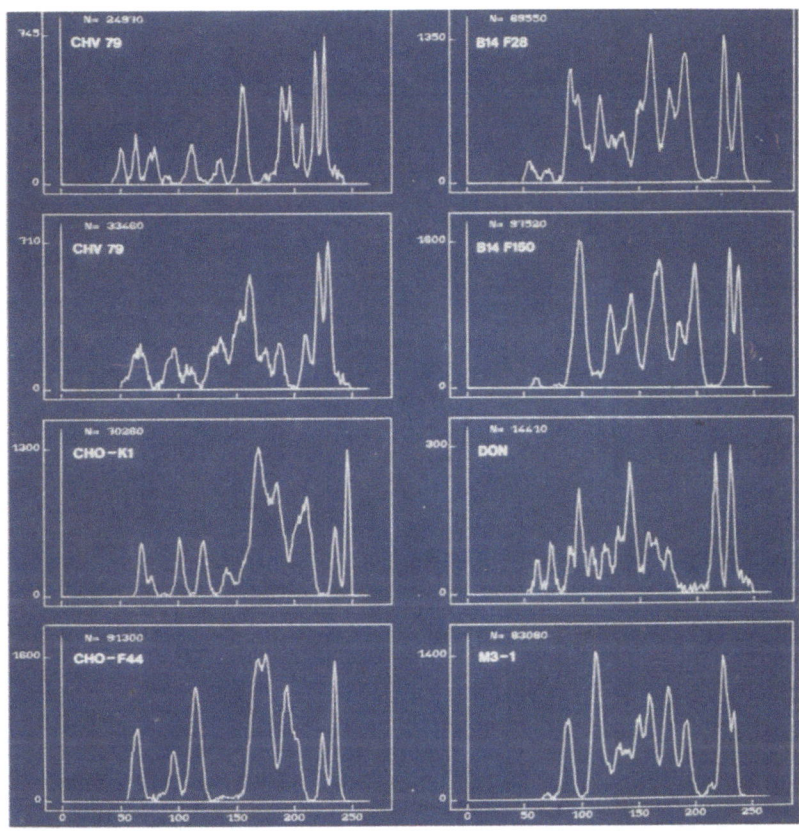

Dipl.-Phys. Michael Stöhr
Dr. Karl-Josef Hutter
Project Group Cytometry and Chromosome Sorting, Tumor Bank,
Institute of Experimental Pathology

Fig. 35
Distribution curves of the chromosome sets shown in Fig. 33 as present at the end of a flow cytometric analysis. n is the total number of registered chromosomes. The position and level of the peaks is characteristic for each cell line. The differences can be clearly seen

Staff participating

Monika Frank
Gerry Futterman
Prof. Dr. Klaus Goerttler
Hans Peter Götz

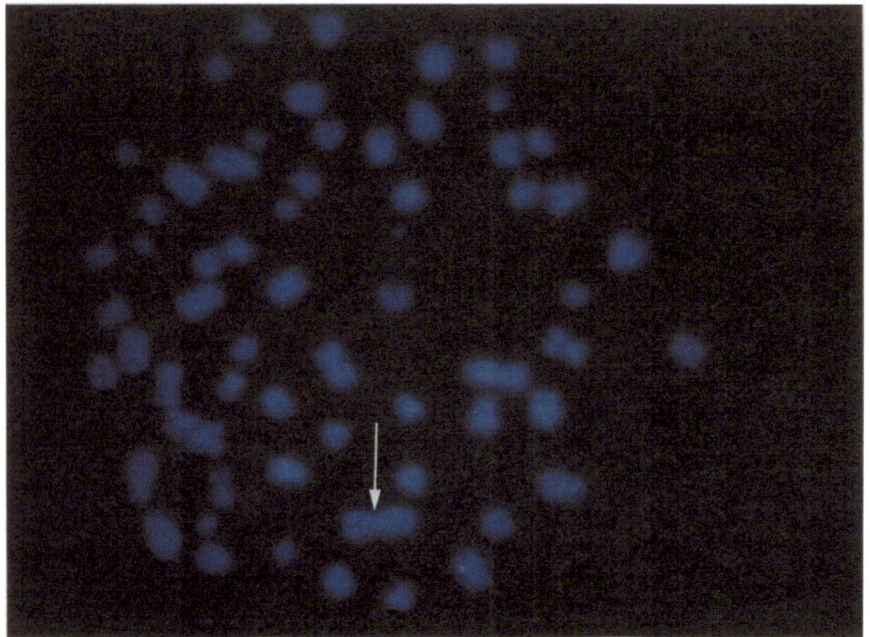

Fig. 36
A typical mitosis of the inoculated tumor (Walker 256 in the rat) investigated. The mitosis contained 63 chromosomes. The marker chromosome is indicated with an arrow. In the flow cytometric analysis, it produces a separate peak with the highest intensity of fluorescence, and can hence be separated very well from the remaining chromosomes

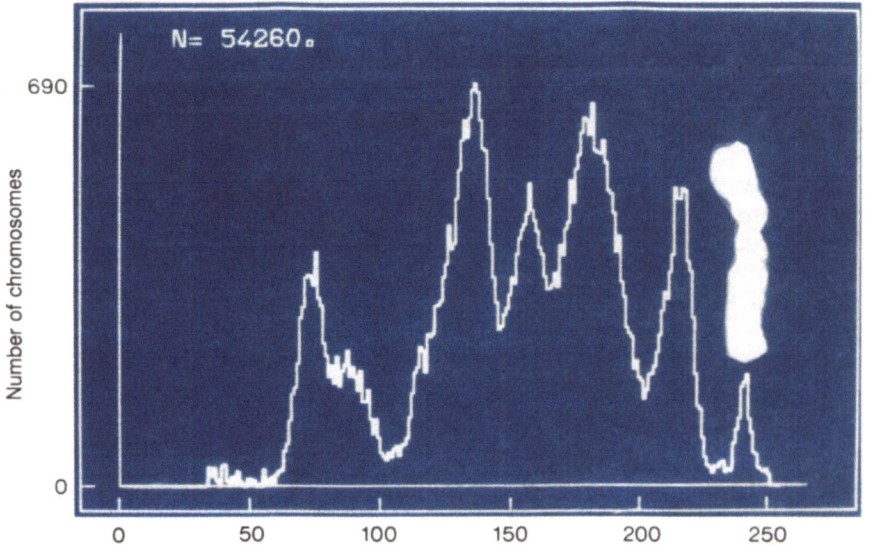

Selected publications

A Flow Cytometric Study of Chromosomes from Rat Kangaroo and Chinese Hamster Cells
M. Stoehr, K.-J. Hutter, M. Frank, G. Futterman and Kl. Goerttler
Histochemistry 67, 179–190 (1980).

Assignment of snRNA Gene Sequences to the large Chromosomes of Rat Kangaroo and Chinese Hamster Isolated by Flow Cytometric Sorting
N. Blin, M. Stoehr, K.-J. Hutter, A. Alonso and Kl. Goerttler
Chromosoma 85, 723–733 (1982).

Chromosomes for Molecular Hybridization
G. Langer, N. Blin and M. Stoehr
Histochemistry 80, 469–473 (1984).

Detection and Separation of the Submetacentric Marker Chromosome of the Walker (W-256) Carcinoma Using Flow Cytometry and Sorting
K.-H. Hutter and M. Stoehr
Histochemistry 82, 469–475 (1985).

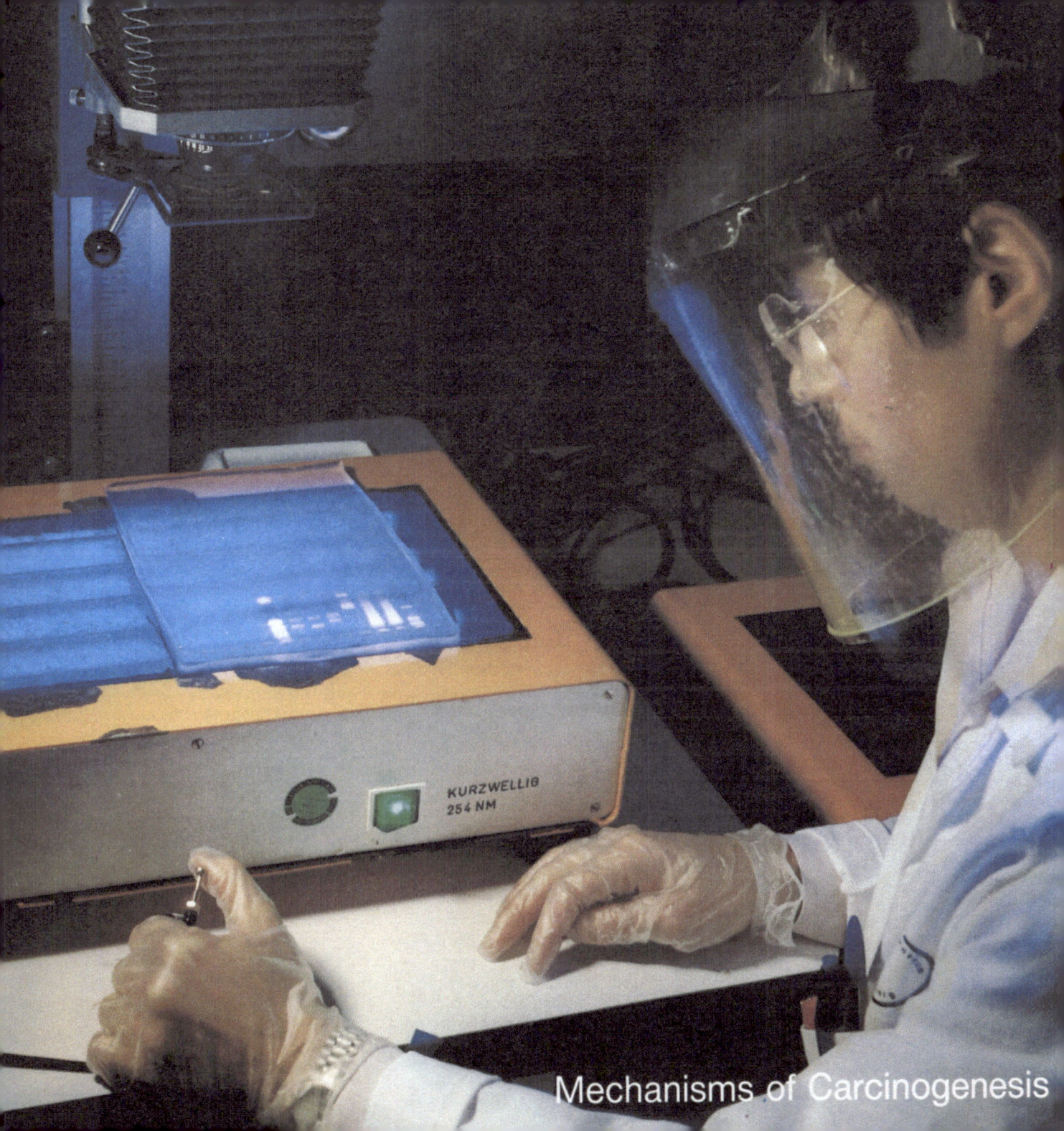

Mechanisms of Carcinogenesis

KURZWELLIG
254 NM

# Mechanisms of Carcinogenesis

The research focused on "mechanisms of carcinogenesis" is concerned with the fundamental question as to how and why cancer arises. The research projects grouped together here thus have a common concept. Despite all diversity of the experimental approaches, this concept can be described as follows: Model reconstruction of the transformation of a normal cell into a cancer cell under deliberately chosen conditions which allow as complete as possible an observation of the molecular processes leading to cancer development. Experimentation with cancer-inducing rays, chemical carcinogens as well as tumor viruses are in principle equivalent. It is indeed appropriate to experiment with different agents, since cancer is not caused by a single factor but by many causes, and this must be borne in mind in experimentation.

We know that the stepwise transformation of a normal cell is accompanied by a multiplicity of biochemical dysregulations, defence reactions and functional deficits which are finally manifested in morphologically detectable alterations. The diversity of these symptoms can be analyzed and brought into a rational context only by cooperation of various disciplines. Cell biologists, molecular biologists, biochemists, virologists and pathologists, to mention only a few, share this work. Although remarkable discoveries have recently been made in this way, it is so far not yet apparent how the problem of cancer as a whole might be solved.

There will probably not be any patent solution, if only because cancer ist not a homogenous disease, but comprises a multiplicity of pathological processes which always end in malignant cell proliferation. In view of the situation, a su-perficial observer might arrive at the conclusion that the exploration of the mechanisms of carcinogenesis is a problem of secondary urgency and is perhaps indeed a hopeless enterprise; one would be far more likely to arrive at the finishing post if one could locate and eliminate the cancer-inducing factors in the human environment which are so far unknown. This is doubtless an ambitious objective even if it appears doubtful whether this can ever be achieved in view of our living habits. However, it is to be borne in mind that purposeful searching for cancer-inducing agents is only possible if the searching scientist has previously sharpened his perception for the particular biochemical and toxicological properties of the agents which are to be discovered. In other words, the scientist must have criteria available with which he can sort out for detailed examination the potentially dangerous factors among the large number of environmental factors which appear to be unremarkable. The following example may document how the study of the mechanism of carcinogenesis provides useful criteria for earlier recognition of carcinogenic substances than would be possible in unconditional testing of all substances under suspicion.

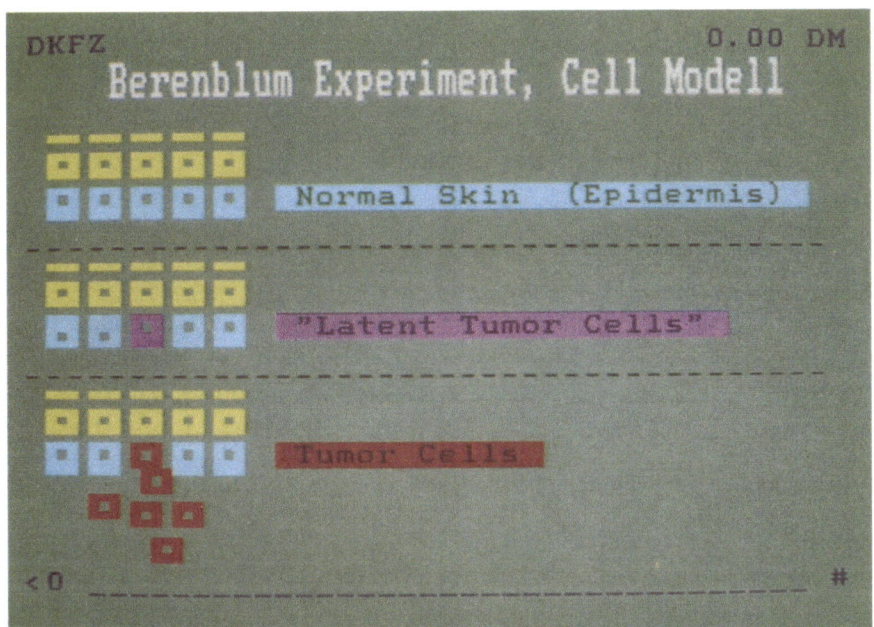

Fig. 37

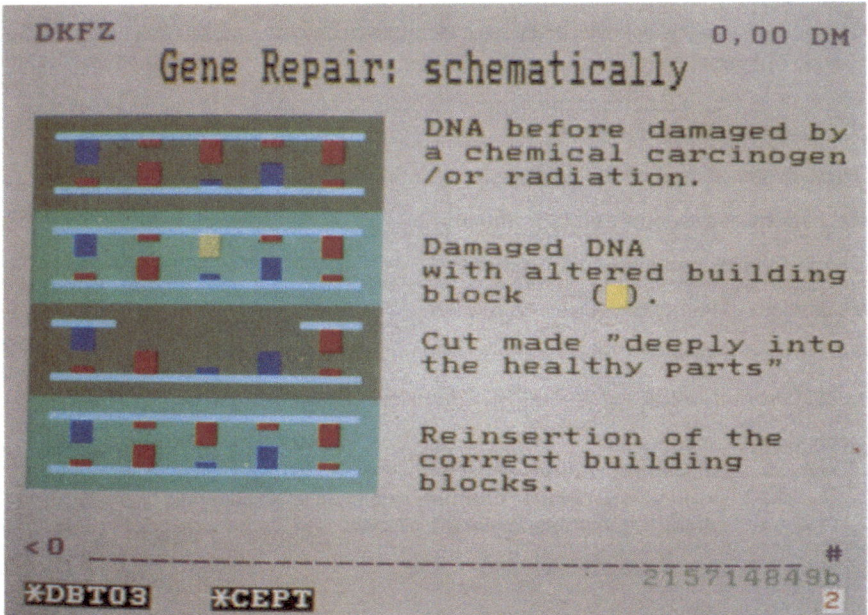

Fig. 38

In the 1960's, it was observed in Britain that highly carcinogenic substances bind more frequently to the deoxyribonucleic acid (DNA) of the genetic material than weak carcinogens. A precise examination revealed that the covalent binding of carcinogenic substances to DNA might indeed be a key reaction in the transformation of normal cells into cancer cells and that these substances have certain chemical properties in common: by themselves or after prior activation in cell metabolism, they must possess attachment groups which enable binding with the DNA. If a cell with genetic material damaged in this way starts to divide, then copying errors (mutations) occur in the replication of the DNA. This may be the point of departure of malignant transformation.

Research on tumor viruses has recently provided a major increase in knowledge in this regard in that it allowed identification of special genes (oncogenes) the activation of which appears to be of decisive significance for carcinogenesis. Although there are indications that such "cancer genes" are altered by mutations in the course of chemical carcinogenesis, we do not yet understand the molecular mechanisms which are necessary for such a genetic defect to be manifested as malignant growth. However, it appears to have been proved that cancer is indeed a "disease of the genes" even if it is not so much a genetic disease.

It is to be emphasized that there is no satisfactory alternative to rational search for carcinogenic factors (i.e. determined by knowledge of the properties of known carcinogens): nonsystematic testing of the many new chemicals which industry produces daily as well as other possible causes would be too tedious and too expensive.

Knowledge of the mechanisms of carcinogenesis is also a precondition for the development of a rational therapy designed to prevent such transformation or destruction of the transformed cells. It is logical that only the knowledge of cellular reaction (regulation) principles and disorders of these principles occurring in the course of malignant transformation opens up possibilities for a specific therapeutic intervention. Many cytostatics used clinically today were developed in this way, but are still subject to great disadvantages (e.g., severe side effects) because of lack of precise knowledge of carcinogenic mechanisms.

Overall, it can be stated that only the study of mechanisms of carcinogenesis creates the foundation of knowledge on the basis of which risk factors can be specifically looked for and means of therapy sought.

## Research Activities Focused on Mechanisms of Carcinogenesis

Sequential analysis of the neoplastic transformation of epithelial and mesenchymal cells

Prenatal induction of cellular thesaurismoses

Cellular and molecular mechanisms of hepatocarcinogenesis

Contribution to the mechanistic aspects of tumor promoters

Regulation of key enzymes metabolizing foreign substances by protein kinases and the effect of carcinogens on the protein-phosphorylating regulation apparatus of the cell

Attempts to quantify chemical carcinogenesis with selected acetyl aryl triazenes

Metabolism and activation of cytostatic and carcinogenic triazine compounds

N-nitro and aromatic nitro compounds

Ultimate carcinogens – reaction with DNA

Influence on N-nitrosamine carcinogenesis by anticarcinogens

Conjugate formation by N-nitrosamines

Organotropy – extrahepatic activation

Metabolism and mechanism of action of initiators of carcinogenesis, polyfunctional aromatic hydrocarbon type

Metabolism and biochemical mechanism of initiation promoters of carcinogenesis, polyfunctional diterpene type

Biochemistry of epidermal hyperplasia

Mechanism of action of tumor promoters

Search for endogenous tumor promoters

Mechanism of keratinocyte transformation

Biochemical analysis of DNA repair defects in xeroderma pigmentosum (XP cells)

Induction of biological functions ("SOS function") by carcinogens

Mechanism of oncogenesis by herpes simplex virus and cytomegalyvirus (HCMV). Latency and persistence of these viruses in vitro and in vivo.
1. Structure and function of virus- and tumor-specific components;
2. Characterization of human syncytial retrovirus

Molecular biology of papillomaviruses

Search for oncogens

Genetic variance of human pathogenic herpes viruses

Limitation of viral proliferation by variant virus particles in HSV

Herpes virus DNA replication

Neurovirulence and latency of HSV in the animal model

Role of papilloma viruses in human tumors

Genome structure and gene expression of human papilloma viruses

B-lymphotropic papova virus

DNA amplification and tumorigenesis

Investigations on virus-host cell interactions of the Epstein-Barr virus

Primary resistance to viral infections

Immuno-regulatory factors of helper and suppressor cells

Surface structures of T lymphocytes and their significance in the regulation of the immune response

Mathematical models of carcinogenesis

## 3.1 Cancer of the Cervix Caused by Viruses? New Aspects of Carcinogenesis and Early Diagnosis

by Lutz Gissmann

It is generally assumed today that the various forms of cancer are not elicited by one event, but that certain substances act repeatedly and that various factors must coincide. Thus, clearly elevated frequencies can be observed in the case of some tumor forms in certain families or populations, which is probably due to the influence of genetic factors combined with noxae from the environment. In view of the occurrence of certain tumors in some geographical regions and the simultaneous presence of certain substances in the environment, a causal correlation between such substances (carcinogens) and the corresponding form of cancer can be inferred. However, this does not by any means entail that all persons who are exposed to the noxious substances also develop cancer, as of course all heavy smokers for example do not develop lung cancer, although the probability of this is about ten times greater for them than for nonsmokers. It hence appears meaningful to refer to cancer risks instead of cancer-inducing factors.

Indications for an involvement of viruses in tumor diseases may result when certain virus types are likewise very widespread in regions with a high cancer incidence, and when the infection usually occurs at an especially early age. In view of such observations and further epidemiological studies, a connection between the hepatitis B virus and

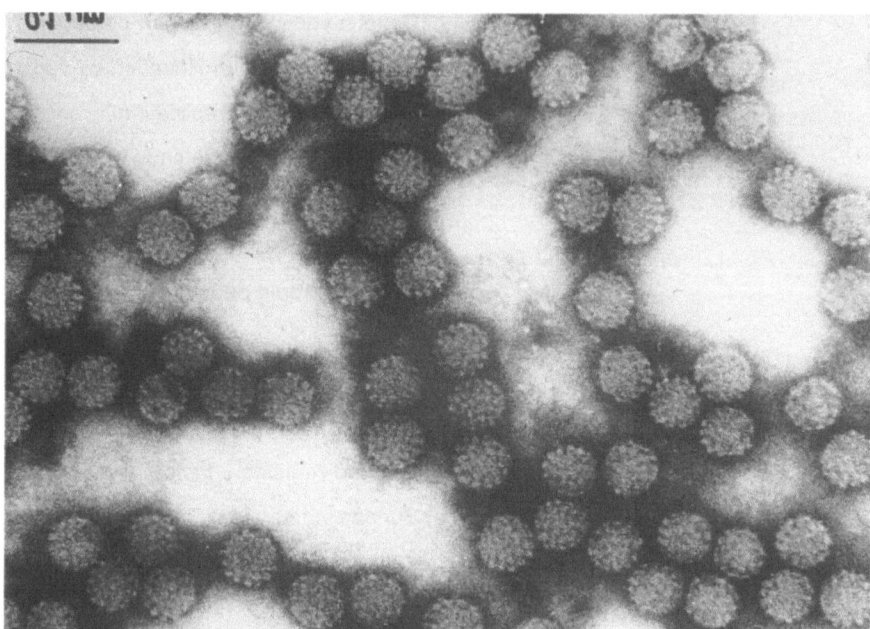

Fig. 39
Papillomaviruses in the electron microscopic picture

hepatocellular carcinoma could be shown in Central Africa and South East Asia. Otherwise, if there is no such correlation between tumors and viral infections, it cannot be concluded that viruses are causal factors in cancer diseases since decades may often pass between the infection as the suspected triggering event and the occurrence of the disease. The causal relationship with an infectious event can then no longer be established. Diseases transmitted by sexual contact are an exception, although a chain of infection can, in this case, no longer be constructed after years. However, a raised risk of infection can be inferred in persons with several sexual partners. Apart from incorrect answers, which are possible under certain circumstances in response to questions about sexual habits, this risk of infection can be established even after years.

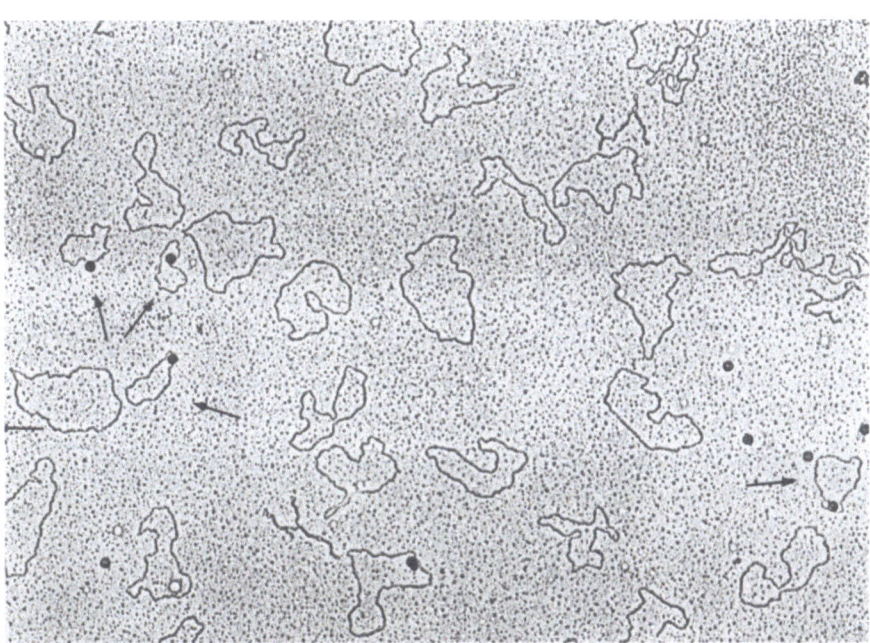

Fig. 40
Papillomavirus desoxyribonucleic acid

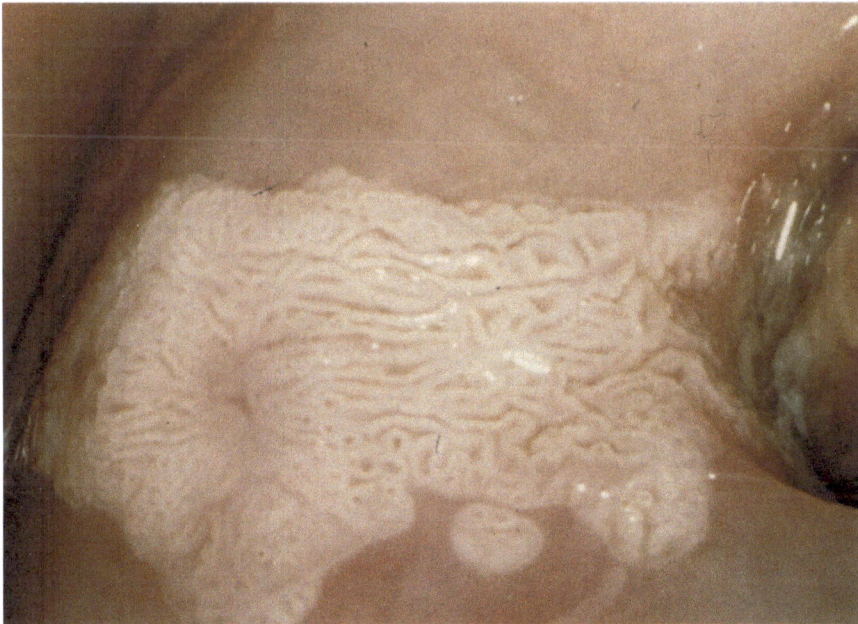

Fig. 41
Alterations in the uterine cervix (dysplasia) photographed by means of a lens in a colposcope

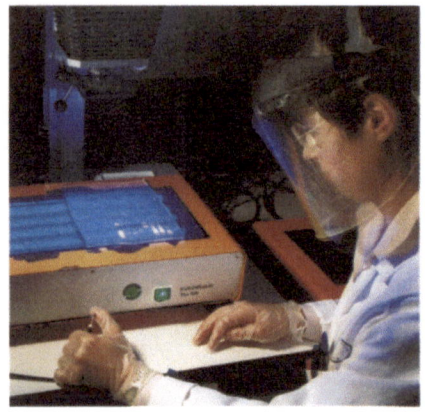

Fig. 42
Virus DNA rendered visible after electrophoresis and staining with a dye. Short-wave ultraviolet light causes it to fluoresce

In the development of cancer of the uterine cervix, the role of infection has been discussed for years. These speculations were occasioned by epidemiological investigations which revealed that the tumor incidence in women living under poor social conditions and in countries with a low standard of hygiene is two to five times higher than in corresponding comparison groups. Furthermore, the early time of the first sexual intercourse as well as the number of sexual partners entail a risk for tumor development. Indeed, new investigations were able to show that women de-

veloped cervical carcinomas significantly more frequently when their husbands had either had contact with various other partners or when wives from an earlier marriage also had this tumor. As candidates for an agent transmitted by sexual intercourse, which might be involved in tumorigenesis, two different viruses have been considered for several years: the herpes simplex virus (HSV) and the human papilloma viruses (HPV). Both have been clearly identified as the cause of various venereal diseases. The papilloma viruses cause condylomata acuminata on the external sexual organs

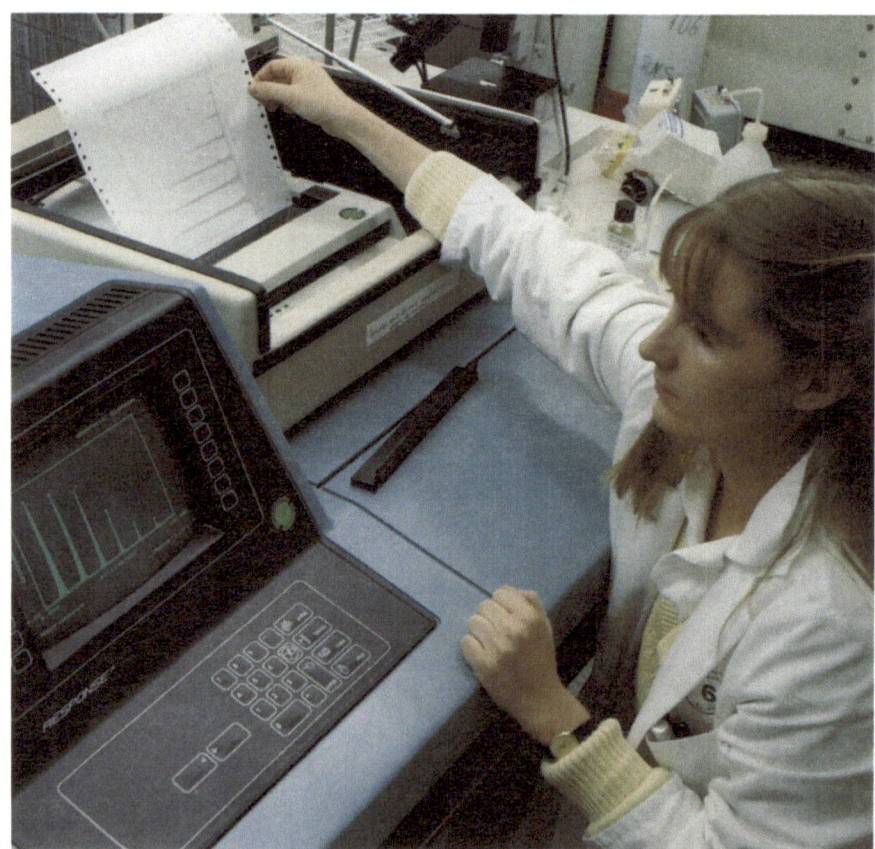

Fig. 43
Determination of the DNA content of a tissue sample with a spectrophotometer

Fig. 44 a–f
Regular investigation of the cell smear by the pathologist (Papanicolaou test) serves to prevent the development of cervical cancer. A possibility of supplementing and modifying the early diagnosis investigation is the identification of papillomaviruses in the woman's cell smear. Papillomaviruses, their identification and evaluation may serve as additional diagnostic markers.

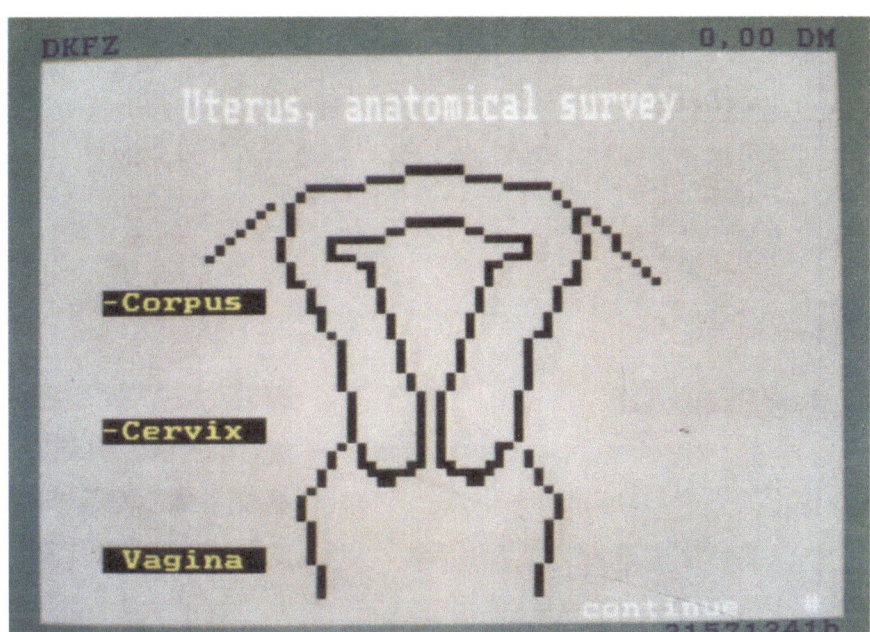

Fig. 44 a

Fig. 44 b

or the flat atypical condylomas of the uterine cervix. Whereas the latter frequently occur together with dysplastic alterations which develop with a certain probability into carcinomas in situ and invasive carcinomas, the alterations caused by HSV cannot be regarded as tumor precursors. The indications for a correlation of this virus and tumorigenesis are not very convincing. Raised HSV-specific antibodies found in earlier investigations in cervical carcinoma patients as compared to the normal population served as the main argument for a role of this virus in the genesis of the tumor. This could not be confirmed in a recent study. In addition, the virus or parts of it could never be detected reproducibly in the tumors themselves.

In the case of the papilloma viruses, the following arguments for an involvement in the genesis of cervical carcinoma are to be mentioned:

1. Certain animal papilloma viruses, e.g., the rabbit papilloma virus or bovine papilloma virus, cause cancer under natural conditions or in animal experiments and are able to transform cells in tissse culture into cancer cells.

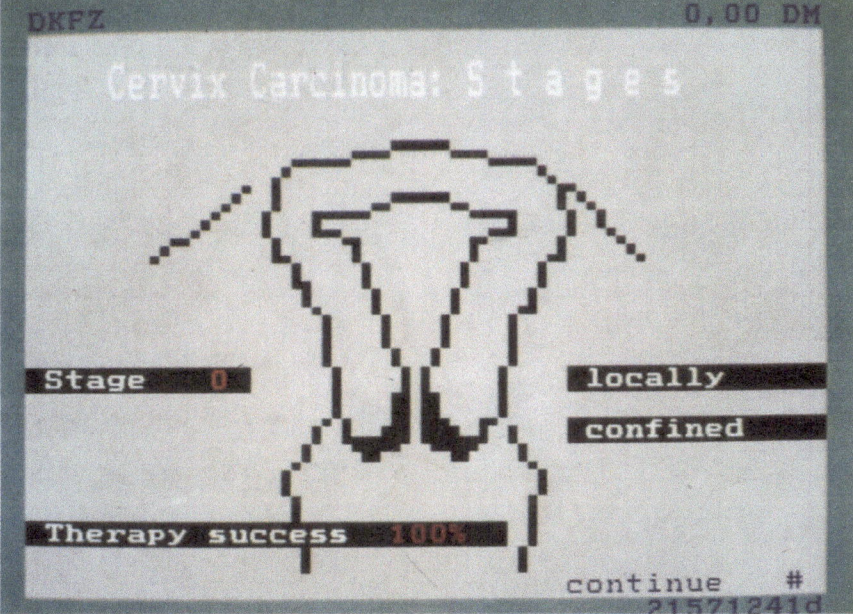

67

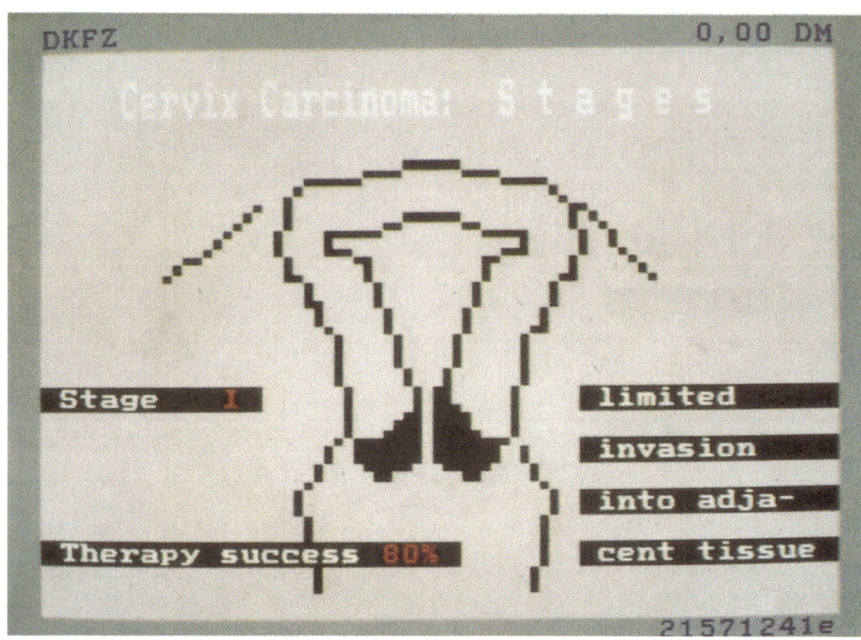

Fig. 44 c

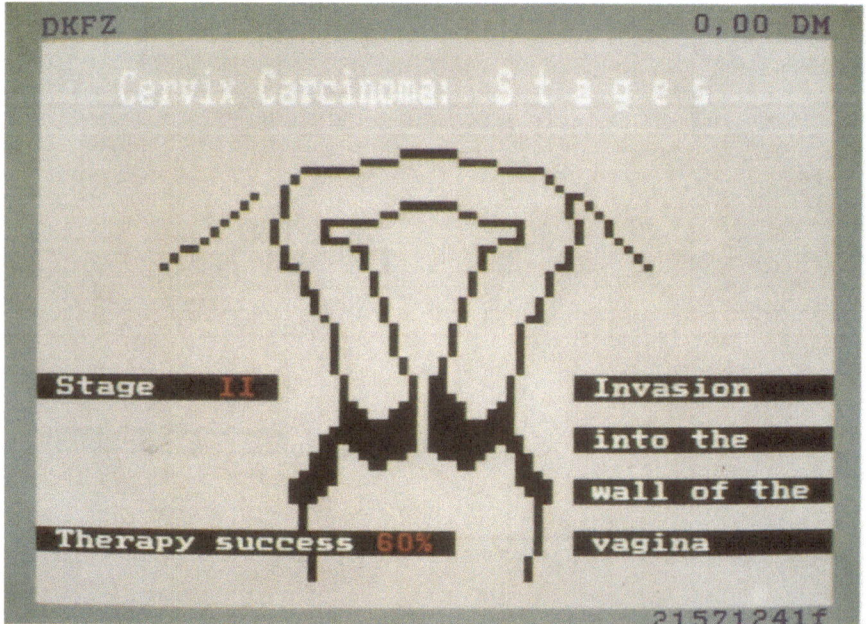

Fig. 44 d

2. Some of the initially benign human papillomas, in which papilloma viruses are regularly demonstrated, can be transformed under certain conditions, e.g., after irradiation with X-rays.

Despite intensive searching, no papilloma virus particles could be demonstrated in tumor cells of cervical carcinomas. However, this is not surprising if it is considered that, as a rule, viruses destroy the cells in which they proliferate and that this property is not compatible with permanent cell growth. However, it is to be assumed that viral deoxyribonucleic acid (DNA) remains in the tumor cells and should also be expressed if the virus is responsible for switching on and maintaining the malignant growth.

A special kind of nucleic acid hybridization has proved its effectiveness for the detection of viral DNA in tumor cells. For this purpose, the DNA from the tissue sample to be analysed is extracted by means of protein-digesting enzymes and phenol, cleaved with restriction enzymes and separated in agarose gels. After transfer to nitrocellulose membranes, a virus-specific sequence can be detected by binding the radioactively labelled papilloma virus DNA with subsequent autoradiography.

Since papilloma viruses do not grow in cell culture and since the concentration of the virus particles in the corresponding epithelial proliferations is often very slight, it was necessary to clone the DNA of the different papilloma virus types by means of genetic engineering methods. The DNA thus obtained after proliferation in Escherichia coli can be radioactively labelled and is thus available for the hybridization reaction mentioned above.

An analysis of roughly 150 different benign condylomata acuminata revealed that more than 95% contain the deoxyribonucleic acids of the closely related virus types HPV 6 or HPV 11. In the case of cervical carcinomas, HPV 11 could only be detected in one out of 33 biopsies investigated. On the other hand, papillomatous types not known up to that time (HPV 16 and HPV 18) could be identified under "nonstringent", i.e. less specific conditions. After cloning their DNA, the so far negative tumors were once more investigated in the hybridization. Now about two thirds of all cervical carcinomas were indeed positive for HPV 16 or HPV 18. In a further 25% of the carcinomas, one or several papilloma viruses not yet identified could be detected, so that 90% of the cervical carcinomas investigated contain papilloma virus DNA. Since HPV 16 and HPV 18 can only be rarely detected in the benign condylomata acuminata (in 3% of the biopsies investigated), we suspect that an infection with these viruses entails a higher tumor risk for a patient than contact with HPV 6 or HPV 11.

Dysplasias of the uterine cervix which may contain both HPV 6 or HPV 11 (39%) as well as HPV 16 or HPV 18 (20%) are of special interest in this connection. It is known that if such alterations are not treated, they may lead to an invasively growing cervical carcinoma in a certain percentage (10–20% in various investigations), although nothing can be stated about the development of an individual dysplasia on the basis of the cell smear. Thus the determination of the papilloma virus type might be important as an additional parameter in cancer prevention.

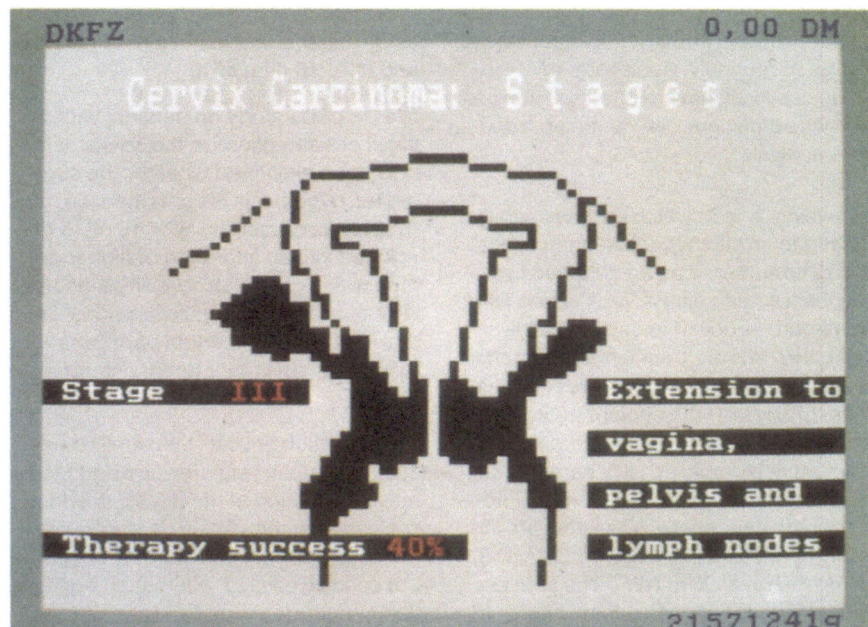

Fig. 44 e

Fig. 44 f

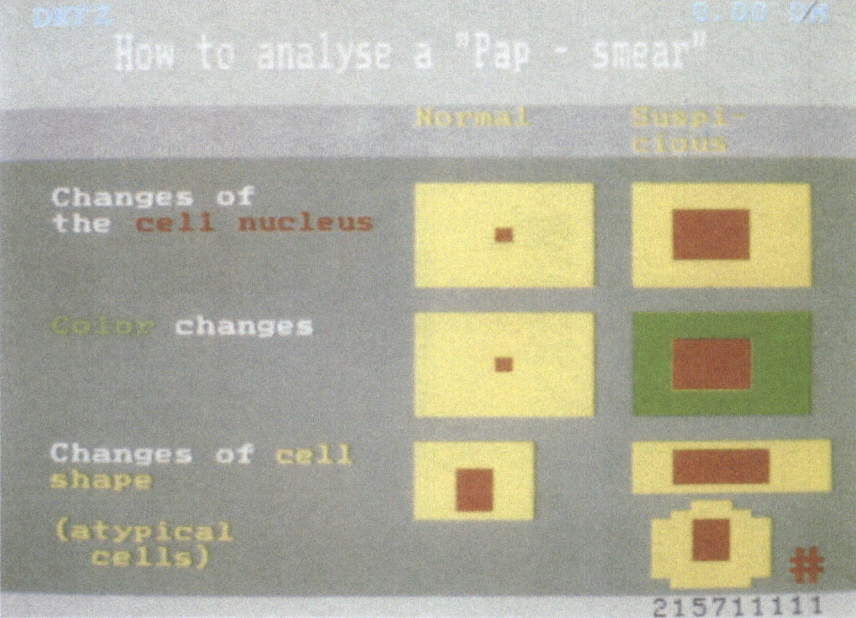

However, the method of DNA hybridization described above is too elaborate to be used routinely. Apart form this, the biopsies available are often too small to provide sufficient DNA for an appropriate analysis.

However, a test, which we have established for in situ hybridization of epithelial cells such as can be obtained in a cervical smear, allows virus typing with minimum trouble (Fig. 45 b). For this test, the cells are transferred into buffer solution, sucked up on a nitrocellulose filter and lysed with sodium hydroxide. In consequence of this treatment, the radioactively labelled HPV samples can bind specifically in the presence of appropriate sequences. The filters are initially hybridized with HPV 11 DNA and exposed on an X-ray film. The subsequent incubation of the same filters al-

lows detection of these viruses in the same material with a mixture of HPV 16 and HPV 18 (Fig. 45 a).

In a progress study on patients with slight cell alterations in the smear, it is now to be examined whether the suggested hypothesis is confirmed, i.e. that dysplasias caused by HPV 16 or 18 developed into an alteration of higher degree with a greater probability than the HPV 6- or HPV 11-positive lesions, i.e. that infection with certain papilloma viruses entails a higher tumor risk for a patient.

The detection of viral DNA could thus attain diagnostic significance and facilitate the decision of the doctor (besides evaluation of the smear) as to whether the patient is only to be further observed in a specific case or whether an operation should be carried out.

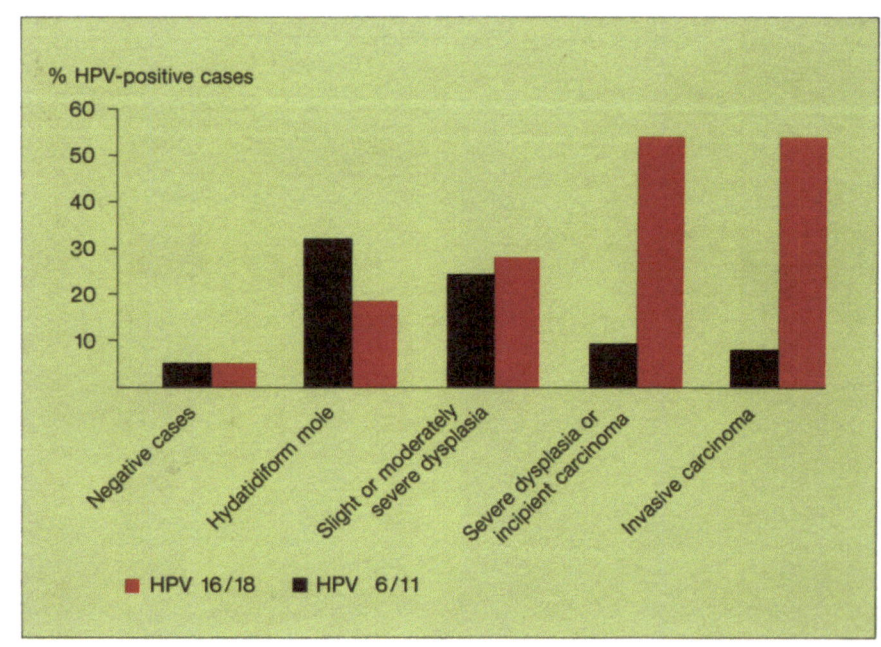

Fig. 45 a
Frequency of different papillomaviruses in smears from the uterine cervix

Although, of course, the high correlation of the occurrence of certain papilloma viruses with the development of malignant cervical carcinomas by no means proves a causal relationship; it renders it very probable. The suspected connection between a virus infection and a tumor disease would afford a means of preventing this disease by vaccination. Indeed, such vaccinations are already being carried out today in some areas with a high epidemic level of hepatitis B virus and simultaneous frequent occurrence of liver cancer (see above). A decline in the tumor incidence in the vaccinated population might be regarded as further strong evidence for the role of the virus in the development of this cancer.

At the present time, a vaccination against certain papilloma viruses is not yet possible, but it might probably be considered in a few years.

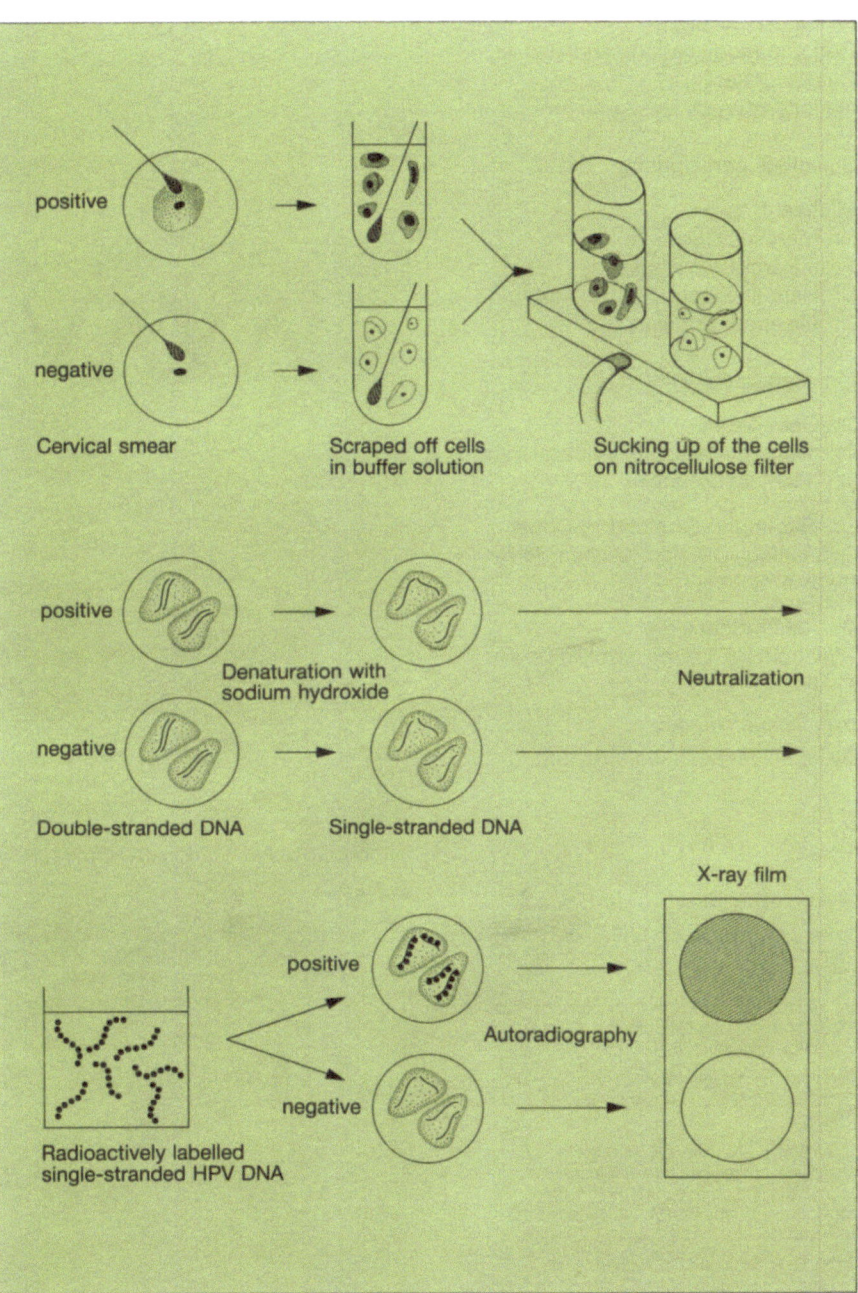

positive

negative

Cervical smear

Scraped off cells in buffer solution

Sucking up of the cells on nitrocellulose filter

positive

negative

Double-stranded DNA

Denaturation with sodium hydroxide

Single-stranded DNA

Neutralization

X-ray film

positive

negative

Autoradiography

Radioactively labelled single-stranded HPV DNA

Fig. 45 b
Production of filters to demonstrate papillomavirus DNA in uterine cervical smears

Prof. Lutz Gissmann
Genome Modifications and
Carcinogenesis,
Institute of Virus Research

Scientists participating

Michael Boshart
Dr. Matthias Dürst
Prof. Harald zur Hausen
Dr. Hans Ikenberg
Dr. Elisabeth Schwarz

In collaboration with

Dr. Gerd Gross
Dermatology Division, Freiburg University Medical School

Dr. Elke-Ingrid Grußendorf-Conen
Gynecology Division, Aachen University
Medical School

Dr. Achim Schneider
Gynecology Division, Ulm University
Medical School

Prof. Dieter Wagner
Diakoniekrankenhaus, Freiburg

Selected publications

Jones, E. G., Mac Donald, I., Breslow, L.: Study of
epidemiologic factors in carcinoma of uteri cervix.
Amer. J. Obstet Gynecol. 76, 1–10 (1958).

zur Hausen, H.: Papillomaviruses and their possible
role in squamous cell carcinoma. Curr. Top.
Microbiol. Immunol. 78, 1–30 (1977).

Report of the Surgeon General, Washington.
Cancer Incidence in Five Continents Vol. 4 (IARC)
(1982).

Gissmann, L., de Villiers, E. M., zur Hausen, H.:
Analysis of human genital warts (condylomata
acuminata) and other genital tumors for human
papillomavirus type 6 DNA. Int. J. Cancer 29,
143–146 (1982).

Crum, C. P., Ikenberg, H., Richart, R. M., Gissmann,
L.: Human papillomavirus type 16 and early cervical
neoplasia. New Engl. J. Med. 310, 880–883 (1983).

Fig. 46
Demonstration of specific DNA by means of a
radioactively labelled DNA sample. The two strands
of DNA can be separated by increase in the temperature or the pH value. Under suitable conditions, the
single strands join up again (hybridization)

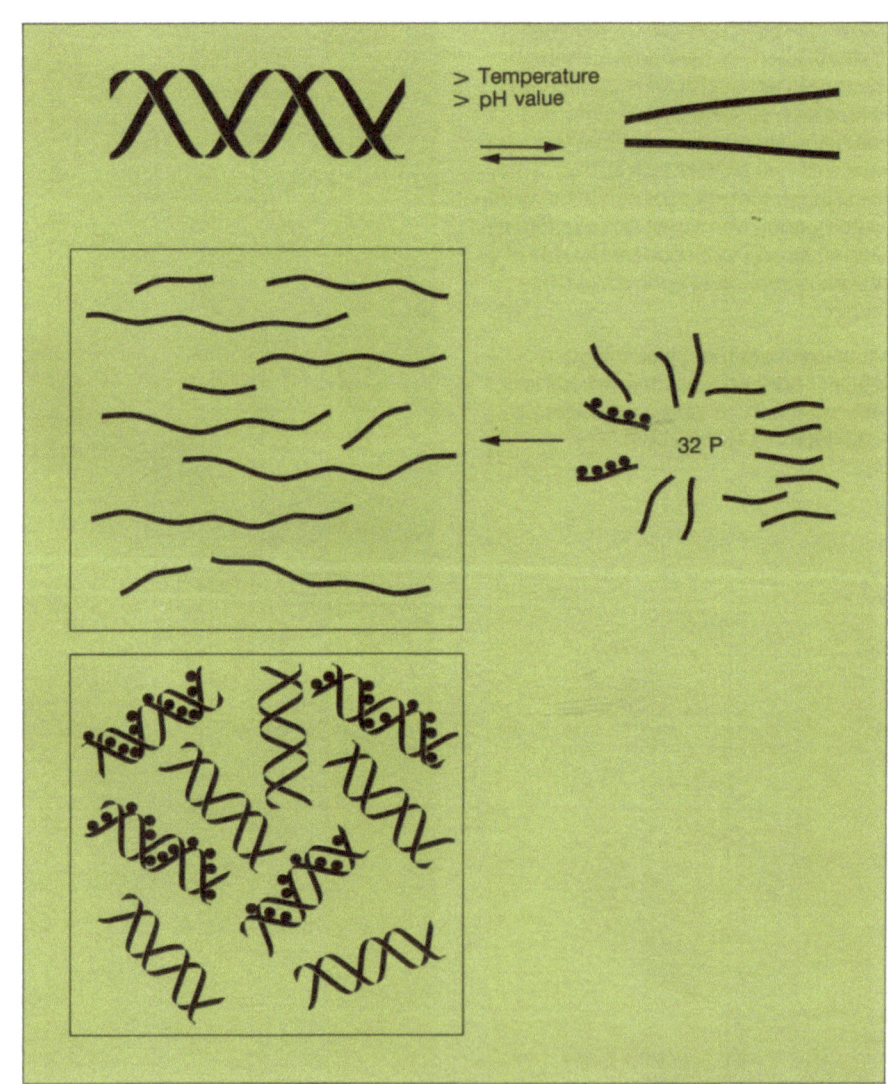

Fig. 47
Demonstration of specific DNA (e.g. viral molecules) in a mixture of cellular DNA by means of "Southern blood hybridization". The viral DNA is first of all made visible by autoradiography

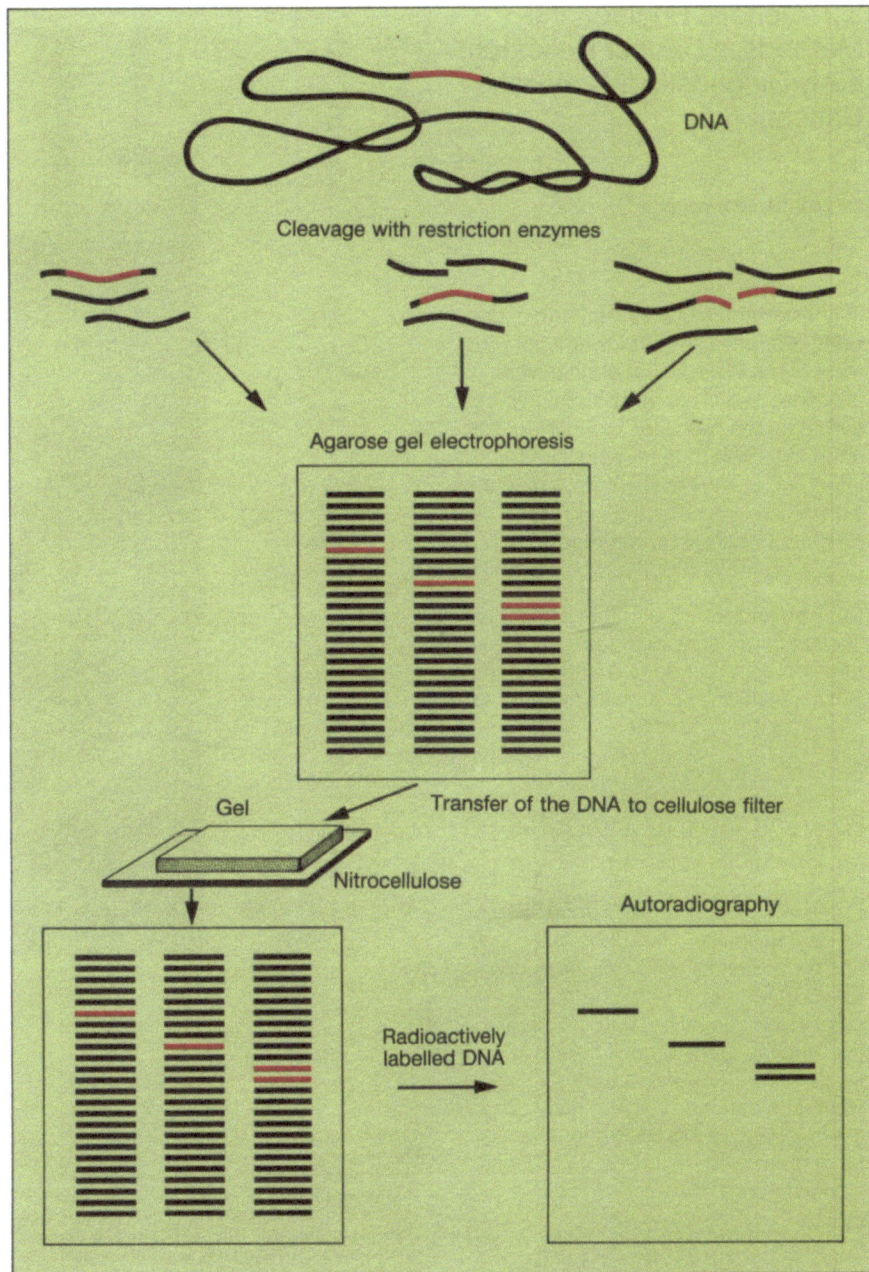

DNA

Cleavage with restriction enzymes

Agarose gel electrophoresis

Gel

Transfer of the DNA to cellulose filter

Nitrocellulose

Autoradiography

Radioactively labelled DNA

Dürst, M., Gissmann, L., Ikenberg, H., zur Hausen, H.: A papillomavirus DNA from a cervical carcinoma and its prevalence in cancer biopsies from different geographic regions. Proc. Natl. Acad. Sci. USA 60, 3812–3815 (1983).

Gissmann, L., Wolnik, L., Ikenberg, H., Koldovsky, U., Schnürch, H. G., zur Hausen, H.: Human Papillomavirus type 6 and 11 DNA sequences in genital and laryngeal papillomas and in some cervical cancer. Proc. Natl. Acad. Sci. USA 80, 560–562 (1983).

zur Hausen, H.: Herpes simplex virus in human genital cancer. Int. Rev. Exp. Pathol. 25, 307–325 (1983).

Boshart, M., Gissmann, L., Ikenberg, H., Kleinheinz, A., Scheurlen, W., zur Hausen, H.: A new type of papillomavirus DNA, its presence in genital cancer biopsies and in cell lines derived from cervical cancer. EMBO J. 3, 1151–1157 (1984).

Gissmann, L.: Papillomaviruses and their association with cancer in animals and in man. Cancer Surveys 3, 161–181 (1984).

Gissman, L., Boshart, M., Dürst, M., Ikenberg, H., Wagner, D., zur Hausen, H.: Presence of human papillomavirus (HPV) DNA in genital tumors. J. Invest. Dermatol. 83, 26s–28s (1984).

Ikenberg, H., Gissmann, L., Gross, G., Grußendorf-Conen, E.-I., zur Hausen, H.: Human papillomavirus type 16 related DNA in genital Bowen's disease and in Bowenoid papulosis. Int. J. Cancer 32, 563–565 (1984).

Vonka, W., Kanka, J., Jelinek, J., Subrt, I., Suchanek, A., Havrankova, A., Vachal, M., Hirsch, I., Domarazkova, E., Zavadova, H., Richterova, V., Naprstkova, I., Dvorakova, V., Svoboda, B.: Prospective study on the relationship between cervical neoplasia and Herpes Simplex Type-2 Virus. I. Epidemiological characteristics. Int. J. Cancer 33, 49–60 (1984).

Gissmann, L., Schwarz, E., Cloning of papillomavirus DNA. In: Developments in molecular virology, Vol. 5, Recombinant DNA pp 173–197. Y. Becker (ed.) Martinus Nijhoff, Publishers, Hingham, Ma. (1985).

## 3.2 Genetic Engineering Methods in Cancer Research: Early Diagnosis of Cervical Cancer

by Günter Krämmer

In consequence of a viral infection, the body produces antibodies against proteins of the virus. Using purified viral proteins, the serum of a patient can be tested for the presence of virus-specific antibodies and thus for a possible viral infection. Conversely, animal antisera, with which viral particles or proteins can be detected in tissue samples, can also be produced with purified viral proteins.

Such an antibody test might be very important for an early diagnosis of cancer development related to a viral infection. Such a relationship is discussed, for example, in the case of cervical carcinomas: in Germany, roughly 70% of these carcinomas contain deoxyribonucleic acid (i.e. the genetic information) of HPV 16 (human papilloma virus type 16) and HPV 18.

Papilloma viruses are known to induce warts and similar alterations of the skin and mucosae. HPV 16 causes condylomas (flat lesions) of the human mucosa in the genital tract. In the case of the mucosa of the uterine cervix, HPV 16-positive alterations frequently develop into carcinomas. The early discovery of a HPV 16 infection might hence be of great diagnostic and therapeutic significance.

The development of a test for early diagnosis applicable in clinical practice has so far been prevented by the fact that

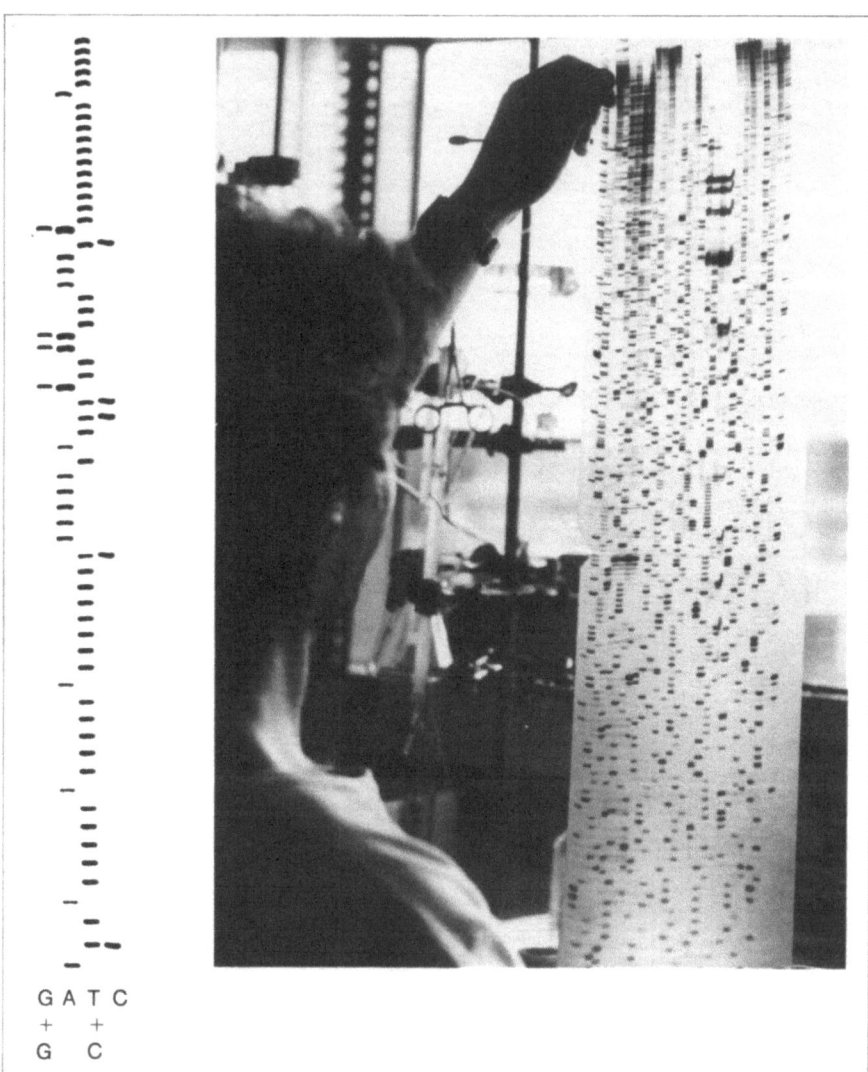

G A T C
+   +
G   C

Fig. 48
The sequence of several hundred bases of a DNA strand can be read off on a "sequence gel". In order to obtain the "sequence gel", from which a detail is shown on the left, a DNA strand is degraded by controlled chemical methods which are specific for one of the four bases respectively. The fragments were then separated according to their length. From the sequence gel obtained in this way, the base sequence can be read off directly. Read from the bottom to the top, this base sequence is here ACTATTTTATTTTTATTTTTTTCAAAAATATCCG, etc. G stands for the DNA component guanosine, A for adenosine, C for cytidine and T for thymidine.

viral proteins are not available: neither can they be isolated from the affected tissues, nor is there a cell culture system in which the virus could be proliferated. In order to be able to obtain appreciable amounts of HPV 16 proteins which could be used as diagnostic agents, the scientists participating in this project are attempting by means of genetic engineering to develop systems in which these proteins are produced by bacteria.

For this purpose, the entire genetic information of the virus (which is coded in its DNA as a sequence of four different bases) had to be decoded: the base sequence of the DNA was determined. A HPV 16 DNA clone, i.e. a bacterial strain in which the entire DNA molecule of HPV 16 containing 8,000 bases had been introduced, provided the material. Besides signals, which regulate the translation of the information from the DNA in the proteins, the DNA also con-

tains information for the structure of the proteins themselves. Such regions can be identified from knowledge of the base sequence of the DNA: the DNA of HPV 16 contains at least eight different regions which can possibly code for viral proteins.

## From the DNA Clone to Production of Viral Proteins

First step: Cloning of HPV 16 DNA from a cervical carcinoma.

The entire information on the structure of the proteins composing the coat of the papilloma virus HPV 16 is stored in the DNA of the virus, a double-stranded molecule of 8,000 base pairs. Such a complete viral DNA molecule was cloned from a cervical carcinoma, i.e. transferred to a circular DNA molecule, a plasmid, and proliferated as a component of this plasmid in bacteria.

Second step: Fragmentation of HPV 16 DNA into fragments.

In order to be able to resolve the base sequence of such a long DNA molecule, it was necessary to divide the DNA consisting of 8,000 base pairs into fragments with suitable enzymes and to clone these independently.

Third step: Sequencing of the HPV 16 DNA.

The individual HPV 16 DNA fragments could then be sequenced, i.e. the base sequence was determined with chemical and enzymatic methods. Put back

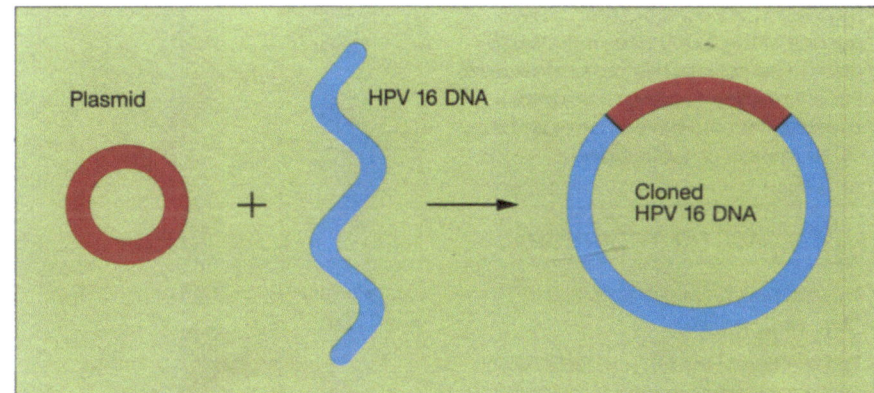

Fig. 49

Fig. 50

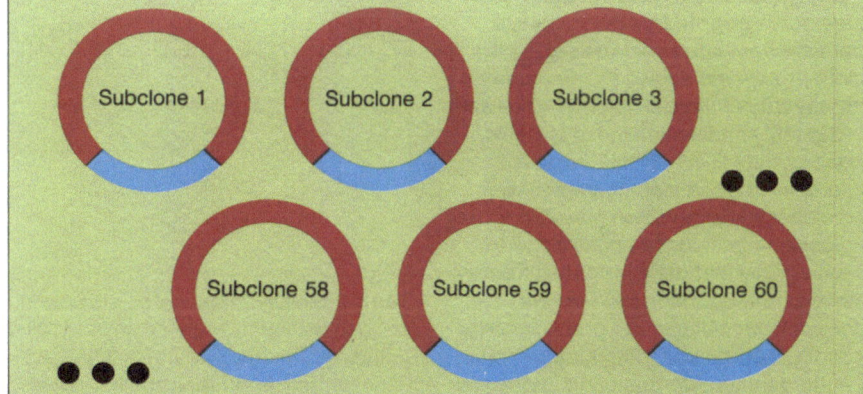

These eight "open reading frames" were recloned in "expression plasmids": they were incorporated into bacterial strains especially constructed for this purpose. In these bacterial strains, the information contained on the HPV DNA is efficiently converted into protein molecules. So far, four virus-specific proteins have been isolated in this way. These four proteins were used to prepare antisera. The suitability of these antisera for recognition of HPV 16 proteins is being tested at present. The next objective is the production of monoclonal antibodies. The development of a specific test system using these antibodies might offer a simple instrument for an early diagnosis of cervical cancer. It is possible that such HPV 16 proteins produced by genetic engineering can also be used as vaccines. Above and beyond their application as diagnostic agents, they might hence also be of significance for cancer therapy or prevention.

together in the correct order, the sequence of the 8,000 base pairs could then be established. In order to visualize the entire base sequence, the detail show here would have to be extended by 10 meters on both sides!

    .....ATTGTGGATAACAGCAGCCT.....
    .....TAACACCTATTGTCGTCGGA.....

Fourth step: Translation of the HPV 16 DNA into proteins.

The regions of the HPV 16 DNA, which contain the information for the protein molecules of the virus, can be identified as "open reading frames" from computer analysis of the base sequence: they are not interrupted by "stop signals", but are translated over their entire length into protein molecules by the enzymatic apparatus of the cell. In order to be able to identify and isolate these proteins, appropriate HPV 16 DNA fragments containing open reading frames were recloned in "expression plasmids". Expression plasmids are constructed in such a way that the information from the incorporated foreign DNA fragment is correctly translated into proteins under control of bacterial transcription signals – the genetic information is expressed.

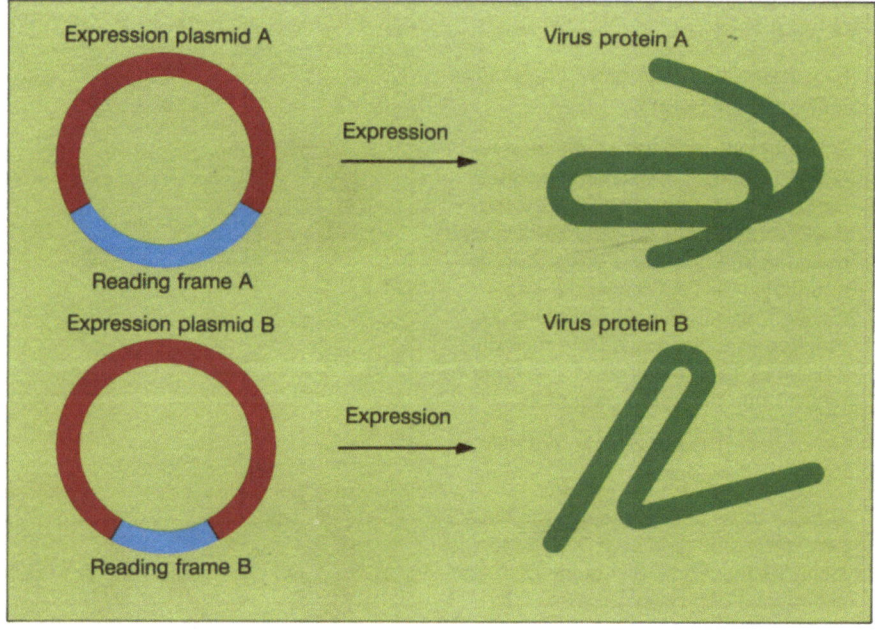

Fig. 51

The proteins synthesized by a bacterial cell can be separated on a gel according to their length (track a and c). If an additional protein is synthesized in the bacterium after introduction of an "expression plasmid", this protein becomes visible as a new band (arrows, track b and d) (Fig. 52).

Dr. Günter Krämmer
Molecular Biology of the Cell I,
Institute of Cell and Tumor Biology

Participating scientists

Dr. Walter Röwekamp
Klaus Seedorf

In collaboration with

Prof. Harald zur Hausen
Prof. Lutz Gissmann
Department Genome Alterations and
Carcinogenesis,
Institute of Virus Research

The HPV 16 DNA clone was isolated by
Matthias Dürst,
Department Genome Alterations and
Carcinogenesis,
Institute of Virus Research

Selected publications

Dürst, M., Gissmann, L., Ikenberg, H., zur Hausen, H.: A papillomvirus DNA from a cervical carcinoma and its prelevance in cancer biopsy samples from different geographic regions. Proc. Natl. Acad. Sci. USA 80, 3812–3815 (1983).

Seedorf, K., Krämmer, G., Dürst, M., Suhai, S., Röwekamp, W. G.: Human papillomvirus type 16 DNA sequence. Virology 144 (1985).

Seedorf, K., Krämmer, G., Röwekamp, W. G.: Human Papilloma Virus Type 16 DNA: Expression of open reading frames in E coli.

Howley, P. M., and Broker, T. R. (ed.) in Papilloma Viruses, Molecular and Clinical Aspects, UCLA Symposia on Molecular and Cellular Biology, New Series, Vol. 32, 1985.

Fig. 52

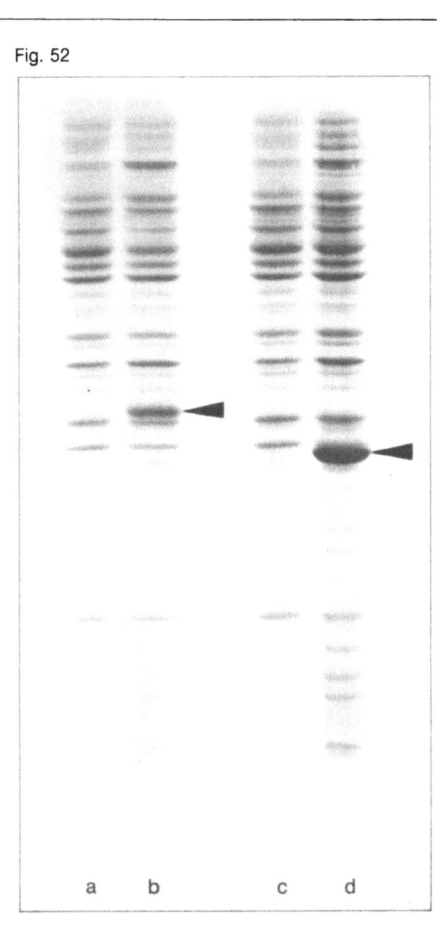

## 3.3 The Liver: a Filter System for Circulating Tumor Cells

by Rudolf Süss and Margarete Malter

What happens when foreign cells are injected into a rat, for example, erythrocytes from another animal, e.g., from a sheep or a human being? Within a few minutes, the foreign "wrong" cells which were quite out of place in the rat were trapped by the liver. The liver proved to be the most effective filter organ of the body.

Tumor cells should actually also be "wrong" cells for a body. We, therefore, posed the question: can the liver perhaps also trap tumor cells and remove them from the circulation? This question is of eminent practical significance. A primary tumor only becomes dangerous if tumor cells migrate and spread throughout the entire body via the bloodstream or the lymphatics and form tumor colonies (metastases) in the most diverse organs.

In purely theoretical terms, the liver should indeed be able to filter tumor cells which have detached from a tumor and which have entered the circulation. As a large organ, which is in the middle of the circulation between large vessels, a great volume of blood flows through it (1.5 liters per minute).

We have proved that leukemia cells (blood cancer cells) are not only arrested in the liver, but that they are also destroyed there. L. Weiss has shown that melanoma cells ("black" tumor cells) are decimated in their passage through the liver (shown schematically in Fig. 53). The liver can thus indeed act as a filter for tumor cells.

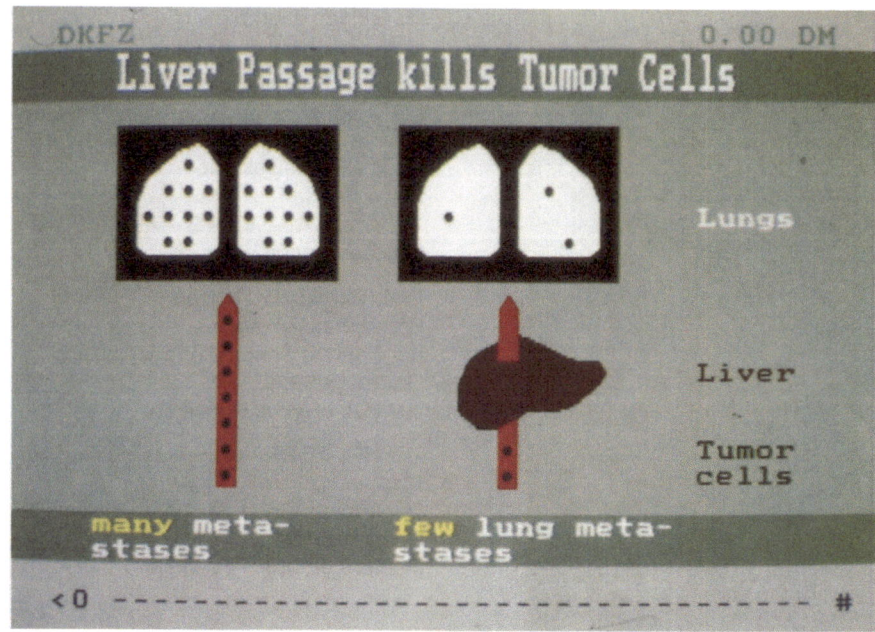

Fig. 53

We then asked ourselves: how does the liver destroy the arrested tumor cells? Does it perhaps crush them in its narrow vessels? In order to obtain clarity on this question, we observed a "living" rat liver under the microscope (intravital microscopy). In this technique, the vessels can be illuminated with a strong light source; an endless stream of red blood corpuscles and white blood corpuscles is seen rolling along the vessels. At some sites, above all in the small vessels, macrophages are seen. In the liver, they are called Kupffer cells. These cells can be readily recognized when very small latex beads are injected into the rat. These beads are ingested by the Kupffer cells and can then be clearly seen in the interior of the cells.

After the Kupffer cells were identified, tumor cells were injected into the rat. These appeared in the visual field of the microscope, and we observed how some of the tumor cells were intercepted by the Kupffer cells and remained attached to them. However, we never directly observed a destruction of a tumor cell. Nevertheless, we suspected that the liver kills tumor cells by means of its macrophages or Kupffer cells (all names for the same cells). This conclusion was not very bold, since it has been known for a long time that macrophages deriving from the peritoneal cavity can kill tumor cells.

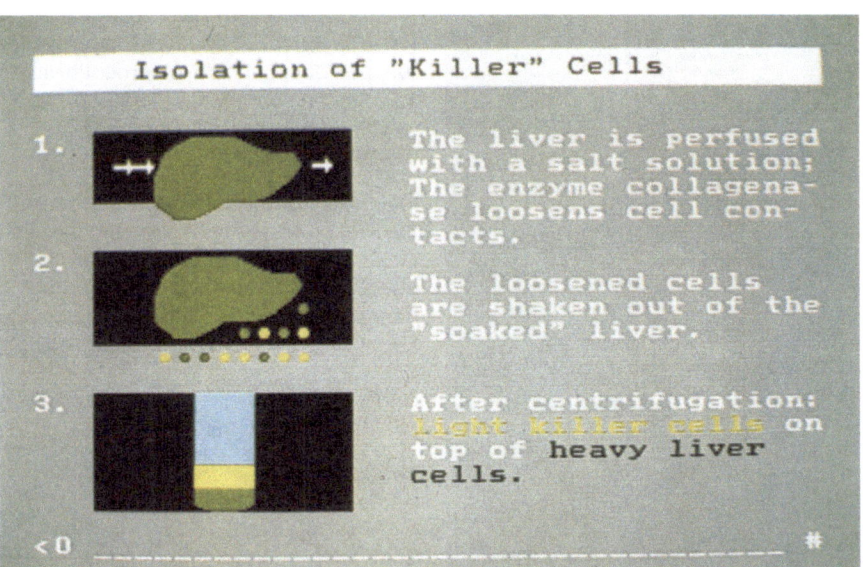

Fig. 54

radioactivity counter. In Fig. 55, this process is shown schematically (cytotoxicity test, from Kytos = cell; toxicity = poisoning, killing).

As expected, the macrophages from the liver were indeed able to kill tumor cells in the test tube. However, there was a surprise: when we eliminated the macrophages with a trick (treatment with quartz particles), tumor cells were still being killed. Our cell preparations evidently contained yet other cell species which are not macrophages but which can nevertheless kill tumor cells. Such tumor killer cells are well known from other organs (e.g., spleen or blood). We have described them in more detail for the first time in the liver.

In order to prove that macrophages are indeed responsible for killing tumor cells, they first of all had to be isolated from the liver.

The liver consists mainly of parenchymal cells. These carry out the actual work of the liver: storage of glycogen as energy reserve, detoxication of chemical substances. Besides the liver parenchymal cells, there are also cells which line the vessels (endothelial cells) and finally also cells located in these vessels, like the Kupffer cells just mentioned.

Figure 54 shows very crudely how the liver is divided into individual cells: first of all, the liver is perfused with a saline solution in order to free it from blood. Afterwards, an enzyme solution (collagenase) is perfused through the liver which loosens the connections between

the cells. The liver is "softened" after a short time and is then carefully shaken out in a saline solution. The individual cells of the liver then separate. The cells are precipitated in a centrifuge: the heavy parenchymal cells at the bottom of the centrifuge tube, and the lighter macrophages above them.

The cells responsible for killing the tumor cells were then easily identified: the macrophages isolated from the liver were mixed with tumor cells in the test tube and kept for a few hours at 37 °C in the incubator. During this time, the macrophages drill holes in the wall of the tumor cells; the tumor cells leak. If they had been labelled with a radioactive compound before the experiment, then this radioactive compound would also run out. It is collected and measured in a

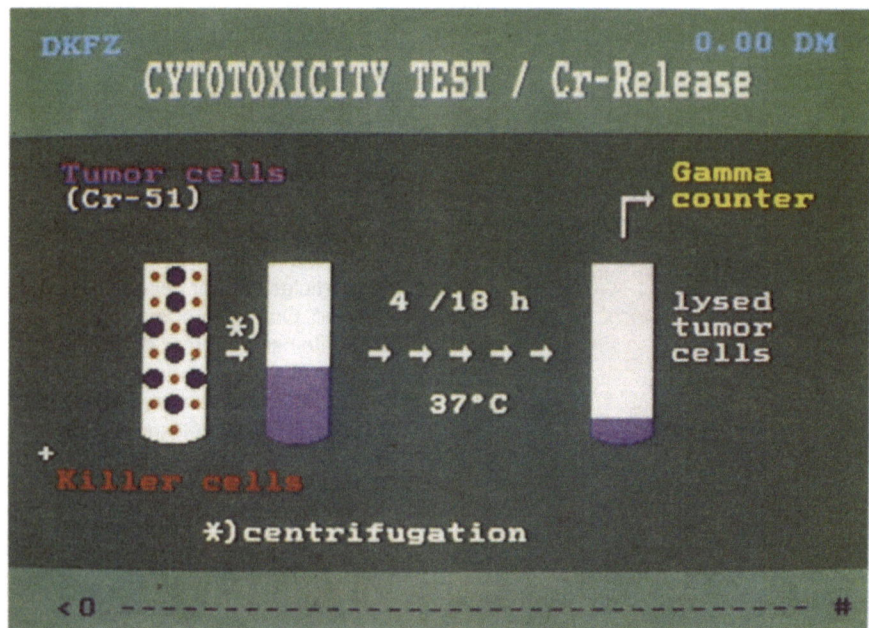

Fig. 55

Our estimates show that the liver is the largest reservoir of macrophages and "natural killers" in the body. This means that the liver is very well equipped to kill off circulating tumor cells.

Recent observations suggest that the liver also contains T killers. Besides this, we found cells which produce anti-bodies (B cells). Finally, the liver (and this has already been known for a very long time) produces complement, a substance which plays a crucial role in the destruction of cells by antibodies.

The liver thus possesses all the conventional weapons of immune defence. For tumor cells circulating in the vascular system, the liver becomes a fatal trap.

However, this trap does not always function: almost half of all people who die of cancer have metastases in the liver (10% of them in fact die in consequence of the resulting liver damage). The liver can filter out and kill tumor cells from the circulation, but a single tumor cell, which is able to lodge in the liver and is overlooked by the defence system, is sufficient to develop a metastasis. This shows that there are limits to the tumor cell defence system of the liver. If this defence system could be appreciably strengthened, the number of metastases in the liver, but also in other organs, should markedly decrease.

In first trials, is has been shown that the natural defence system of the liver is pre-programmed, but that it is also entirely able to adapt to external stimuli: classical stimulators (such as Corynebacterium parvum) can activate the tumor defence of the liver. The liver defence system also appears to adjust its function during the development of liver tumors: the number of its "natural killers" (and thus its killing capacity) increases considerably.

The flexibility of the defence system of the liver gives rise to the hope that ways and means will be found of supporting it effectively in its function of eliminating metastasizing tumor cells so as to counteract the development of metastases.

Dr. Rudolf Süss
Dr. Margarete Malter

Project Group Cancer Encyclopedia
Institute of Experimental Pathology

Staff participating

Rainer Kühnlein

Selected publications

Cohen, S. A., Salazar, D., Nolan, J. P.: Natural cytotoxicity of isolated rat liver cells. J. Immunology 129, 495–501 (1982).

Burkart, V., Friedrich, E.: Intravital microscopy of the perfused liver: RES 32, 269–272 (1982).

Burkart, V., Malter, M., Süss, R., Friedrich, E.: Liver as a tumor cell killing organ: Immunol. Comm. 13, 77–81 (1984).

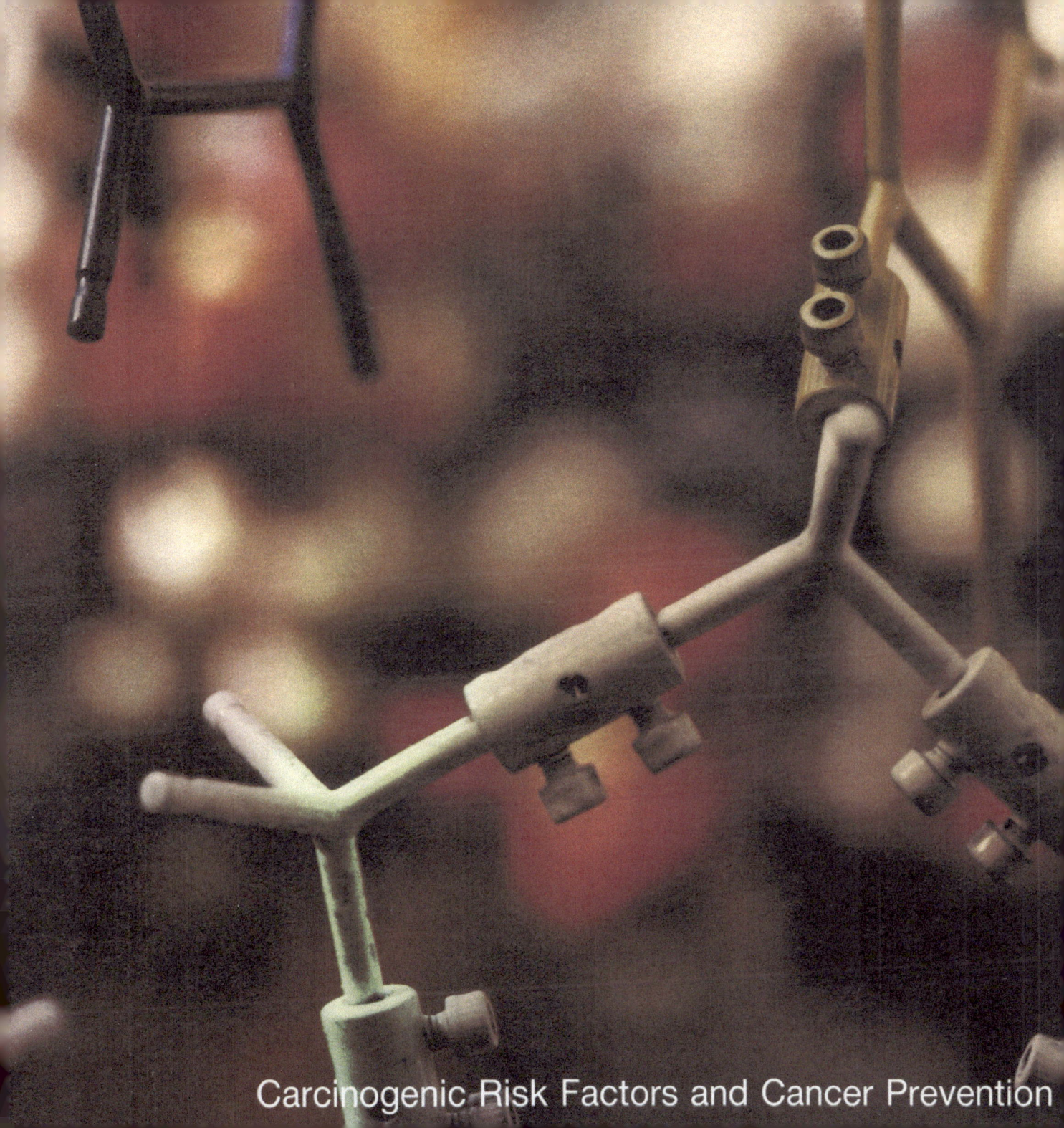

Carcinogenic Risk Factors and Cancer Prevention

# Carcinogenic Risk Factors and Cancer Prevention

The assumption that cancer in human beings is largely caused and triggered by environmental factors is undisputed today. Such carcinogenic factors include chemical substances, high-energy physical rays and viruses. Recognition and determination of such factors is the precondition for preventive measures.

## Methods of Research on Causes of Cancer

Environmental influences on the incidence of cancer were initially identified by investigations of occupational risks of small groups of people.

However, animal experiments (with major limitations also suitable tests for alterations in genetic material, mutagenicity test) remain the basis of the theoretical and practical exploration of carcinogenic environmental factors and of the verification of findings in humans. On the other hand, data on the occurrence of chemical carcinogens, the action of which was discovered in animal experiments, are leading increasingly to specific epidemiological investigations in man. Both approaches are hence jointly represented in this research focus.

Fig. 56

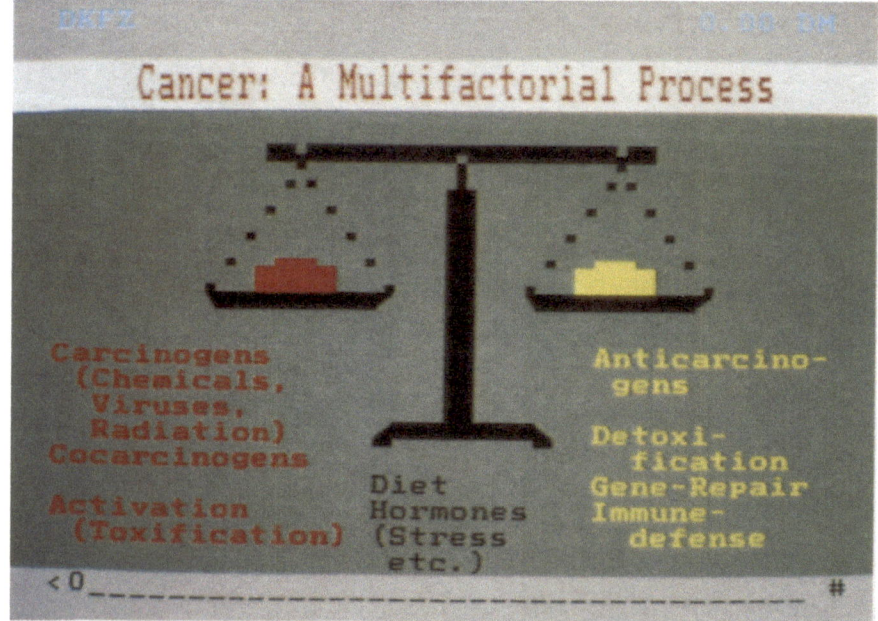

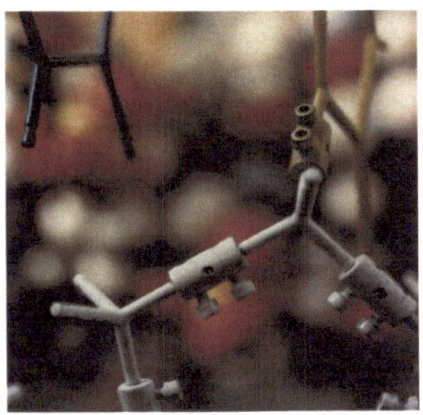

Fig. 57
View into a model of the DNA. Here the decisive alterations accure which initiate the formation of a cancer cell, e.g. under the influence of a chemical carcinogen

cinogenic up to now. These include physical factors, chemical compounds and also biological factors (viruses). For methodological reasons, it is appropriate to distinguish these factors, and such a subdivision is also carried out in this research focus.

## Viruses as a Cause of Cancer

The tumorigenic action of viruses is documented by animal experiments; oncogenic viruses produce tumors in animals. In human beings, a virus has so far not been identified with certainty as the sole carcinogen. With its capacity to remain latent in the human body throughout life, the herpes simplex virus has a characteristic property of oncogenic viruses containing desoxyribonucleic acid. On the basis of

seroepidemiological immunological and molecular biological findings, this virus has been suspected to be involved as a causal factor in the development of uterine cancer since the beginning of the 1970s. In addition, this virus appears to have a particular relation to the central nervous system. For this reason, the question of a herpes virus etiology is discussed in brain tumors. It must, of course, be asked why germs like the herpes simplex virus occurring everywhere show a selective frequency, for example in the tissue of brain tumors. It will also have to be investigated whether the regular detection of an organism can reveal a causal correlation as in the already known models of carcinogenesis in animals due to oncogenic viruses. The initially selective investigation of tumor tissue for the presence of the vi-

## Environmental Factors in Carcinogenesis known so far

Factors, which cause a transformation of tissue cells into tumor cells with a higher frequency than would be expected from spontaneous biological alterations, are designated as carcinogens. Analogous to this, the more frequent occurrence of tumor diseases in experimental animals or in certain human population groups in the presence of one or several carcinogenic factors can be rated as an indication of a causal effect. In these terms, experiments either serve as a confirmation of epidemiological findings or occasion the investigation of risk groups.

On the basis of such approaches, carcinogenic substances of the most diverse structure have been discovered or at least identified as potentially car-

Fig. 58

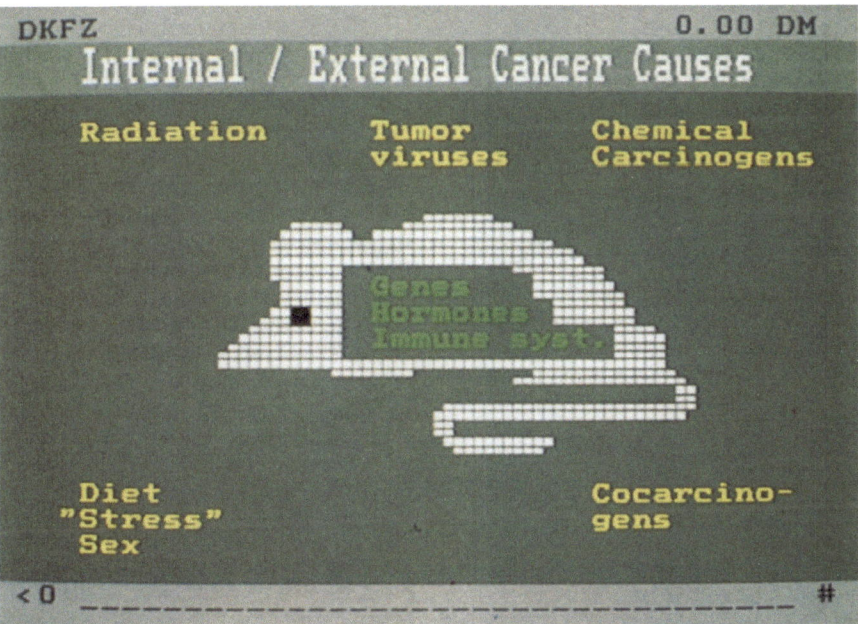

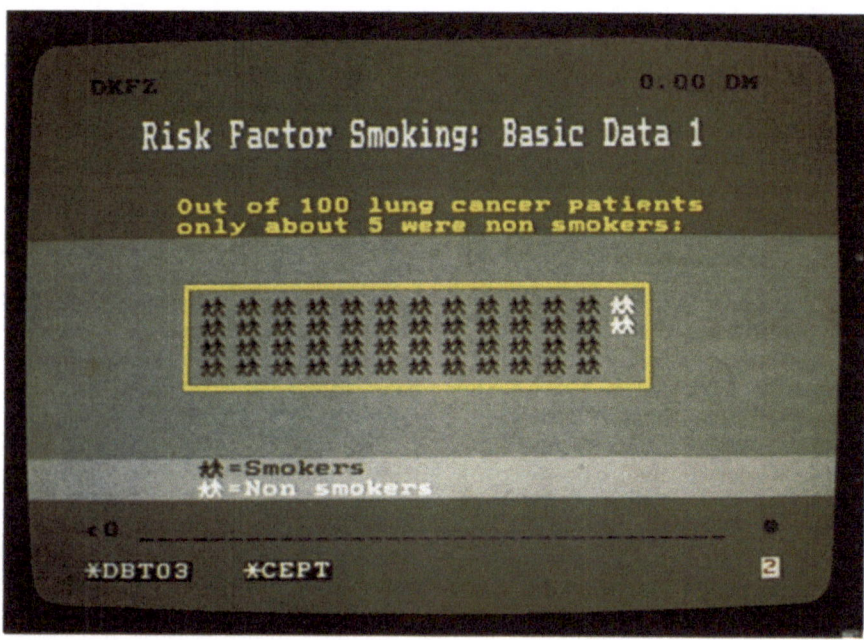

Fig. 59

ruses must be followed by epidemiological investigation of the relationship of virus traces (serological antibodies) and tumor incidence in the population. To characterize a final causal correlation, it will be necessary to detect the virus in the tissue before occurrence of the tumor.

The situation is also similar for other carcinogenic viruses as the hepatitis B virus and certain papilloma viruses; the latter are a further focus of studies at the German Cancer Research Center.

## Chemical Carcinogens

Certain chemical substances may be either widespread in the environment (ubiquitous), or geographically restricted or localized and hence associated with an exposure which can be determined (occupational groups, nutritional habits). Besides the recognition of isolated factors or substance groups, additive or synergistic effects are of very great significance (synergism = interaction of several factors), since they probably occur very much more frequently as compared to single effects and since a monocausality in carcinogenesis can only very rarely be assumed.

The occurrence and formation in the environment of already suspected carcinogens has been established by means of analytical methods. This enables an es-

timation of the exposure of a population group to such factors. Together with the investigation of the incidence of disease, this can give important information for prevention and early prognosis. This avenue of research (e.g. the identification of nitrosamines and their analysis) is pursued by the German Cancer Research Center on an international basis. Systematic animal experiments with in some cases very elaborate methods (e.g. inhalation) are concerned both with the relationship between chemical structure and carcinogenic action and with dose-effect relationships. Such data are necessary preconditions for risk estimations for environmental carcinogens. These studies are supplemented by investigations on synergistic and modifying effects in chemical carcinogenesis.

Substances, which may induce cancer under certain conditions (so-called cocarcinogens) and which intensify the action of carcinogenic factors, can be identified by means of experiments and analysed by biochemical methods in such a way that inferences can be made with regard to the carcinogenic action from the structural details. Screening programs lead to an estimation of the quantitative significance of such factors in the overall exposure of human beings in their everyday environment. Such systematic investigations are expected to provide important information for epidemiological cancer research which will be included these in the analysis of the interaction of diverse factors.

## Radiation Cancerogenesis

The follow-up examination of the final fate of about 5,000 patients, in whom the radioactive x-ray contrast medium Thorotrast (a colloidal solution of thorium dioxide) had been used for diagnostic reasons from 1935 to 1948, was investigated in an epidemiological study of the German Cancer Research Center. This study serves above all to gain more information on dose-effect relations of radiation cancerogenesis in man. The objective of this study requires strict maintenance of a follow-up scheme. From a total of about 2,000 dead patients registered so far the causes of death have been established; patients who are still alive are being constantly followed up. A pseudorandomly selected control group (matched for sex and age) is followed according the same scheme.

This is the rare case of an iatrogenic carcinogenesis (caused by medical intervention). Its investigation can provide important knowledge about the radiation to which present and future generations may be exposed.

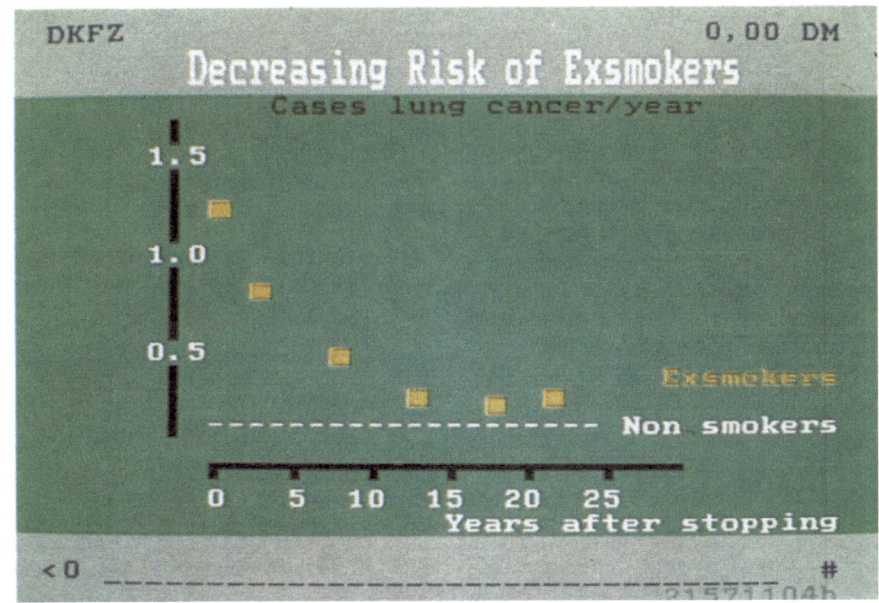

Fig. 60

Fig. 61

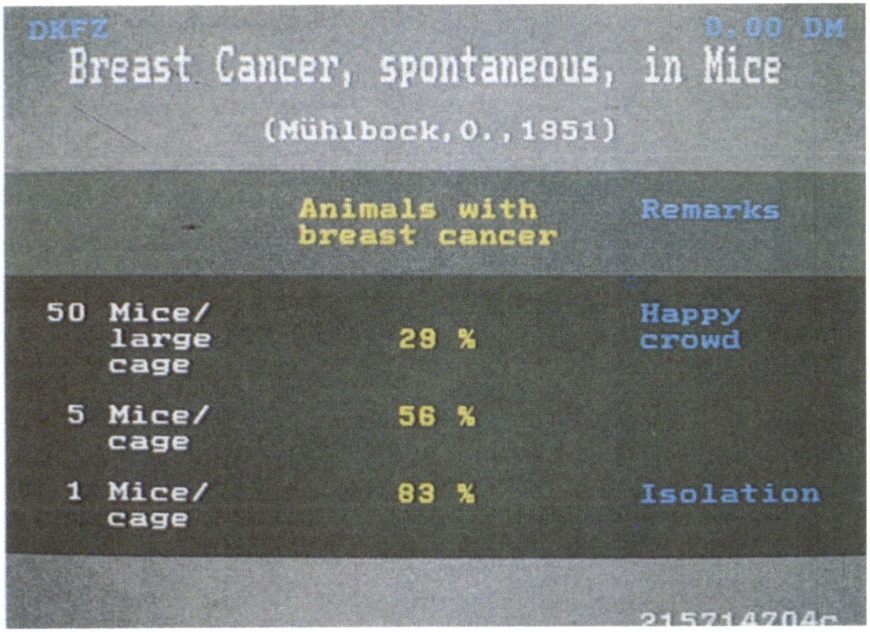

85

## Cancer Epidemiology

Despite the familiar difficulties of cancer epidemiology in the absence of cancer registries in the Federal Republic of Germany, this important field will be extended and intensified in the near future in the German Cancer Research Center. Modern analytical epidemiological investigations will be carried out to an increased extent; specific prospective investigations and intervention studies are also planned on an international basis.

## Research Activities focused on Cancer-Inducing Factors and Cancer Prevention

Radiation protection dosimetry

Chemical carcinogenesis

Investigations of chemical carcinogens for biological effects in various short-term test systems

Toxic, teratogenic and carcinogenic action of various chemical substances, heavy metals with particular environmental relevance as well as viruses in perinatal animal trials

Investigation of the carcinogenic action of metal dusts of alloys containing nickel

Comparison of the etiological mechanisms and the possibility of influencing tumors induced in the digestive tract in rats in the perinatal or adult phases of life

Occupational exposure to nitrosamines

Biological monitoring of nitrosamines

Analysis of nonvolatile N-nitroso compounds

Quantification of endogenous nitrosation and precursors of N-nitroso compounds

Tumor promoters of the diterpene ester type as cancer risk factors

Early molecular and cellular parameters of chemical hepatocarcinogenesis

Application of hepatocarcinogenic substances to evaluate their risk

Influence of drugs and foreign substances on chemical carcinogenesis

German Thorotrast study

Investigations on radiation-induced carcinogenesis

Epidemiological bone tumor registry; Working Group Bone Tumors

Descriptive epidemiological studies

Analytical epidemiological studies

Clearing House for On-Going Research in Cancer Epidemiology

Statistical methods for planning animal experiments taking into account the course of the tumor process

Statistical models in carcinogenesis and cocarcinogenesis

## 4.1 Cancer and Nutrition

by Rudolf Preußmann

What is the scientific basis of the thesis of correlations between food habits and cancer risks? In the following, I should like to find answers and would want to emphasize that I do this from the viewpoint of experimental research on carcinogenesis; it may be that the epidemiologist or the nutritional scientist will arrive at somewhat different results and interpretations of the facts.

The basis of all reflections is the largely accepted theory that the majority of cancer cases in men are the result of chronic toxic effects and are caused by environmental influences in the widest sense. There is no doubt that the diet is quite a crucial environmental factor for human beings. Adults consume about 2.5 kg of "chemicals" in the form of proteins, carbohydrates, fats, minerals, trace elements, vitamins, aroma substances and other animal and plant constituents. It is thus justified to enquire whether food in general and individual nutritional habits in particular may induce or promote cancer.

In 1981, the British epidemiologists R. Doll and R. Peto presented a comprehensive review of the causes of cancer. The distribution over various causal factors is shown in Table 1.

The authors expressly designate the percentages given for the causes as working hypotheses. These are estimates of the main factors in carcinogenesis in humans which are subject to appreciable uncertainties. The significance of "foodstuffs" defined as food

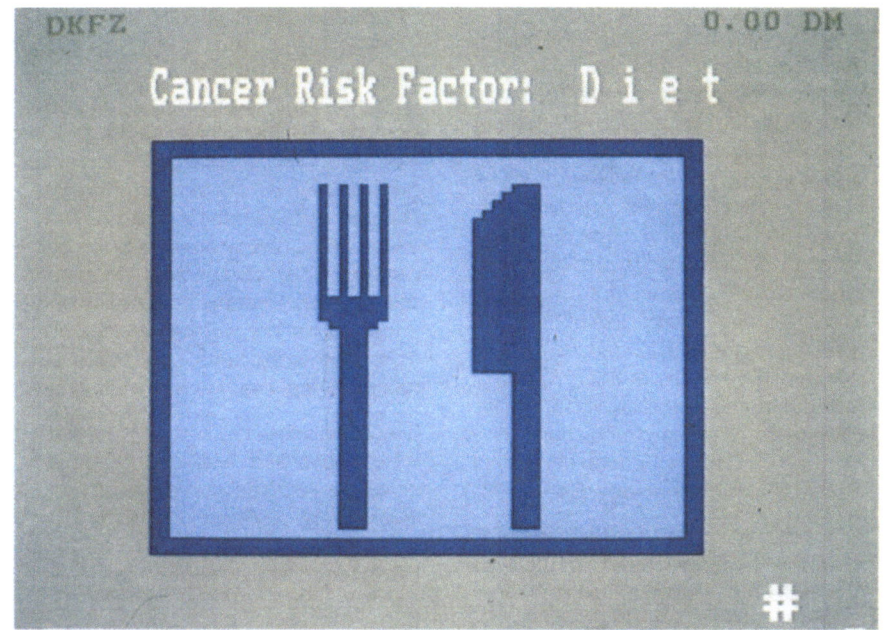

Fig. 62

Tab. 1 Causes of cancer in humans. Working hypotheses according to R. Doll and R. Peto, Journal of the National Cancer Institute 66, 1191–1308 (1981), modified

| factors | % cancer deaths best estimate | range of justifiable estimates |
|---|---|---|
| foodstuffs | 37 | 10–75 |
|   food | 35 | |
|   water and air | 2 | |
| tobacco | 30 | 25–40 |
| alcohol | 3 | 2–4 |
| reproductive and sexual behavior | 7 | 1–13 |
| occupation | 4 | 2–8 |
| geophysical factors (sunlight) | 3 | 2–4 |
| medication and medical treatments | 1 | 0.5–3 |
| industrial chemicals | less than 1 | less than 1–2 |
| food additives | less than 1 | – 5–2 |
| infections (viruses, bacteria, parasites) | 10? | 1–? |
| unknown | ? | ? |

plus air and water is evident; besides tobacco, they assume a central position. In contrast to tobacco, however, the enormous range of variation of possible estimated values shows the many uncertainties inherent in such values due to major gaps in knowledge, particularly in the food sector. However, it remains to be observed that human nutrition often gives rise to problems with regard to carcinogenic factors in the widest sense. An expertise of the US-National Academy of Sciences published in 1982 on the problem "Diet, Nutrition and Cancer" arrives at similar conclusions (German translation: Ernährung und Krebs, Federal Ministry of Research and Technology, Bonn, 1984).

For systematic reasons, it is meaningful to subdivide the discussion of the available data into epidemiological and experimental data.

## Epidemiological Investigations

The very voluminous literature is complex, frequently contradictory and often confusing for the critical reader. Doll and Peto note that "nutrition and cancer is a chronic source both of frustration and excitement for epidemiologists". The evident difficulties derive from the complexity both of food and of human nutrition, but also from the complexity of the causes of cancer. It is known that, apart from a few exceptions, cancer in man has many causes, i.e. it is multicausal.

It must be accepted that up to now there is no precise and reliable proof, based on epidemiological surveys, that cancer is caused by nutritional factors in humans, and even definite information on this is rare despite intensive research and intensive discussion of the question.

The main reason for this regrettable situation is the often underestimated difficulty in exactly determining nutritional habits. Even within a comparable population, people live on very different, types of food. The establishment of nutritional habits, mostly by enquiring about fat, meat or vegetable consumption, provides only a very rough idea about actual consumption habits. In epidemiological case control studies, nutritional behavior is determined in that eating habits are explored three days or one week before the interview. However, the relative certainty in such questions is deceptive: amongst the factors eliciting cancer, dietary habits of 20–40 years ago are of crucial importance. However, we all change our individual dietary habits in the course of time. General eating habits have also changed over such a long period. Consumption of meat, eggs, fat, sugar and in particular of vegetables and fruit has increased, and the consumption of cereal products, potatoes and pulse has decreased. Such "global" changes are not necessarily reflected in alterations in individual consumption. Finally, it is very important that the quality of foods has changed both in the positive and in the negative sense due to the introduction of new technologies in industrial and household food preparation, the introduction of foods capable of being stored, of food "from cans" and, finally, due to the influence of microbiological and environmental chemical contaminations.

The difficulties for retrospective epidemiology are evident. The inherent problems are hard to solve.

In the method of case control studies, the food habits of cancer patients are investigated. An attempt is made to find retrospective reasons for the cause of the disease, compared to patients who have not developed cancer (the control group). As already mentioned, a major problem here is our inability to carry out sufficiently precise measurements of nutrition. In correlation (or ecological) studies, the frequency of cancer (mostly in relation to a certain organ) is related to possible causal factors, in the specific case to food habits. In such studies, large populations, inhabitants of the country, racial or religious groups, emigrants in the old and new home country or indeed industrial countries and developing countries are investigated and their general nutritional habits compared with differences in cancer morbidity or mortality.

Nutritional characteristics mostly derive from statistical figures for per capita consumption of the variously categorized foods which derive either from production or from consumption data. Such studies evidently iron out the heterogeneity of nutrition between individuals as well as the individual variation of eating habits; they often make untenable assumptions with regard to a homogeneity of the diet of larger populations which does not exist. Accordingly, the results of such studies can only be translated with difficulty into the causes of cancer in an individual. It is hence not surprising that the results of correlation studies are very often not confirmed by case-control studies and vice versa. Correlation studies are of great importance in the formation of hypotheses for further research. However, they will hardly ever be able to prove causal relationships (although they are unfortunately only often used for this purpose).

After these brief descriptions of relevant epidemiological methods and their disadvantages, I should like to mention some selected important results. It appears to me to be more reasonable to take individual constituents of the food and not individual cancer localization, since this makes it easier to include experimental results to support epidemiological findings. The data for this essentially derive from the monograph of the US National Academy of Sciences already mentioned.

## Fats

In correlation studies, the most distinct indications of correlations between cancer and food have been obtained between fats and the raised risk of tumors of the breast and the intestines. In some cases, but by no means always, these have also been confirmed by case-control studies. In animal experiments, raised fat contents in the food influence the incidence of tumors after prior initiation with chemical carcinogens (colon, breast) or the number of spontaneous cancers. The available data from both research sectors make it probable that fats do not initiate tumors, but accelerate their manifestation.

## Protein (Animal)

Although there are some indications for a raised risk of cancer (breast, intestines, possibly pancreas) in high meat consumption, these are mostly not confirmed in case-control studies. However, as a rule there is a high correlation between a high uptake of animal protein and fat so that the effects can probably be attributed to fats. Experimental studies on the influence of protein on chemical carcinogenesis are contradictory.

## Carbohydrates

Most epidemiological and experimental studies provide indications that carbohydrates do not play any role in carcinogenesis.

Fig. 63

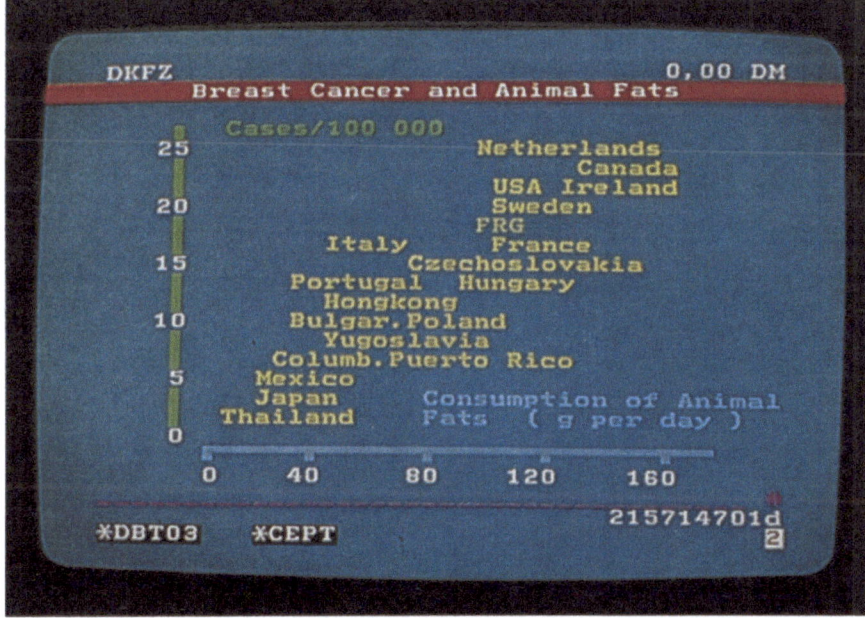

89

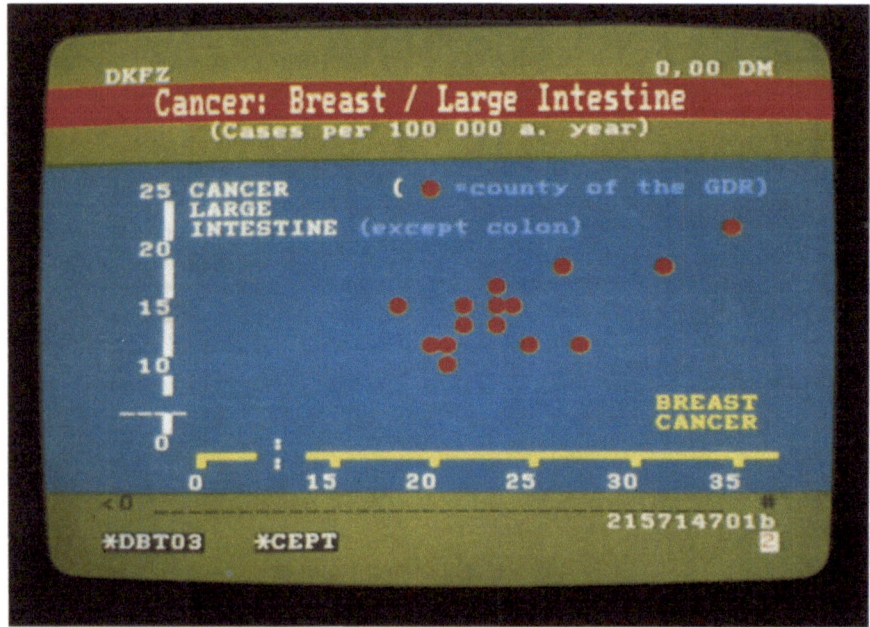

Fig. 64

## Roughage (Celluloses, Lignins, Pentosans, etc.)

Roughage, or fiber, mainly occurs in vegetables, fruit and whole grain products. Reduced uptake of these substances is alleged to raise the risk of intestinal cancer. However, both types of epidemiological studies have provided results which neither confirm nor refute the hypothesis. The available experimental studies also do not solve the problem at present. In the future, more attention must be paid to specific fiber constituents and not to their total content.

## Vitamins

Vitamin A has recently attracted great interest with regard to its role in the process of carcinogenesis. Epidemiological studies indicate a correlation between the genesis of epithelial tumors in the lungs, urinary bladder and larynx and deficiency of vitamin A or its precursors (carotinoids or synthetic retinoids) which occur preferentially in green and yellow vegetables. Some if not all experimental studies confirm a certain inhibitory effect of vitamin A on chemically induced epithelial tumors. Vitamin A modifies the differentiation of epithelial tissue. Its role is likely to consist in an inhibition of tumor growth. The original enthusiasm with regard to vitamin A anticarcinogenesis has given way to the observation formulated as follows at a

specialist conference: "There is at present no basis for the notion that vitamin A protects against cancer, and there is practically no evidence justifying additional administration of vitamin A in the diet." (Science 223, 1161, 1984).

Vitamin C (ascorbic acid) and vitamine E (alpha-tocopherol) inhibit the formation of carcinogenic N-nitroso compounds from amine precursors in the food and nitrite in the human stomach. This will later be briefly reported on.

The findings on the influence on carcinogenesis (probably not its induction) by groups of food constituents such as fats, proteins or certain vitamins described above are a good basis for further specific investigations. In particular, further investigations must be more differentiated with regard to individual fat constituents (especially in high fat intake); thus, for example, the question is to be examined whether the formation of oxygen radicals greatly emphasized by B. Ames and the resulting lipid peroxidation may play a role here, especially as a tumor promoter.

In principle, even in the near future epidemiological investigations of certain foods or their constituents will suffer from the fact that it is probably impossible to find two reasonably similar populations whose diet differs over a long period in only one factor to be investigated.

To summarize, and considering many further investigations not mentioned here, I conclude that epidemiological indications on correlations between nutrition and cancer are in all very vague and by no means conclusive. In my opinion, on a purely epidemiological basis, the value of a 35% involvement of nutrition in the causes of cancer in man estimated by Doll and Peto is by no means tenable. The question whether experimental investigations will provide more information is thus to be examined.

## Experimental Investigations

We have seen that the observational-descriptive methods of epidemiology produce a blurred picture which is unsuitable for documenting causal interrelationships. In contrast to this, experimental data illuminate details of an overall picture very clearly, i.e. they produce a kind of pointillist picture. Here, the difficulty is to construct a convincing overall picture from exact individual findings.

In the discussion of experimental findings on the topic, it is appropriate to start from mechanistic concepts of carcinogenesis. Afterwards, one can subdivide relevant investigations into the following subareas, as shown in Table 2.

In the following, I shall concentrate on the possibilities 1 and 2 listed in the Table, since there are exact analytical measurements of the occurrence of chemical carcinogens in the diet (although these are subject to fluctuations and also do not by any means cover the exposure in this regard completely and without gaps in knowledge), and there is also a generally accepted theory of carcinogenesis in the initial phase (J. A. Miller, Cancer Research, 30, 559ff., 1970). Quantitative measurements are already rare in the second topic group, the formation of carcinogens in the body itself. The remaining possibilities mentioned are usually only (and sometimes little) founded working hypotheses for which there are empirical data but no comprehensive theory. This is especially characteristic for the area of promotion

Tab. 2 Hypotheses or facts according to which nutrition can influence cancer incidence. After R. Doll and R. Peto, National Cancer Institute 66, 1191–1308 (1981), modified

| Possibilities | Examples |
|---|---|
| 1. Ingestion of carcinogens in the diet | 1. Food contaminated with carcinogens <br> 2. "Natural" carcinogens occurring in plant products <br> 3. Carcinogens produced in the preparation of food <br> 4. Carcinogens produced by micro-organisms in stored foods |
| 2. Influence on the formation of carcinogens in the body | 1. Uptake of substrates for endogenous carcinogen formation (e.g. nitrite/nitrate and secondary amines for nitrosamine formation) <br> 2. Alteration of the bacterial intestinal flora (and thus of the capacity to form carcinogenic metabolites) <br> 3. Alteration of the uptake or excretion of cholesterol or bile acids (and thus the formation of carcinogenic metabolites in the intestine) |
| 3. Influence on the transport as well as activation and detoxication of carcinogens | 1. Alteration of the concentration or duration of contact in the intestine (dietary fiber) <br> 2. Induction or inhibition of enzymes which determine carcinogen metabolism <br> 3. Deactivation or prevention of the formation of carcinogen metabolites (SH compounds, selenium, beta-carotene and antioxidants) |
| 4. Promotion of transformed cells | 1. Influence on stem cell differentiation <br> 2. Stimulation of proliferation |
| 5. Obesity | 1. Estrogens produced in the adipose tissue after the menopause |

at present intensively discussed (i.e. the promotion of transformed cells or pre-neoplastic cell areas) which is also being worked on experimentally (area 4, Tab. 2). Besides an acceleration of growth, the substances which are regarded as promoters also bring about an inhibition in some cases. An "anticarcinogenesis" by inhibition of the activation of genotoxic carcinogens by metabolism in the body or by interception of ultimate carcinogens is possible (area 3). These possibilities of inhibition of the processes of carcinogenesis are of crucial significance for primary prevention, but are only in exceptional cases so far advanced that intervention studies are justifiable in man. There is no doubt that more research is necessary here.

## Carcinogen Contaminants in the Food

By far the greatest problems with regard to potential carcinogens in the food result in the case of undesired and more or less unavoidable contaminations.

## 1. Polycyclic Aromatic Hydrocarbons

Polycyclic aromatic hydrocarbons (PAH) of the 3.4-benzpyrene type are a group of widespread environmental carcinogens which are formed in the incomplete combustion of organic material and are hence emitted, e.g., from petrol engines or industrial and domestic burners. Members of this class of substances show a potent carcinogenic effect in animal studies on local application, e.g., on the skin; in oral application, the effect on the stomach is rather weak.

Figure 65 gives an overview of the main sources of exposure through food according to the data from Fritz. It is evident that the main exposure derives from plant foods and results from the

sedimentation of air pollution with PAHs; it can be proved that, with increasing vicinity of the cultivated areas to PAH emitters, the contamination of plant food increases. A second group of contaminated foods are smoked and highly roasted products. However, they contribute less to the overall exposure than the first group mentioned.

If one compares the present exposure data to the tumorigenic doses effective in animal trials, one arrives at a very rough estimate of a safety factor of 1,000 in the oral uptake of PAHs.

For 3,4-benzpyrene there is a highest allowed amount of 1 ppb (µg/kg) in smoked meat products in the Federal Republic of Germany. A similar regulation for plant food would be desirable in order to avoid peak exposures.

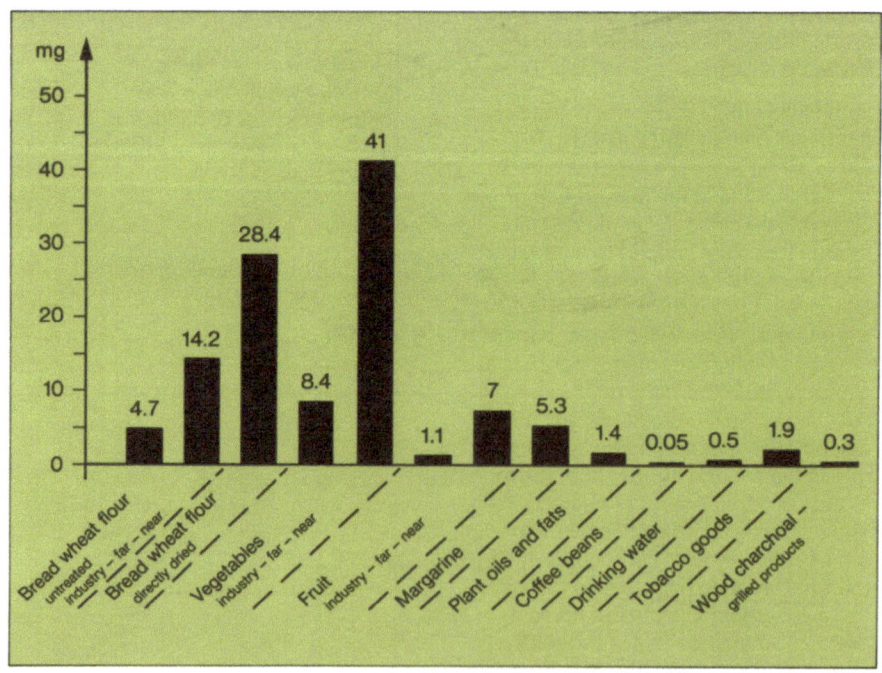

Fig. 65
Estimated amount of the 3,4-benzypyrene ingested per capita with food in the course of 70 years

Tab. 3 Aflatoxin content of foods (selection)

| Product | Sample number | positive % | of these more than 10 ppb |
|---|---|---|---|
| Peanuts | 316 | 11 | 7 |
| Peanut flips | 62 | 24 | 12 |
| Almonds, undecorticated | 124 | 4 | 2 |
| Almonds, ground, chopped | 144 | 25 | – |
| Marzipan | 12 | 25 | – |
| Persipan | 16 | 25 | – |
| Peanut butter, cream | 12 | 1 | 1 |
| Cereals | 283 | 2 | 2 |

## 2. Halogenated Pesticides and Polychlorinated Biphenyls

A number of chlorinated hydrocarbon pesticides such as DDT, HCH, aldrin, dieldrin, lindane are difficult to evaluate with regard to their carcinogenic action despite intensive research. At a high dosage, they regularly produce liver tumors in mice, but show mostly little or no activity in other animal species. The application of such data to man is hence difficult, especially since epidemiological investigations on occupational exposure have not revealed convincing indications of a carcinogenic action in man. Substances of this class are hence often classified as epigenetic carcinogens, and a threshold value in exposure below which there is no health risk is regarded to be possible.

Polychlorinated biphenyls (PCBs) are used industrially in various applications, especially as condenser and hydraulic fluids. Like the chlorinated hydrocarbon pesticides, PCBs have an extraordinary persistence in the environment. At a very high dosage, PCBs produce liver tumors in mice and in some experiments also in rats; epidemiological studies have not provided hard evidence. In view of the high persistence of these halogenated substances, their occurrence in food is not remarkable. Since application of halogenated pesticides has been largely prohibited and production of PCBs has been stopped, there has been a marked decline in human exposure in recent years. This trend will continue. Apart from rare exceptions, the present exposures are far below the highest amounts specified as tolerable by the WHO.

## 3. Aflatoxin

Aflatoxins are metabolic products of molds (especially of Aspergillus flavus) which can grow on practically all foods under favorable conditions such as high temperature and high relative humidity. Aflatoxin $B_1$ is the most potent hepatocarcinogen known today. In some tropical countries, a direct correlation of the level of aflatoxin uptake via the food and the incidence of liver cancer in the population is known. In temperate climate zones and with the predominantly high food hygiene prevailing, on the other hand, high exposures to these mycotoxins appear to be relatively rare and are restricted to con- taminated nuts and cereal products. Some of the available data, which appear to be representative at present for Western industrial countries, are listed in Table 3.

For the total content of aflatoxins in the individual foods, a maximum of 10 ppb is valid in the Federal Republic of Germany.

## 4. Protein Pyrolysis Products

Very recent investigations by Sugimura et al. have shown that in pyrolysis (intense dry heating) of amino acids and proteins, highly mutagenic (i.e. altering the genetic material) reaction products are formed. In some cases, their chemical structure could be elucidated (Fig. 66).

First investigations revealed that representatives of this class of substances also have a carcinogenic action in animal studies. In the food, such substances might be formed in roasting, toasting, and grilling foods containing proteins even if the temperatures are very much lower under the usual conditions in the kitchen than in the model trials. Only a few analytical investigations are available. Appropriate analytical methods for the detection of trace amounts of substances will have to be further developed. A series of further investigations will be necessary to clarify whether there is a risk to human health and, if so, how great it is.

## 5. Nitrosamines

N-Nitroso compounds (especially nitrosamines) are a group of highly potent chemical carcinogens. They are characterized in that, depending on their chemical structure, the mode of appli-

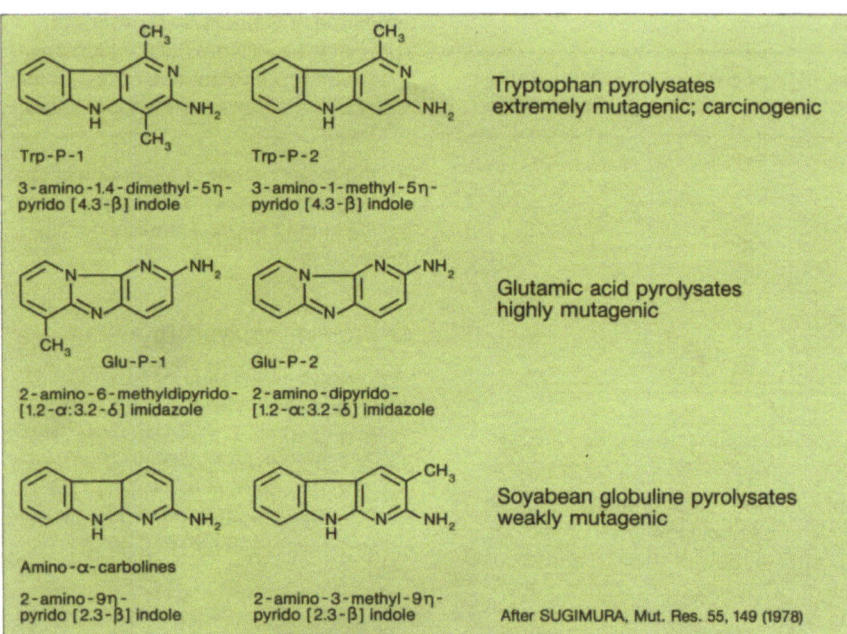

Fig. 66
Protein pyrolysis products

Trp-P-1

3-amino-1.4-dimethyl-5η-
pyrido [4.3-β] indole

Trp-P-2

3-amino-1-methyl-5η-
pyrido [4.3-β] indole

Tryptophan pyrolysates
extremely mutagenic; carcinogenic

Glu-P-1

2-amino-6-methyldipyrido-
[1.2-α:3.2-δ] imidazole

Glu-P-2

2-amino-dipyrido-
[1.2-α:3.2-δ] imidazole

Glutamic acid pyrolysates
highly mutagenic

Amino-α-carbolines

2-amino-9η-
pyrido [2.3-β] indole

2-amino-3-methyl-9η-
pyrido [2.3-β] indole

Soyabean globuline pyrolysates
weakly mutagenic

After SUGIMURA, Mut. Res. 55, 149 (1978)

cation, the dose and the animal species, they can produce malignant tumors in practically all major organs of the animal body. In their histological structure, they often resemble the clinical pictures familiar in man. A carcinogenic action in man must be regarded as very probable.

The doses required to induce tumors in animal experiments are in some cases very low. In chronic feeding trials, amounts of about 10 µg/kg dimethyl nitrosamine (NDMA) in the daily feed was still effective. The extraordinary efficacy of these substances is also characterized in that a single dose of 0.3 mg can still produce tumors in rats. Other nitrosamines are somewhat less active.

Our group recently concluded an analysis of almost 3,000 food samples on the German market. The selection of the samples was representative on the basis of average consumption figures in Germany contained in the Nutrition Report of 1976. Table 4 gives a short synopsis of all the results. Only three nitrosamines, namely N-nitrosodimethylamine, N-nitrosopyrrolidine (NPYR) and N-nitrosopiperidine (NPIP) were found more or less regularly, whereas all other possible volatile nitrosamines were observed only in extremely rare cases. As is to be seen from Table 4, the two cyclic nitrosamines NPYR and NPIP occur in concentrations of more than 0.5 ppb only in 3% or 2% of the samples, i.e. relatively rarely. On the other hand, dimethylnitrosamine was found in 30% of all samples, and 6% of these samples contained more than 5 ppb.

Tab. 4  Nitrosamines in foods on the German market (1978)

| ppb | NDMA | NPYR | NPIP |
|---|---|---|---|
| less than 0.5 | 70% | 97% | 98% |
| 0.5–4.9 | 24% | 2% | 1% |
| more than 5 | 6% | 1% | 1% |

Total number of the investigated samples: 2,826 samples, from 169 kinds of food.

Part of the overall results is shown in detail in Table 5.

For meat and meat products, our results confirm our own previous investigations and data from the published literature, i.e. that only samples treated with nitrite or nitrate (i.e. cured) are contaminated with nitrosamines. Of almost 400 samples investigated, 118 proved to be positive in the range from 0.5–4.9 ppb, and nine were positive for NDMA in a concentration in excess of 5 ppb. For NPYR, 27 samples were above the limit of detection up to 4.9 ppb, and 24 samples were over 5 ppb with a maximum value found of 45 ppb. As a rule, the concentration of NDMA is not raised by heating cured meat products. On the other hand, the content of NPYR can increase considerably on heating. Thus, for example, the mean value rose in the case of ham from 1.2 ppb in unheated samples to 14.2 ppb after roasting. The results in cheese are likewise to be seen

Tab. 5 Nitrosamine contents of meat and sausage as well as cheese

| Food | n | Nitro-samines | less than 0.5 ppb | 0.5–4.9 ppb | more than 5 ppb | $x_{max}$ ppb |
|---|---|---|---|---|---|---|
| Meat and sausage | 395 | NDMA | 268 | 118 | 9 | 12 |
| | | NPYR | 345 | 27 | 24 | 45 |
| Cheese | 208 | NDMA | 159 | 48 | 1 | % |

in Table 5. Of 208 investigated samples, 23% proved to be positive for NDMA in the range from 0.5–4.9 ppb, only one sample with 5 ppb being above this range.

However, the most surprising result of the investigation presented here was the regular contamination of beer with NDMA. The results are shown in Table 6.

As a whole, we have analysed 199 samples from bottled, canned and barrel beer including imported beers and

found that 141 of the samples (= 66%) contained NDMA. The mean value of all samples investigated was 2.5 ppb. The maximum of 68 ppb was found in a special beer, a "smoked beer". A classification according to the beer types showed that Pilsener beers, export beers and top-fermented light beers showed a relatively low contamination with NDMA. The higher values were found either in beers with very high original wort content such as strong beers or in dark beers.

Tab. 6 Nitrosodimethylamine in beer: comparison of the content before and after introduction of modified kiln-drying procedures

| Beer type | 1978/79 | | | | 1981 | | | |
|---|---|---|---|---|---|---|---|---|
| | n | % positive (more than 0.5 ppb) | Mean value ppb | Max-imum ppb | n | % positive less than 0.5 ppb | Mean value ppb | Max-imum ppb |
| Pilsener | 54 | 65 | 1.2 | 7 | 169 | 24 | 0.43 | 6.5 |
| Export | 42 | 67 | 1.2 | 7 | 179 | 26 | 0.39 | 2.0 |
| Light strong beer | 25 | 76 | 1.9 | 8 | 38 | 26 | 0.42 | 1.6 |
| Top fermentation, light | 22 | 23 | 6.2 | 1 | 19 | 5 | 0.32 | 0.7 |
| Top fermentation, dark | 25 | 76 | 2.7 | 11 | 21 | 24 | 0.96* | 7.0 |
| Dark export and strong beer | 22 | 68 | 6.0 | 47 | 25 | 32 | 0.51 | 4.0 |
| Smoked beer (from roasted malt) | 9 | 100 | 18.0 | 68 | 3 | 100 | 1.50 | 2.0** |
| All types | 199 | 66 | 2.5 | 68 | 454 | 24 | 0.44 | 7.0 |

* not representative.
** values from 1980.

In order to find out the reasons for the nitrosamine contaminations in beer, we divided the entire brewing process into 12 stages and analysed each individual stage for its nitrosamine content in 1978/79. This was carried out with five different kinds of beers and the result was fairly unequivocal. It was shown in all cases that the malt was the source of the nitrosamine contamination, whereas all other stages of the brewing process make practically no contribution to this contamination. Systematic investigations on the causes of this contamination clearly revealed that direct heating in the malting kiln is the main source: the high $NO_x$ content of the drying air heated with gas is the nitrosation agent which reacts with dimethylamine (probably from hordenin and gramin of the malt) in the drying material to form NDMA. By reduction of the $NO_x$ content of the drying air by suitable technical procedures or by other methods (e.g., sulphuring), NDMA in the malt and thus in the beer can be greatly reduced. After the introduction of such measures, very much lower NDMA values were shown in a new investigation carried out in 1981 in 454 beer samples. The recommended guide value of 0.5 ppb NDMA in beer and 2.5 ppb in malt can be maintained.

In more than 2,000 samples of all other foods, e.g., bread, cereal products, fish, milk and dairy products, potatoes, vegetables, fruit, drinks, etc., our investigation only very rarely showed the occurrence of volatile nitrosamines, in each case at concentrations near the limit of detection of the methods.

The results elaborated allow a calculation of the average daily uptake of volatile nitrosamines from the diet in the Federal Republic of Germany. These calculations are based on the mean per capita consumption figures for the various foods listed in the Nutrition Report of 1976. The calculations relate to male adult subjects. This is shown in Table 7. In Table 8, these data are broken down in percentages.

## Naturally Occurring Carcinogens in Plant Foods

It has been known for a long time that toxic substances are not only of anthropogenic origin, but this is readily forgotten today. A series of natural carcinogenic constituents in plants are known and may pass into human food. The most important representatives of naturally occurring carcinogens will be briefly listed here. The relevant carcinogenicity data derive from animal experiments.

Tab. 7  Main per capita daily intake for male adults (1979 or 1981) calculated according to the mean per capita consumption (Nutrition Report 1976)

| Food | Consumption (g) | Nitrosamine | µg/per capita 1979 | 1981 |
|---|---|---|---|---|
| Beer | ~ 560 | NDMA | 0.7 | 0.2 |
| Meat and sausage products | ~ 210 | NDMA | 0.1 | 0.1 |
| | | NYPR | 0.1 | 0.1 |
| | | NPIP | 0.01 | 0.01 |
| Cheese | ~ 30 | NDMA | 0.01 | 0.01 |
| Other | ~ 150 | NDMA | ~ 0.2 | ~ 0.2 |
| Total | | NDMA | ~ 1.1 | ~ 0.5 |
| | | NPYR | ~ 0.1–0.15 | ~ 0.1–0.15 |

Tab. 8  Contribution of individual food to total daily intake of NDMA (1.1 µg/head 1979, 0.5 µg/head 1981)

| Food | % by weight in consumption | % of the total exposure to NDMA 1979 | 1981 |
|---|---|---|---|
| Beer | 24 | 64 | less than 40 |
| Meat and sausage products | 10 | 10 | 20 |
| Cheese | 1 | 1 | 2 |
| Other | 25 | 25 | 40 |

Pyrrolizidine alkaloids from Senecio, Crotataria and Heliotropium may enter human food as contaminants. Safrol, isosafrol and estragol, which occur as aromatic oils in many plants, were added from time to time as sassafras oil in the USA to root beer as a flavoring. Some hydrazine derivatives, e.g., N-methyl-N-formylhydrazine, 4-methyl-phenylhydrazine) are constituents of the mushrooms Agaricus bisporus and By-romitra esculenta which are regarded as edible. Bracken (Pteridium aquilinum) which is used as a salad, e.g., in Japan, contains a carcinogen the structure of which has not yet been completely clarified. Cycasin is a carcinogenic constituent of many Cycadaceae which also serve as food in the tropics as palm sago meal. Quercetin and coumarin, which are widespread flavonoids, show mutagenic action, but their carcinogenic potential cannot yet be appraised.

All these plant carcinogens very probably have no significance as risk factors for large populations; however, they may be important in regionally limited areas when specific consumption and living habits prevail in this region.

To point out the complexity of the interrelationships here: plants naturally also contain a series of substances which may exert an anticarcinogenic action in the widest sense. The following are perhaps the most important: vitamin E (alpha-tocopherol) and vitamin C (ascorbic acid) which inhibit endogenous nitrosamine formation, e.g., in the stomach, beta-carotene and carotinoids.

## Formation of Carcinogens in the Body

The formation of nitrosamines in the human gastrointestinal tract is probably of greatest significance here. Precursors are nitrosable amines, which may be widespread in human nutrition either as natural constituents of the food or as contaminants, and, on the other hand, nitrosating agents such as nitrite and nitrate under reducing conditions. Endogenous formation (e.g., within the body) of N-nitroso compounds must be accepted as an established fact today. It is unique for this specific group of carcinogens, since it is not known up to now that any other carcinogenic substance can be formed in a simple chemical reaction in the human body itself from nontoxic precursors which occur in the food.

The in vivo formation of N-nitroso compounds has been documented in very many experimental examples. It would be going too far here to list all facts as evidence for this assertion.

A major difficulty in evaluation is that, in contrast to the occurrence of nitrosamines in the food, their endogenous formation cannot be quantified at present. In this field, nitrosamine research is working intensively at present. A further important research field in this direction is endogenous nitrite formation. Investigations of our own study group as well as of American scientists have shown that nitrate ingested with the food may be partially excreted again via the salivary glands into the oral cavity after absorption and distribution in the blood. Nitrate can be reduced to nitrite by the bacterial flora of the oral cavity. This nitrite formed in the oral cavity is then swallowed with the saliva and serves as a nitrosation agent in the stomach (Fig. 67). According to these investigations, the nitrite concentration in the saliva is directly correlated with the level of nitrate uptake via the food. All plant foods are relatively rich in nitrates. Especially high nitrate contents are found in root vegetables, e.g., beetroot, radish.

Fig. 67
Flow diagram of gastrointestinal nitrate circulation

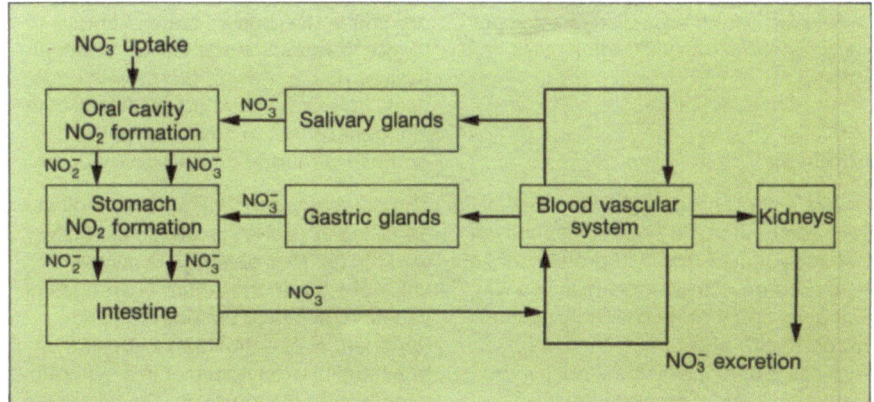

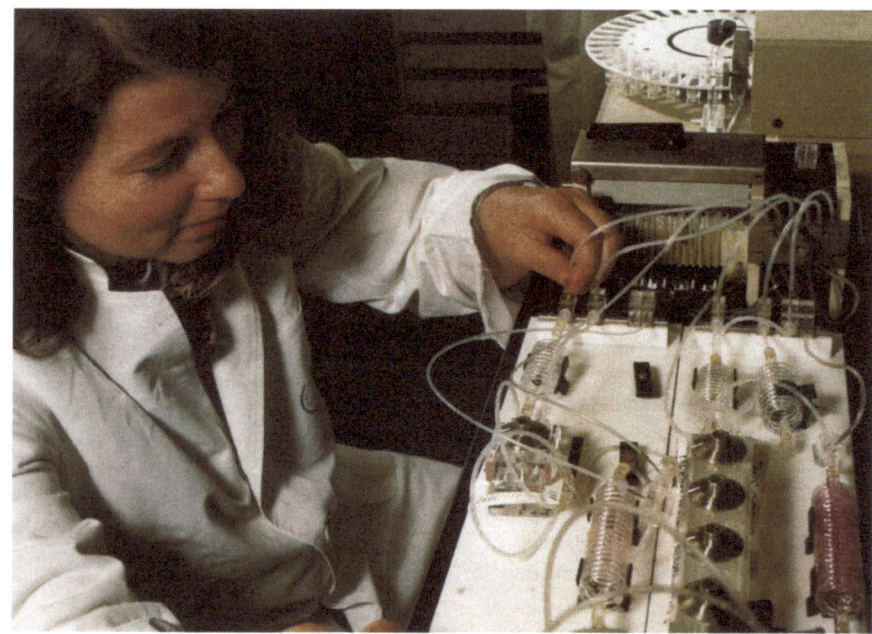

Fig. 68
With an automatic analysis instrument, foods and saliva samples are investigated for their content of nitrite and nitrate

At present, the possibility of formation of potentially carcinogenic metabolites from cholesterol and bile acids by alteration of the normal bacterial flora of the intestine must be designated only as a working hypothesis. However, raised fat intake and lower fiber content of the diet in Western countries is discussed especially in connection with colon carcinoma.

## Additives

Finally, a short note on additives. § 8 of the Food Law of the Federal Republic of Germany states that it is prohibited
- to prepare or treat food in such a way that its consumption is likely to damage health and
- to sell foods of which the consumption is likely to damage health.

The precept of § 8 can be readily applied in deliberate additions to foods, e.g., of colorants and preservatives in that additives are prohibited in principle (§ 11), and that only those substances are permitted by statute which are both necessary and toxicologically harmless according to the present state of knowledge. New knowledge also occasionally gives rise to new problems with additives, for example the controversial carcinogenic effect of amaranth or the problem of nitrites already mentioned.

The percentage of 1 % for food additives specified in Table 1 is related exclusively to the nitrite problem. The negative value of – 5 % in the column of ranges of variation relates to the possible antitumor effect of antioxidants such as butylated hydroxytoluene. In a synoptic expertise on the situation, Shubik (Preventive Medicine, 9, 167–202, 1980) also arrives at the view that additives make no measurable contribution to the incidence of cancer in Western countries.

To summarize the experimental findings relating to nutrition and cancer, it should be emphasized that carcinogenic substances can occur in certain foods. However, it is to be emphasized even more strongly that the amounts of these substances are generally low to very low. The problem in evaluating risks is that every single exposure considered in isolation will hardly occasion acute anxiety. However, it is very difficult to evaluate the overall risk resulting from the sum of the individual risk factors, because our knowledge with regard to synergistic (additive or potentiative) effects and modifying factors (inhibitory and/or promoting) is inadequate. The overall picture is thus also blurred here despite a precise knowledge of details.

However, in my opinion the experimental findings do not constitute a secure foundation for the estimate of Doll and Peto, according to which more than a third of all cases in cancer are due to nutritional causes.

I am convinced that there is no reason for acute concern. However, this does not by any means imply that everything possible has been done in order to eliminate potential risk factors. Both science and the lawgiver must do more in this regard.

## Nutritional Recommendations of the US National Academy of Sciences

The provisional dietary recommendations for minimizing the risk of cancer presented by the Academy in 1982 after a synoptic appraisal of all data comprise:

1. Reduction of the proportion of saturated and unsaturated fats to a maximum of 30% of the calorie content of the diet.
2. The importance of fruit, vegetables and whole serial products, particularly as sources of roughage, is emphasized.
3. The consumption of pickled and heavily salted foods should be restricted.
4. Alcoholic drinks should only be consumed in moderate amounts.

In principle, the Academy justifies these recommendations, which in some cases have been severely criticized as scientifically unfounded, by saying that they can at least do no harm.

In general, it can be recommended that risks present should be distributed as far as possible and thus reduced by as diverse and varied a diet as feasible without onesidedness.

Prof. Rudolf Preußmann
Environmental Carcinogens,
Institute of Toxicology and
Chemotherapy

Selected publications

Miller, J. A., Miller, E. C.: Chemical Carcinogenesis: Mechanism and Approaches to Control. J. Natl. Cancer 47, V. (1971).

Teuteberg, H. J.: The General Relationship between Diet and Industrialisation. Europ. diet from preindustrial to modern times. H. Elbory und R. Forster, Ed., Karger Torchbooks (1975).

Habs, M., Schmähl, D.: Diet and Cancer. J. Cancer Res. Clin. Oncol. 96, 1–10 (1980).

Preussmann, R.: Vorkommen und Bedeutung chemischer Carcinogene in der menschlichen Umwelt. In: Maligne Tumoren. Ed. Schmähl, D., Aulendorf, Württ., Editio Cantor, 160–202, (1981).

Doll, R., Peto, R.: The Causes of Cancer. J. Natl. Cancer Inst. 66, 1191–1308 (1981).

Natl. Acad. of Sciences, Natl. Research Council: Diet, Nutrition and Cancer, Natl. Acad. Press, Washington, D.C. (1982).

Palmer, S., Bakshi, K.: Diet, Nutrition and Cancer: Interim Dietary Guidelines. J. Natl. Cancer Inst. 70, 1153–1170 (1983).

Heyns, K.: Lebensmittel und Ernährung im Rückblick. In: Wie sicher sind unsere Lebensmittel?, Heft 102 der Schriftenreihe des Bundes für Lebensmittelrecht und Lebensmittelkunde, B. Behrs Verlag Hamburg, 22–65 (1983).

Ernährung und Krebs. Symp. der Dt. Ges. für Ernährung. Wiss. Verlagsges., Stuttgart (1983).

Ames, B. N.: Dietary Carcinogens and Anticarcinogens. Science 221, 1256–1264 (1983).

Byers, T., Graham, S.: The Epidemiology of Diet and Cancer in: Advances in Cancer Res., Vol. 41, 1–69 (1984).

## 4.2 Nitrosamines at the Workplace

by Rudolf Preußmann
and Bertold Spiegelhalder

N-Nitroso compounds are amongst the most potent carcinogenic substances tested so far in experimental animals. In particular, they are characterized by a pronounced organ-specific activity and by extraordinarily low doses. It is possible to produce tumors selectively and specifically in practically all major organs. A carcinogenic action in man has been demonstrated recently both in medical application of nitrosourea chemotherapeutics and in the development of buccal cavity cancer in tobacco chewers. However, comparative studies also indirectly indicate that metabolism in human and animal organs is very similar. A carcinogenic action of N-nitroso compounds must thus also be assumed in man.

Numerous investigations show that nitroso compounds occur in the human environment in many areas, including foods, tobacco, cosmetics, etc. In addition, there is no doubt today that a serious problem of occupational exposure to nitroso compounds is present in certain branches of industry. Since the occurrence of nitrosamines in the air of workplaces in the rubber industry became known, we have carried out a total of 23 measurement campaigns in 18 factories of 15 different manufacturers in a large-scale study. Nitrosamines could be detected in all cases. In particular, N-nitrosodimethylamine (NDMA) and N-nitrosomorpholine (NMOR) were regularly found. The concentration in the air varied between 0.1 and 380 µg/m³.

However, the concentrations mainly varied in the order of range of 1 to 10 µm/m³ air. In most cases, the higher values were detected in the field of final manufacture, quality control and in the tyre store. This is attributable to permanent degassing from the end products of nitrosamines formed during production.

In the rubber industry, chemicals containing amines are used as accelerators for vulcanization. During the production process, the amines can be converted into nitrosamines. Other rubber chemicals such as nitrosodiphenylamine or nitrite salt baths act as nitrosation agents: they release nitrogen oxides ($NO_x$), which then convert the amines or amine derivatives used into nitrosamines. However, not only rubber chemicals play a role as nitrosation agents. Increased nitrogen oxide concentrations in the air caused by transport vehicles with combustion engines and in particular by the exhaust fumes of gas-driven fork lift trucks convert the amines into nitrosamines.

High nitrosamine concentrations were also measured in tube manufacture. Here, the highest value in a vulcanization room was 130 µg nitrosodimethylamine/m³ air. As shown by a check of the formulation, a readily nitrosatable vulcanization accelerator had been mixed with a nitrogen oxide-releasing retarder in the rubber mixture. The nitrosamine concentration in the air could be reduced to 1 to 5 µg/m³ by exchanging the retarder.

In the technical rubber article industry, diverse rubber chemicals are used due to the wide range of products. The spectrum of nitrosamines found is correspondingly wide: Nitrosodimethylamine (NDMA), nitrosodiethylamine

(NDEA), nitrosodibutylamine (NDBA) as well as nitrosopiperidine (NPIP) were detected at working places. The result of the investigations in the working area of salt bath vulcanization facilities were especially striking. In such facilities, the rubber comes into direct contact with a nitrite salt bath during vulcanization. If the rubber vulcanized in this way contains nitrosatable accelerators, nitrosamine concentrations of up to 40 µg/m³ air are found. In one case, mixtures were used which did not contain any nitrosatable chemicals and the nitrosamine concentration/m³ air was correspondingly low, i.e. less than 0.1 µg.

The highest measured nitrosamine levels were found during personal monitoring in injection moulding and curing of conveyor belts. The values were 90 µg nitrosodimethylamine and 380 µg nitrosomorpholine/m³ air.

By substituting accelerators as well as by various preventive measures, a reduction of the nitrosamine exposure (which was in some cases drastic) could also be attained in other production areas.

Cooling fluids, which are used in practically all metalworking processes such as polishing, drilling, milling, rolling, grinding or cutting, contain amines or amine derivatives as corrosion inhibitors, as well as emulsifiers.

Nitrite, which is added as corrosion inhibitor in amounts up to 30%, acts as a nitrosation agent with formation of nitrosamines.

As revealed by the investigation of numerous coolant lubricants, several nitrosamines can be detected. The concentrations found were between 10 and 20 mg/kg. In working with coolant lubricants, the nitrosamines are incorporated mainly by inhalation of oil mist and via the skin. A possibility of monitoring an exposure consists in the the detection of nitrosodiethanolamine (NDEIA) in the urine.

In the first studies in a grinding shop, urine from over 270 workers was investigated for the content of NDEIA. More than 60% of the urines contained NDEIA in amounts up to 100 μg/l.

The need for systematic "monitoring" of exposure at the place of work was first detected in recent years. The restricted number of studies available so far should, if anything, be regarded more as a starting signal than as an adequate collection of data for an estimation of the risk. For such appraisals, it is necessary to establish representative data banks in which the individual level of exposure is combined with prospective epidemiological studies. By means of such combined studies, it might then become possible to show the direct connection between exposure and the risk of cancer.

Animal experimental data document that air concentrations from 70 μg/m$^3$ nitrosodimethylamine can already induce tumors in rats. In some cases, nitrosamine concentrations at workplaces in the rubber industry were in the same concentration range. We hence regard it as absolutely necessary to reduce the exposure to these very strong carcinogens as far as possible by the application of new technologies and new formulations, and thus also to put into practice the principle of primary prevention in corresponding industrial fields.

Prof. Dr. Rudolf Preußmann
Dr. Bertold Spiegelhalder
Environmental Carcinogens
Institute of Toxicology and
Chemotherapy

Selected publications

Spiegelhalder, B., Preußmann, R.: Occupational nitrosamine exposure. 1. Rubber and tire industry. Carcinogenesis 4, 1147–52 (1983).

Spiegelhalder, B., Preußmann, R.: Biological monitoring in the metal working industry. N-Nitroso Compounds, IARC Scient. Publ. No. 57, 943–946, Lyon (1984).

## 4.3 Cancer by Inhalational Exposure – Questions and Problems

by Reinhold G. Klein

Many cancer researchers have repeatedly expressed the suspicion that more than half of the malignant tumors occurring in humans are caused by environmental influences. The following questions are posed:

a) What noxae in our environment play a role in the development of cancer?
b) Are single noxae effective alone or must several factors coincide?
c) In what way do the noxae pass into the body and according to which mechanisms does the transformation of a cell take place when malignant neoplasias occur often only decades after an exposure phase?
d) May other factors, e.g., viruses, play a role in this process?

The style of life is today regarded as a very major factor favoring cancer. Besides a specific exposure (E = dependence on the place of work, the area of residence, contact with certain substances), a certain predisposition (D = disposition, i.e. special hereditary or acquired genetic features) and the factor age (A) can be formulated:
cancer = exposure plus predisposition plus age
(Prof. Dr. Dietrich Schmähl in: Federal Environment Office, Reports 2/83, Appraisal of the risk of small doses of carcinogenic substances for humans, Erich Schmidt Publisher, 1983).

The familial, the social and the geographic environment also play a role which is not to be underestimated. Nutritional habits, the occupational situation and a more rural or urban environment will doubtless have an influence on the biological interactions in a living body in the course of time.

The significance of such influence is not based on a pure supposition, but can be illustrated by impressive data, as shown by pictorial representations of actuarial statistics, as, for example, in the Cancer Atlas of the Federal Republic of Germany. This shows a "landscape of cancer deaths" in the individual counties and cities (Becker, Frentzel-Beyme and Wagner, Springer Verlag 1984). However, in principle such surveys do not allow causal conclusions, since a number of action parameters, which still cannot be clearly assessed today, are involved in the development of these differences in cancer mortality. It is by no means admissible to select a single, apparently plausible factor, e.g., air pollution, and to relate it on its own to the number of cancer deaths. A correlation suspected in this direction must under all circumstances first be demonstrated with recognized scientific methods which allow a logical appraisal with regard to the causality of the effects, since otherwise misinterpretations of serious extent would result without disclosure of the real interrelationships responsible. Besides foods and drinks, of which the daily consumption is of the order of several kilograms, the respiratory air constitutes a medium which depends on the site of residence and which is "ingested" in the same way by all persons in a certain environment. The air volume, which with the average way of life comes into very close contact with the body of an adult human being after thorough cleansing on the ciliary hairs of the airways, amounts to 20,000 l daily, corresponding to a mass of 25 kg. The noxae contained in this air pass via respiration into the interior of the body and are trapped and stored there and accumulated for decades (fine fiber dust, carbon particles, certain aerosols).

Experimental inhalation toxicology in collaboration with related medical, biological, chemical and physical disciplines has to investigate the qualitative and quantitative processes of the absorption of volatile substances and size-deposition relationship of airborne particles in the lungs, the accumulation in the respiratory organs as well as the metabolic fate and lung clearance and elimination mechanisms in humans, animals and theoretical models.

Numerous carcinogenic substances such as the intensively investigated polycyclic aromatic hydrocarbons, e.g., benz(a)pyrene, have been investigated for their carcinogenic potential in animal experiments and in certain occupational groups in man. It has been shown that the presence of substances, which are hardly aggressive biologically such as finely ground iron oxide (hematite), fine fiber dusts or, for example, volatile constituents of cigarette smoke with and without condensate components in the airways, is sufficient to increase the activity of a carcinogen which is simultaneously present even at a low dose. Such experiments on the combination effect of noxae, which attempt to explore the synergism, the interaction of influence parameters, can only be carried out with a few meticulously deselected substance groups because of the large number of possible noxa combinations. Dr. Walter Jens Zeller and collaborators from the Institute of Toxicology and Chemotherapy of the German Cancer Research Center have demonstrated

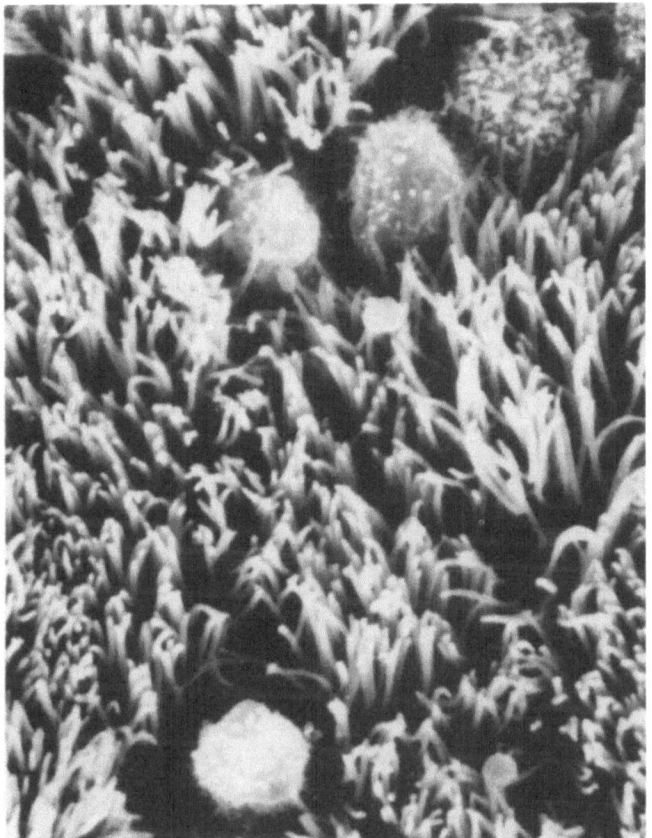

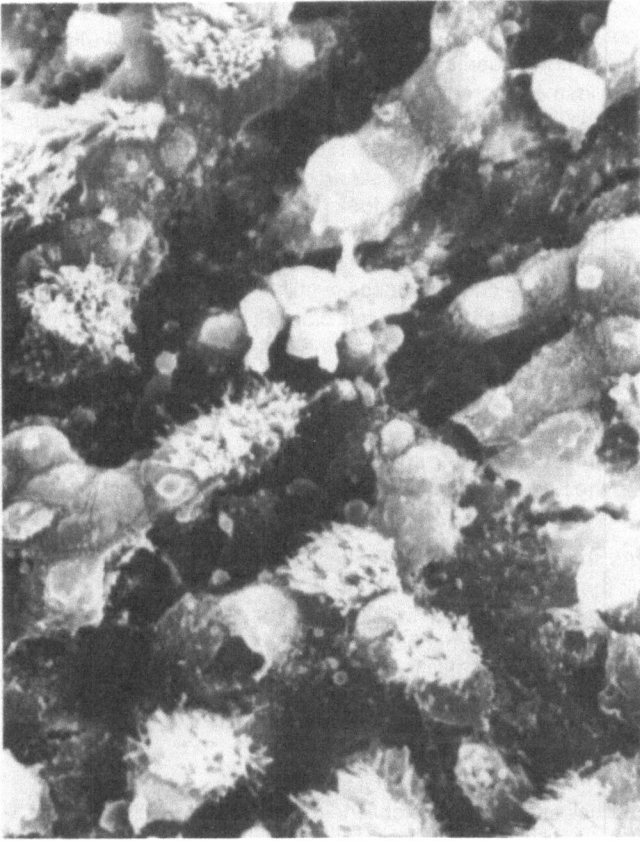

Fig. 69
The mucosal surface of hamsters shows a very differentiated picture with diverse cell processes. Ciliary hairs are freely motile in relation to each other (magnification × 1000)

Fig. 70
On the other hand, the tracheal mucosa of the animals treated with $SO_2$ shows a pronounced fibrosis with numerous irregular cells without differentiated cell processes (magnification × 660)

that not only the tobacco smoke condensate but also the volatile constituents of cigarette smoke exert a synergistic carcinogenic action on the respiration organs of the Syrian Golden hamster: small amounts of benz(a)pyrene were introduced into the respiratory tract of hamsters where they produced a quantifiable carcinogenic reaction. By simultaneous inhalation of cigarette smoke, from which the tar constituents which contain carcinogenic hydrocarbons had been removed in special filters, the number of tumors was significantly raised. This can be implied from the fact that even the volatile components of the smoke and those of conventional filter cigarettes (apart from cigarettes with active carbon filters) are not held back and must be inferred to exert a carcinogenic action in the hamster lung.

At the symposium of the Federal Health Office on inhalation toxicology in Berlin in 1984, similar conditions were discussed in a mixture of substances of

103

which the overall effect likewise could not be predicted on the basis of the individual constituents of the mixture: certain leather impregnation agents from sprays. In the use of this leather spray, some potentially fatal accidents due to inhalation of the spray mist had occurred when the application took place in closed spaces. The toxicological mechanisms of this potentiated action of substance combinations are still largely unclarified even in this case. By alteration of the composition, the other sprays which can be purchased today are less dangerous than the preparations used before these investigations. The test trials had been carried out here by the Federal Health Office on chickens and pigeons.

As shown inter alia by the investigations in the Institute of Chemotherapy and Toxicology at the German Cancer Research Center, bronchitis can be produced experimentally in Sprague-Dawley rats by the inhalation of sulfur dioxide in high concentrations. The sulfur dioxide inhalation had a marked inhibitory influence on the rate of transport of particles from the bronchi and the trachea. Scanning electron microscopic photographs shows the obliteration and damage to the surface of the ciliated epithelium induced by the inhaled sulfur dioxide. There are numerous contributions to short-term effects of aerial noxae, but further experiments are urgently necessary, in particular on the long-term influence of noxae and their combinations on the activity and regeneration capacity of the bronchial epithelium, the protective function of the bronchial mucus and the defence capacity of the pulmonary macrophages. These experiments should also be so designed that they do not produce any acute damage in the animal (rat, hamster, ...), and cor-

respond as far as possible to the situation of human beings in their environment. The way, in which a biologically active substance passes into the body, may be crucial for the realization of its toxic and carcinogenic properties. The different sensitivity of the tissue concerned, the elimination and defence mechanisms as well as increased secretion of mucus or conversion of poisons into harmless products which the body can excrete finally determine the activity spectrum of the noxae. However, there are also processes in which the body achieves the opposite effect in its intention of detoxicating an incorporated substance. The body then converts the chemical into the "ultimate carcinogen". This is carried out by certain enzymes, e.g., in the biotransformation of nitrosamines in the liver. The pathway of the

inhaled substance, which is already located in the lungs (in the center of the body), then passes into the bloodstream via an inner surface of the alveolae which is more than hundred $m^2$ in extent in man. It is no longer far to the liver where the "bomb is activated". From the liver, the substance, which has now been transformed into a carcinogenic poison, reaches the target organs in which a cell transformation takes place as a result of which the malignant proliferation can begin after a long time. This quite definitely does not happen with every toxic molecule which enters the body, since otherwise every person who is exposed to tobacco smoke would develop cancer. However, highly effective defence mechanisms quite definitely exist, but we have not yet been able to obtain a detailed picture of how they

Fig. 71

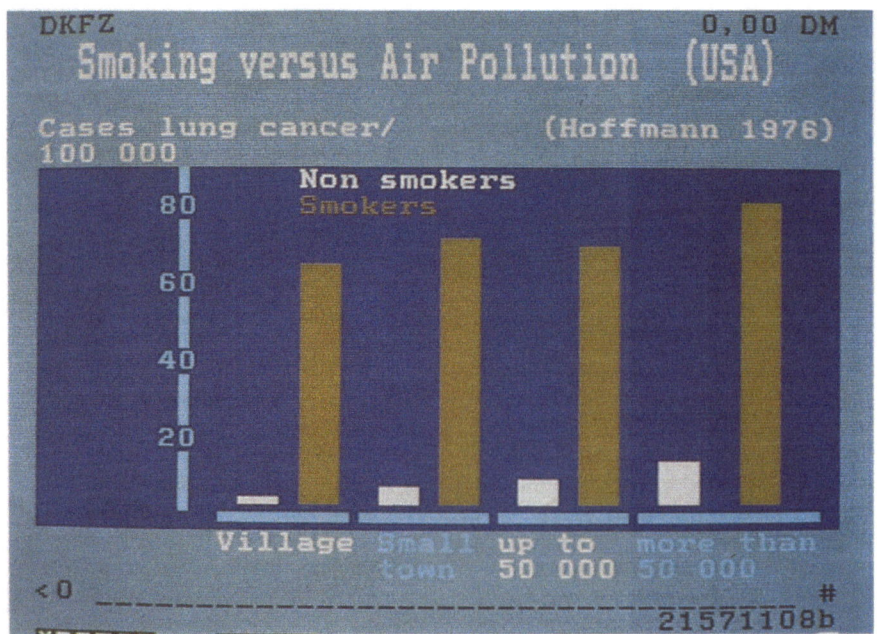

function. For example, we are able to show that nitrosamines, which can be formed at places of work in industry and in the domestic household by chemical reaction of nitrogen oxides of the air or with nitrites and amines in the food or in cutting oils or hydraulic fluids as well as in tobacco smoke (especially in the side stream smoke), can in part be breathed out again from the lungs in the rat. This process depends on the structure of the compound and its physicochemical properties. However, the carcinogenic action of nitrosamines must be rated as very high, since even exceedingly low concentrations in the respiratory air are sufficient to produce tumors in experimental animals with lifelong exposure.

The objective of the experimental approach was not to produce tumors in a short time with very high dosages from which the animals would already have died at a very early stage. On the contrary, the objective was to attain as minimal as possible an acute toxic or injurious effect on the body by exactly dosed, very small, analytically monitored concentrations of nitrosamines in the respiratory air. Only in this way can a parallel to the situation in a human being be inferred. Thus, the long-term action of carcinogens only causes tumors at the end of the natural lifespan of the animals of which the animals rarely die. In the Syrian golden hamster, this may be on average two to three years and in the rat three to four years. By autopsy of the dead animals and histological workup and appraisal of the microscopic tissue sections, it was proved that both benign and malignant tumors had developed.

The procedure presented as an illustration here is designed to achieve a rational scientific goal. In investigations on carcinogenesis, this should consist in attaining conditions which come as close as possible to reality in human beings. This is more informative than "rapid experiments" with high doses of substances which are not only acutely destructive and thus painful for the animals, but also disrupt the structure of biological feedback loops in the body. By the massive buildup of substances, this also brings out of balance the biochemical interaction between the individual organs. The effects of such high doses of substances can be investigated more reasonably and in less time in isolated cells and tissues or perhaps indeed in theoretical biological-mathematical models.

Dr. Reinhold Georg Klein
Carcinogenesis and Chemotherapy,
Institute of Toxicology and
Chemotherapy

Staff participating

Johanna Jäger
Dr. Jürgen Lany, now Bad Friedrichshall, County Hospital
Heidemarie Oberst
Beatrice Schmezer
Peter Schmezer
Dipl. biol. Dr. Liselotte Wesely-Lany, now Bad Friedrichshall, County Hospital

In collaboration with

Prof. Dr. Rudolf Preußmann
Dr. Berthold Spiegelhalder
Department of Environmental Carcinogenesis,
Institute of Toxicology and
Chemotherapy

Prof. Dr. Dymitr Komitowski
Department of Histodiagnostics and
Pathomorphological Documentation,
Institute of Experimental Pathology

Dr. Lutz Edler
Department of Biostatistics,
Institute of Documentation, Information
and Statistics

Prof. Dr. Gerhard Eisenbrand
Dr. Christine Janzowski
Division of Food Chemistry and Environmental Toxicology,
Chemistry Department,
University of Kaiserslautern

Selected publications

Eisenbrand, G., Spiegelhalder, B., Kann, J., Klein, R. G., Preußmann, R.: Carcinogenic N-nitrosodimethylamine as a contamination in drugs containing 4-dimethylamino-2,3-dimethyl-1-phenyl-3-pyrazolin-5-one (Amidopyrine, Aminophenazone), Arzneim. Forsch./Drug Res. 29, 867–869 (1979).

Lany, J., Wesely-Lany, L.: Mukoziliarclearance bei gesunden Ratten und Ratten mit experimentell erzeugter Bronchitis im Hinblick auf die Carcinogenese im Tracheobronchialbaum. Inauguraldissertation, Univ. Heidelberg, Fakultät für Medizin (1980).

Janzowski, C., Klein, R. G., Preußmann, R.: Formation of N-nitroso compounds of the pesticides Atrazine, Simazine and Carbaryl with nitrogen oxides, IARC Sci. Publ. No. 31, N-nitroso compounds: Analysis, Formation and Occurrence, Proc. VIth Internat. Sympos. Budapest, 16–20 Oct. 1979 (1980).

Klein, R. G.: Calculations and measurements on the volatility of N-nitrosamines and their aqueous solutions. Toxicology 23, 135–147 (1982).

Janzowski, C., Klein, R. G., Preußmann, R., Eisenbrand, G.: Nitrosierung von Pestiziden durch Stickoxide in einem Modellsystem, Deutsche Forschungsgemeinschaft, Rundgespräche und Kolloquien, Verlag Chemie, Weinheim (1983).

Klein, R. G.: Carcinogenicity of N-nitroso-acetoxymethyl methylamine (Acetoxymethyl-methylnitrosamine) after inhalation in rats, Toxicology 27, 139–146 (1983).

Schmezer, P.: Quantitative Resorptions- und Exhalationsmessungen mit flüchtigen Nitrosaminen an Versuchstieren, Diplom-Arbeit, Universität Heidelberg, Fakultät für Biologie (1983).

Klein, R. G.: Kombinationswirkung von polycyclischen aromatischen Kohlenwasserstoffen und Schwefeldioxid im chronischen Inhalationsversuch am Syrischen Goldhamster, eingereicht bei Toxicology (1985).

## 4.4 Short-Term Tests for the Investigation of Carcinogenic Substances

by Beatrice Pool

Cancer develops in several phases. The process of carcinogenesis can be triggered off and promoted by factors of predisposition, age and physical, biological or chemical stimuli (exposure). Since specific predispositions cannot be altered, primary cancer prevention can, in the first instance, only entail elimination of carcinogens from the human environment. Prophylactic measures of this kind presuppose that, among the many thousand natural and synthetic substances to which the human being is exposed (via the respiratory air, via the food or via intake of drugs), those substances are identified which exert a carcinogenic action.

### Detection of Carcinogenic Substances with Short-Term Systems

The ability of a substance to produce tumors can be documented experimentally only by animal experiments. Long-term carcinogenesis trials with animals are elaborate and expensive, and several years may be required until results are available which clarify the tumor promoting action of the inducing substance investigated. It is not possible to test all the substances which would have to be investigated for their carcinogenic action with animal experiments, since the necessary laboratories and financial preconditions all over the world are not sufficient.

For this reason, alternative short-test systems are being developed and evaluated for their capacity to distinguish carcinogenic from noncarcinogenic chemicals. Many of these test systems are based on the detection of permanent alterations of the genetic material (mutation) in diverse cells and organisms since similar processes are also closely related with one or several steps of the complex transformation of a normal cell into a tumor cell (Fig. 72).

More than 100 short-test systems have been described so far. These can be roughly subdivided into (a) organisms in which the genetic effect is determined or (b) according to the genetic effects themselves:

Fig. 72
Steps of conversion of a normal into a tumorous cell

### a) Organisms

Tests with microorganisms (bacteria, eukaryonts), in vitro tests (with freshly isolated primary mammalian cells, cell lines, human cells), tests in insects (e.g., Drosophila) and in animals (rat, mouse, hamster).

### b) Genetic Effect

The detection of genetic (DNA) damage (adducts, strand breaks, prophage induction, repair) of mutations in individual genes or whole chromosomes (aberrations, micronuclei, sister chromatid exchanges) and of chromosome sets is possible.

The common feature of all short-term tests is that they provide results in a few days or weeks.

When results are available in short-term tests, potentially dangerous and widespread substances may be given specific further tests in long-term animal experiments. The development of short-term methods was initiated above all by the studies published in 1975 by the Californian researcher Bruce N. Ames and his co-workers. With a remarkable test system (which in the meantime is

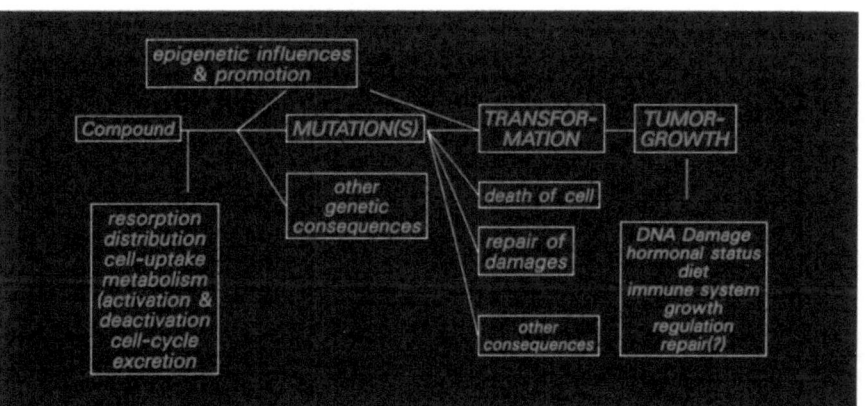

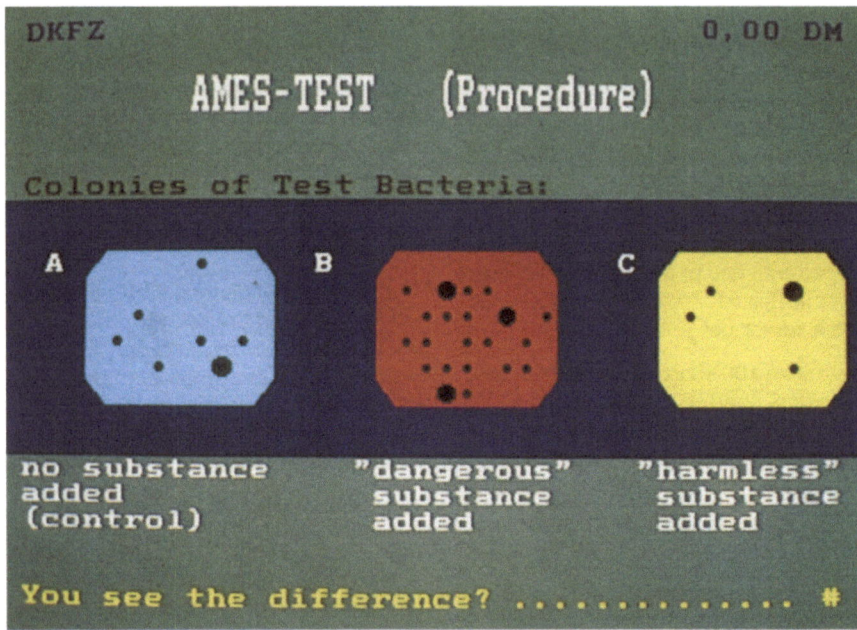

DKFZ　　　　　　　　　　　0,00 DM

## AMES-TEST　(Procedure)

Colonies of Test Bacteria:

A　　　　　　B　　　　　　C

no substance added (control)　　"dangerous" substance added　　"harmless" substance added

You see the difference? ............... #

Fig. 73　　　　　　　　　　　　　　　　Fig. 74

DKFZ　　　　　　　　　　　0.00 DM

## Sister Chromatid Exchange

Duplication　　　　Exchange

A　　　　　　A + B　　　　　　SCE

parental chromo-some　　newly built chromosome (from "red" building blocks)　　Sister Chromatid Exchange: "Harlequine Chromosome"

< 0 ———————————————— #

known as the "classical" Ames test), in which cell fractions to metabolize the substance are placed together with bacteria as indicator organisms for induced mutations, many carcinogenic substances could be identified relatively simply and quickly as mutagenic, i.e. injurious to the genetic material. One of the first publications "Carcinogens are mutagens" was followed by several publications of other study groups indicating that in up to 90% of cases this test could distinguish between possibly carcinogenic and noncarcinogenic substances. In the meantime, the number of carcinogenic substances investigated has become larger. The result of the greater experience, however, is that the originally high predictive value is still valid only for certain groups of substances. According to a new synoptic report, only 63 out of 102 carcinogens (62%) had a mutagenic action. The test has thus lost predictive value.

This error rate is, of course, too high to investigate unknown substances for their carcinogenic action. It should, therefore, be possible to improve the predictive value by using additional short-term systems which may be sensitive to other groups of substances.

This "battery" method entails the pretesting of substances with bacterial test systems, in vitro cell systems and short-term test systems using animals. In the ideal case, the sum of the results from this battery should be used as an indicator as to whether a substance is to be rated as carcinogenic or noncarcinogenic. However, today we are still far away from this objective.

## Restrictions of Short-Term Test Systems

Some of the important reasons why not all carcinogenic substances can elicit alterations in the DNA in the conventional short-term test methods or why the noncarcinogenic substances are identified as positive are summarized as follows:

### Systems for the Metabolism of Substances

Many substances which pass into the body cannot react as such with the genetic information. They must first of all be converted by certain enzymes into an active phase, or substances which are already active can be inactivated in the whole body. The equilibrium between processes of activation and inactivation occurring within an experimental animal or a human being may not always be presented in the in vitro systems of biotransformation.

### Genetic Effect

In short-term test systems, we mainly test whether or not the substance elicits genetic alterations. In long-term trials, we obtain the information actually desired: namely whether or not the substance is carcinogenic. The agreement of the results from the various systems therefore depends on the extent to which the respective genetic alterations which we demonstrate are also actually involved in the carcinogenic action of the substance. However, certain carcinogenic substances exert their tumor-inducing effect without a direct reaction with the DNA (epigenetic influences). Such nongenotoxic substances cannot be detected with the usual short-term test systems for demonstration of genetic alterations. Not all the substances which elicit any genetic alterations exert a carcinogenic action, since only certain (but not all) mutations may be involved in the transformation of a normal cell.

### Pharmacology

For metabolic transformation or as indicator cells the majority of the short-term test systems described apply mammalian material which has been taken from intact animals. In these "in vitro" systems, not all the influences which occur within a mammal (in vivo) may be manifested. For example, the metabolic activities of the microorganisms of the gastrointestinal tract, the interactions between various cells of one or several tissues and the influence of other substances (hormones, food, etc.) are absent. Pharmacological factors of uptake, distribution and excretion may also play a critical role in the carcinogenic effects of substances.

For these reasons, it is necessary to investigate test substances in animals. However, many "in vivo" short-term test methods have the general disadvantage that cells from several organs cannot be analysed, since actual mutations can only be detected in dividing tissues (e.g., bone marrow, white blood cells).

However, numerous carcinogens can produce tumors in very many and very specific organs (lungs, liver, gastrointestinal tract, nervous system, etc.). For this reason, it is necessary to develop short-term in vivo test systems with which different tissues of an animal can be investigated for genetic damage.

## Systematic Test Battery

At the German Cancer Research Center, we are concerned with applying a test battery which counteracts or compensates these restrictions (Fig. 75). By a combination of tests on microbiological systems (e.g. bacteria) with investigations on freshly isolated mammalian cells and by monitoring several compound-induced alterations, substances are investigated systematically for their genotoxic potential. In this regard, the adjacent tests in the figure only differ in one parameter (metabolism, monitored effect, or pharmacology) in each case.

The intact cells can be added to the bacteria as metabolizing system. In addition, DNA damage (DNA single strand breaks) can be demonstrated within these cells. Cells from different organs and animal species can be investigated and the techniques can be extended to the in vivo situation.

- The first cells, in which we have demonstrated substance-induced DNA single strand breaks, are freshly isolated hepatocytes. In contrast to cultivated cells or even to cell fractions, these cells should possess a complete enzyme spectrum.
- Investigations on triggering off selective DNA amplification should provide information on whether a demonstration of this process (which should be involved in carcinogenesis) will be suitable for the detection of carcinogenic substances.
- Specific in vivo investigations are carried out to explore the organ-specific action of carcinogenic substances.

The actual value of a possible prediction of the carcinogenic action of a substance with this test battery can only be established accurately when as many

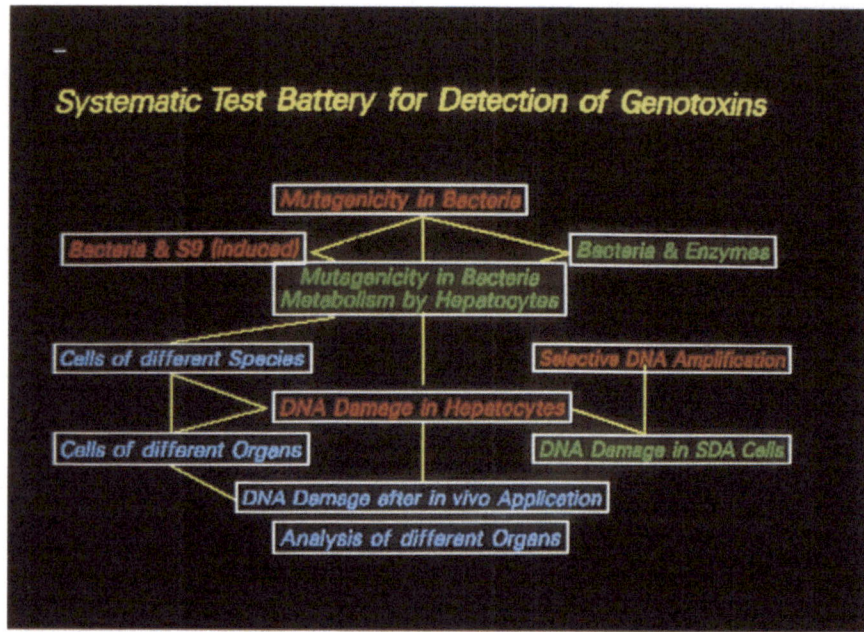

**Systematic Test Battery for Detection of Genotoxins**

- Mutagenicity in Bacteria
- Bacteria & S9 (induced)
- Bacteria & Enzymes
- Mutagenicity in Bacteria Metabolism by Hepatocytes
- Cells of different Species
- Selective DNA Amplification
- DNA Damage in Hepatocytes
- Cells of different Organs
- DNA Damage in SDA Cells
- DNA Damage after in vivo Application
- Analysis of different Organs

Fig. 75
Systematic test battery. S9 = preparation of certain liver enzymes; SDA = selective amplification (proliferation)

different carcinogens and noncarcinogens as possible have been investigated. The coupled systems are, however, now already extremely valuable for clarifying the mode of action of substances.

## Investigations on the Mode of Action of Substances

We are investigating various (mainly carcinogenic) compounds for their genotoxic effects. The compounds either occur in the environment (e.g., in foods, cosmetics, tobacco goods, in the respiratory air), or they are contained in pharmaceutical products. In collaboration with other study groups, not only the genotoxic properties of these substances are to be determined, but detailed information is also to be obtained on biotransformation, pharmacokinetics and other toxicological effects of the substances. These investigations are important for the clarification of mechanisms of tumor induction by carcinogens and are necessary for the estimation of risks for man.

The results obtained with the test battery are considered in the overall evaluation of the substance effects (Fig. 75).

The "direct" mutagenic effect of substances and their action after biotransformation by various systems and cells provide us with information on the mechanisms of toxication and detoxication in the body. The detection of various genotoxic events is important in order to clarify the interaction between the substance (or the intermediate products) and DNA. The in vivo investigations provide information on the pharmacokinetics and the organo-specific effects of the substances.

The mode of action of substances in cells of different animal species and in particular in human beings improves the transferability of results from animals to humans and provides a better basis for risk appraisal.

## Determination of Risk Groups

The recognition of individual risks in persons who come into contact with carcinogenic substances (e.g., tobacco smoke, drugs, occupational factors) has a different basis than the evaluation of the carcinogenic action of a certain substance. To this end, specific exposures, predispositions and early lesions of affected persons must be determined.

Chemical analyses of the circulating air or other samples, e.g., of the food, can provide information on the level of concentrations of one or several known substances in the human environment. Determination of mutagens in body fluids can serve to establish whether certain exposed persons actually ingest genotoxic substances. Furthermore, early effects (e.g., alterations in the chromosomes of white blood cells, DNA or protein adducts) show that ingested genotoxic substances have reacted with autologous material. By recognition of this and other factors it is hoped to delimit exposure and predisposition to such an extent that individual risks of developing cancer can be appraised (Krebserkennung?).

At present, we are investigating urine from persons working with mutagenic and carcinogenic drugs.

By using a sensitive variant of the AMES test (on microtiter plates), the mutagenic action of relatively small amounts of these drugs or their metabolic products in the urine can be demonstrated.

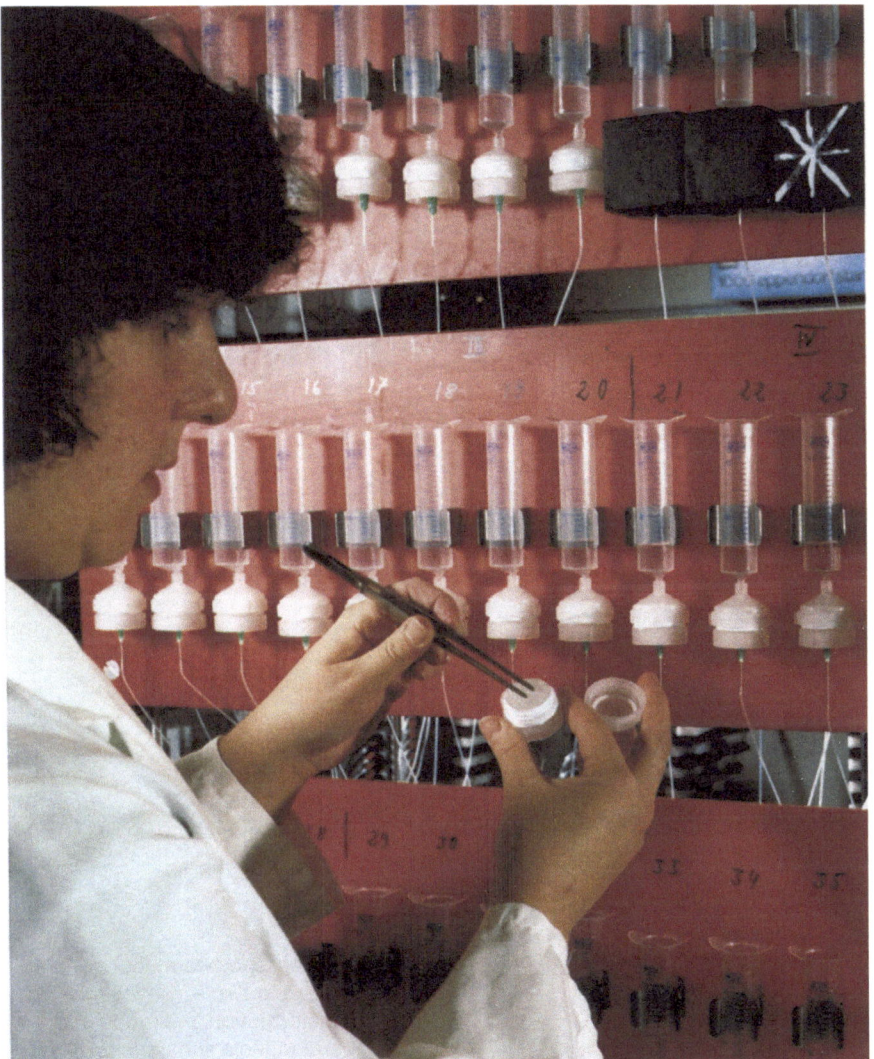

Positive results from these investigations are, in the first instance, used to improve conditions of work so that further exposure of the subjects does not occur. The estimation of the relative risk of such exposures is the objective of further research.

Fig. 76
Damage to hereditary substance by carcinogenic substances is tested here (alkaline elution)

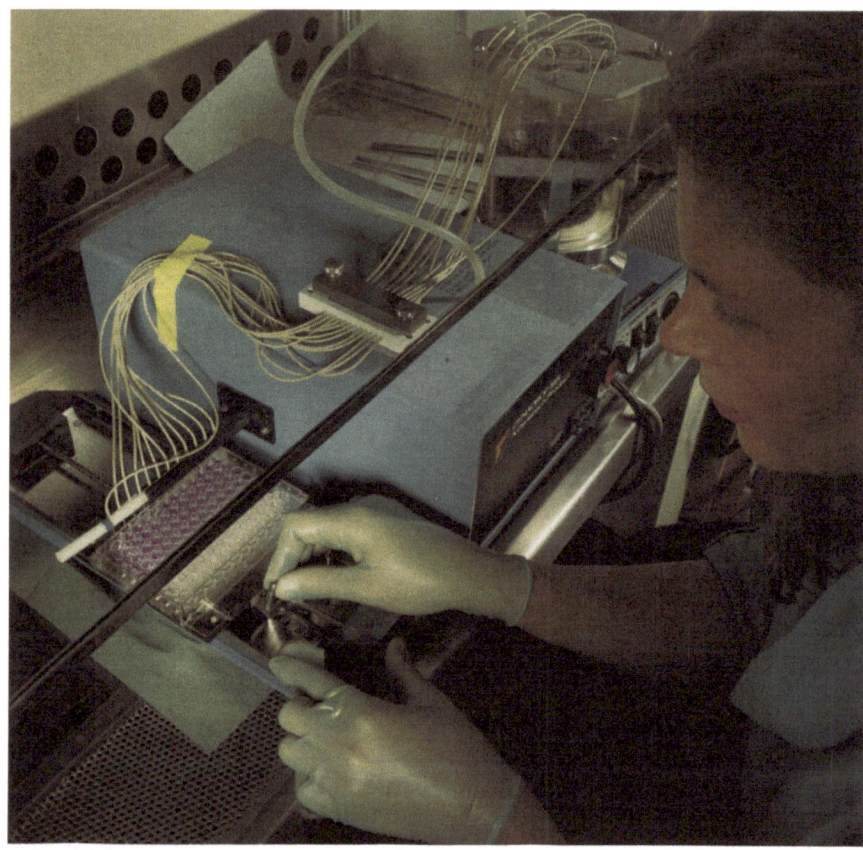

## 4

Fig. 77
With a variant of the Ames' test, mutagenically active cytostatics and their metabolic products can be demonstrated in the urine

## Conclusions

To summarize, short-term test systems may play a central role in investigations on biotransformation and mode of action of carcinogenic substances. It is likewise possible to determine the exposure of individuals by means of this test.

However, systems and batteries of systems must be developed and investigated for their suitability for detection and identification of a possible carcinogenic action of unknown substances.

Priv. Doz. Dr. Beatrice Pool
Carcinogenesis and Chemotherapy,
Institute for Toxicology and
Chemotherapy

In collaboration with

Prof. Rudolf Preußmann
Department of Environmental Carcinogenesis

Priv.-Doz. Dr. Manfred Wiessler
Department of Metabolism of N-Nitroso Compounds,
Institute of Toxicology and
Chemotherapy

Prof. Werner Baltes
Institute of Food Chemistry,
Berlin Technical University

Priv.-Doz. Dr. Bernd Clement
Institute of Pharmaceutics,
University of Freiburg

Prof. Gerhard Eisenbrand
Food Chemistry and Environmental Toxicology, Chemistry Division,
University of Kaiserslautern

Dr. Waltraut Göggelmann
Department of Toxicology,
Gesellschaft für Strahlen- und Umweltforschung
Neuherberg

Priv.-Doz. Dr. Georg Mohn
Department of Radiation Genetics and Chemical Mutagenesis,
State University of Leyden, Netherlands

Prof. Franz Oesch and
Priv.-Doz. Dr. Hansrudi Glatt
Institute of Toxicology,
University of Mainz

Dr. Heinz Renner
Federal Nutritional Research Institute,
Karlsruhe

Selected Publications

Ames, B. N., Darston, W. E., Yamasaki, E., Lee, D.: Carcinogens are mutagens: a simple testsystem combining homogenates for activation and bacteria for detection. Proc. Natl. Acad. Sci (USA) 70, 2281–2285 (1973 b).

Hollstein, M., McCann, J.: Short-Term-Tests for Carcinogens and Mutagens. Mutation Research 65, 133–226 (1979).

Purchase, I. F. H.: ICPEMC Working Paper 2/6. An appraisal of predictive tests for carcinogenicity. Mutation Research 99, 53–71 (1982).

Ashby, J.: The unique role of rodents in the detection of possible human carcinogens and mutagens. ICPEMC Working Paper 1/1, Mutation Research 115, 177–213 (1983).

Harper, B. L., Rinkus, S. J., Scott, M., Ammenhauser, M., Bang, K. M., Lowery, M., Legator, M. S.: Correlation of NCI and IARC carcinogens with their mutagenicity in Salmonella. Nato advanced Sc. Instituts Series V. 60, Ed. by Ameleto Castellani „The use of human cells for the evaluation of risk from physical and chemical agents", Plenum Press, New York (1983).

Maron, D. M., Ames, B. N.: Revised methods for the Salmonella mutagenicity test. Mutation Research 113, 173–215 (1983).

Sina, J. F., Bean, C. L., Dysart, G. R., Taylor, V. I., Bradley, M. O.: Evaluation of the alkaline elution/rat hepatocyte assay as a predictor of carcinogenic/mutagenic potential. Mutation Research 113, 357–391 (1983).

ICPEMC Publication No. 9: Report of ICPEMC Task Group 5 on the differentiation between genotoxic and non-genotoxic carcinogens. Mutation Research 133, 1–49 (1984).

## 4.5 The Cancer Atlas of the Federal Republic of Germany

by Gustav Wagner

Individual attempts to provide synoptic pictures of the geographical distribution of diseases date back several decades. However, only the "National Atlas of Disease – Mortality in the United Kingdom" by the British geographer and epidemiologist Melvin Howe, published in 1970, first stimulated numerous attempts to map the "cancer landscape" of a country or a defined region. Since then, numerous cancer atlases have been published. All of these use official mortality statistics as a data base and show the situation with regard to cancer mortality. Among the numerous relevant publications in recent years, only the cancer atlases of Belgium, Canada, the People's Republic of China, the Netherlands, Italy, Japan, Switzerland, Taiwan and the USA are mentioned here. International, and national congresses on "mapping of cancer", which is the English term for the cartographic presentation of cancer geography, were held in Lyon and Southampton.

The worldwide interest of epidemiologists in the cartographic representation of the geographic pathology of cancer is explained on the one hand by the advances in statistical methodology and computer technology in recent years, which have appreciably facilitated the compilation of cancer maps. On the other hand, it is also due to increasing public awareness that cancer is a curable disease. This has resulted in growing public interest in the extent of malig-

nant diseases in people's own living environment. The publication of the "Cancer Atlas of the Federal Republic of Germany" was not a crazy idea of the authors, but is a contribution to international efforts to improve the registration and description of the geographic pathology of cancer.

Fig. 78

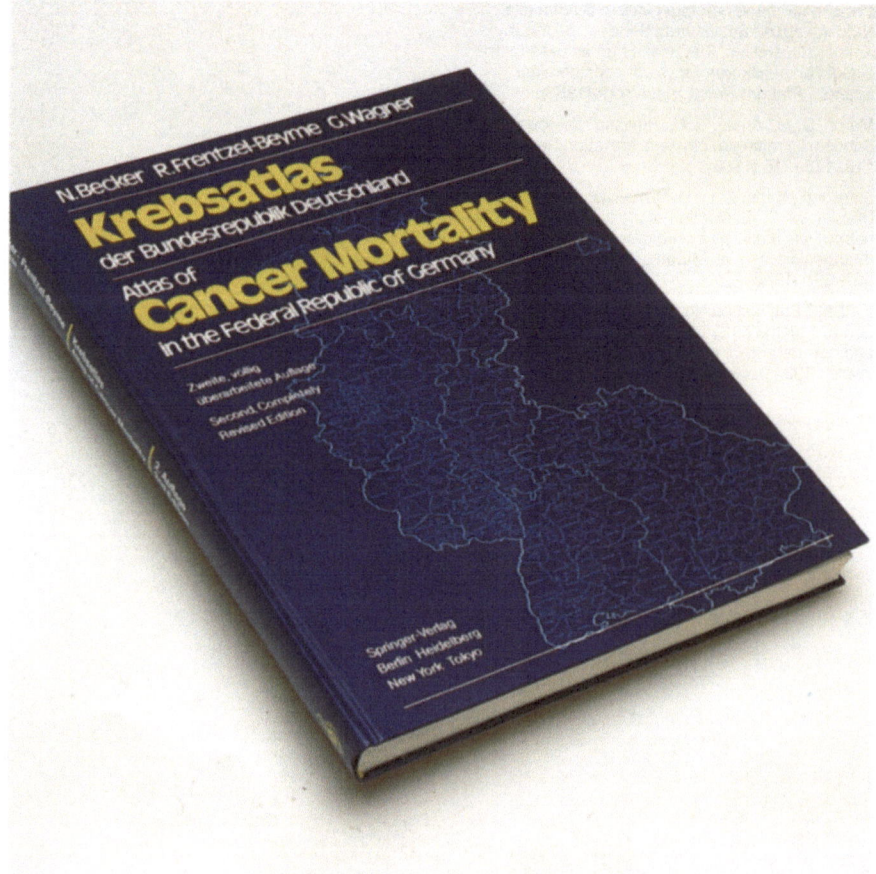

### The Methods

The first edition of the Cancer Atlas, published in 1979, was able to show the situation with regard to cancer mortality in the Federal Republic of Germany only on a very rough raster of the eleven federal states (including West Berlin), since detailed data was not available. This was a disadvantage which the authors had already pointed out at the time.

Substantial efforts were necessary before the authors obtained the cancer mortality data from all state statistical offices with a better regional differentia-

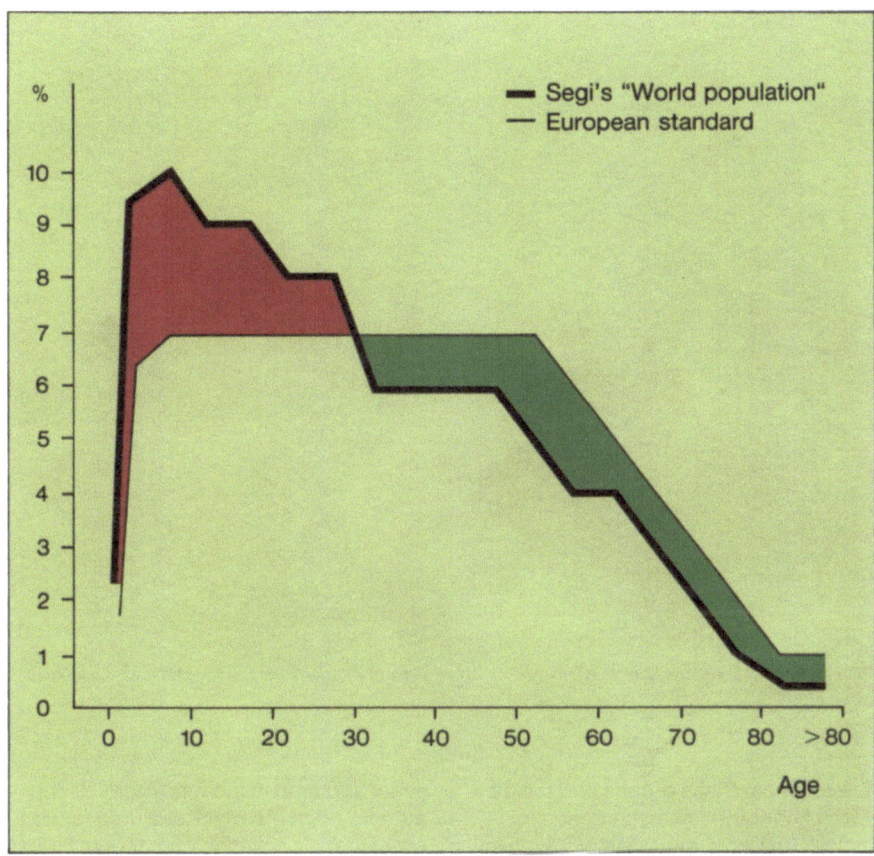

Fig. 79

Because of the differences in the age structure of the populations to be compared, the absolute figures observed can, as a rule, not be used for epidemiological comparisons. The data are hence usually standardized, e.g., as to a "standard" population, and age-standardized mortality rates are calculated. This rate specifies how high the number of cancer deaths per 100,000 population would be if, with the mortality observed in the different age classes, the population to be evaluated had the age structure of the standard population.

Besides various methods of standardization, there are also very many different standard populations. In the interest of as great as possible an international comparability of the figures from the Federal Republic of Germany, we chose the "world population" of the Japanese epidemiologist Segi for this purpose. Since the age structure of this population is younger than, e.g., the "European standard population" (Fig. 79), the age-standardized rates related to this are lower than in relation to the latter standard. Other atlases have chosen different standard populations, and yet other atlases did not calculate any age-standardized mortality rates but the respective ratio of the observed and expected mortality, or variations from an overall mean value.

In addition, in the Federal German Cancer Atlas, a second procedure for calculating the age-standardized mortality was used: the "cumulative mortality rate" suggested by N. E. Day. It is an estimate of the risk that a person will die of a certain disease in the course of a 75 year lifetime if he has not already died from another cause. As a probability generally specified in percent, the cumulative mortality rate is independent

tion (namely at the district level) and broken down according to sex and into five-year age classes. The second edition of the Cancer Atlas of the Federal Republic of Germany described here shows the mortality from 24 different forms of cancer separately for men and women in the 328 counties and municipalities of the Federal Republic on the basis of mean values for the years 1976–1980.

The cancer types were selected primarily on the basis of their incidence. All

tumors with roughly 1,000 deaths per year and more for at least one sex are considered. Cancers, which occur in less than 1,000 cases per year at the moment but are rapidly increasing and are, therefore, of significance in terms of health policy (melanoma and testicular tumors) as well as tumor types, for which an increase was expected but which are in reality decreasing, which is of etiological interest (bone tumors), are included in addition. Furthermore, thyroid cancer is also considered because it reveals a distinct geographical pattern despite a smaller number of cases.

115

of the age structure of a population and is hence generally comparable. It has the disadvantage that it has so far been little used.

The problems of cancer mapping are multifarious in nature. Geographic investigation units of different sizes, noncoincident report periods, reference to different standards, index parameters obtained with different methods of calculation, dissimilar presentation of results, etc. result in substantial difficulties in comparing the data in the atlases published up to now. It is not so simple to make statistical material directly comparable with other materials as the layman may assume.

## The "Landscape" of Cancer Mortality

The Cancer Atlas made it possible for the first time to obtain a differentiated view of cancer mortality based on a more detailed regional breakdown. The color gradations of the maps from red to yellow demonstrate high to moderately high, and from yellow to green moderately low to low cancer mortality rates (a total of five colors).

The maps are unable to "prove" anything and do not have this intention; their objective is an optical representation of geographical differences in cancer mortality which should, if anything, be investigated in more detail.

The maps are accompanied by an explanatory text which compares the data available in the Federal Republic of Germany with those available internationally, also taking into account data on new cases of cancer. In addition, it offers an overview on the knowledge or the best founded hypotheses with regard to the causes of the different cancer forms.

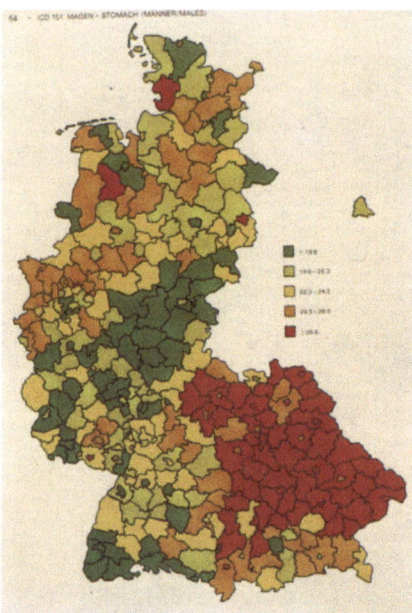

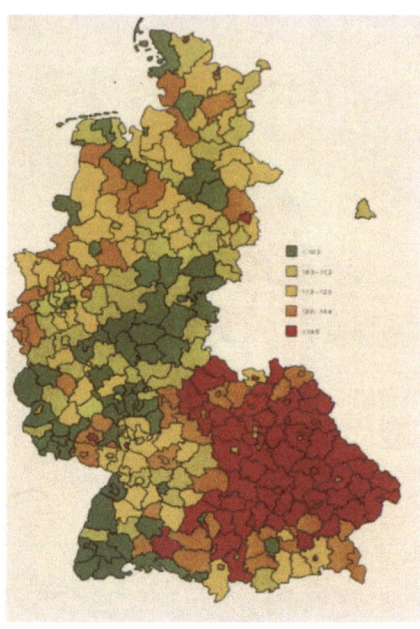

Fig. 80
Rate of mortality from stomach cancer in men. Maps from the Cancer Atlas

Rate of mortality from stomach cancer in women

The text comprises graphs and tables which show, inter alia, the trends for mortality rates to decrease or increase for the respective cancer types. The Cancer Atlas thus represents a detailed documentation on the cancer mortality in the Federal Republic of Germany.

It becomes evident that the highest mortality from lung cancer is present in some conurbations such as the Ruhr area, Berlin, Hamburg, the Saarland and the Rhine-Neckar area, but not in other thickly settled regions.

There is no doubt that smoking is by far the most important risk factor for lung cancer. It must be borne in mind in this regard that smoking was more intensive in municipal conurbations ten to thirteen

years ago than in the rural regions. The authors point out that there is so far no proof that air pollution constitutes an appreciable risk factor.

The atlas further demonstrates that the highest rates of stomach cancer are to be found in the eastern counties of Bavaria and that the moratlity from colon cancer and breast cancer shows a distinct tendency to rise.

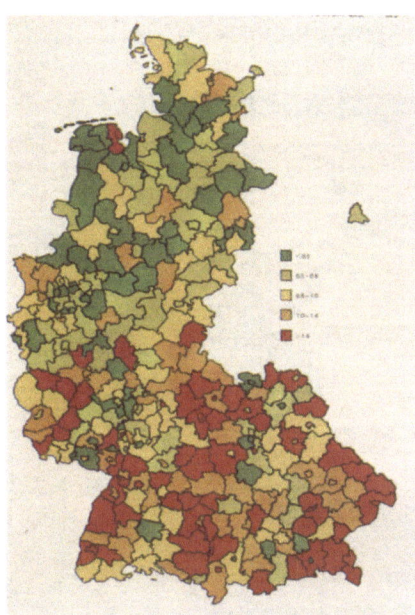

Rate of mortality from thyroid cancer in women

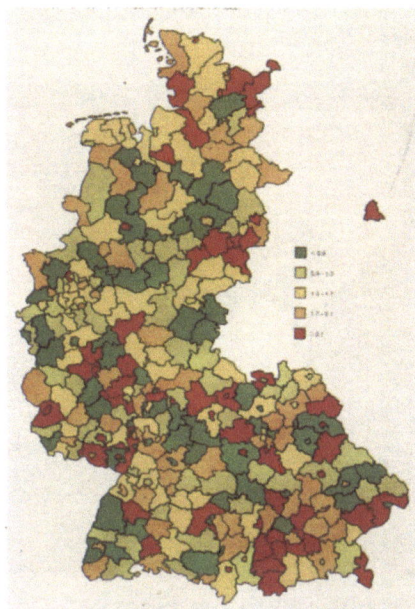

Rate of mortality from lung cancer in men

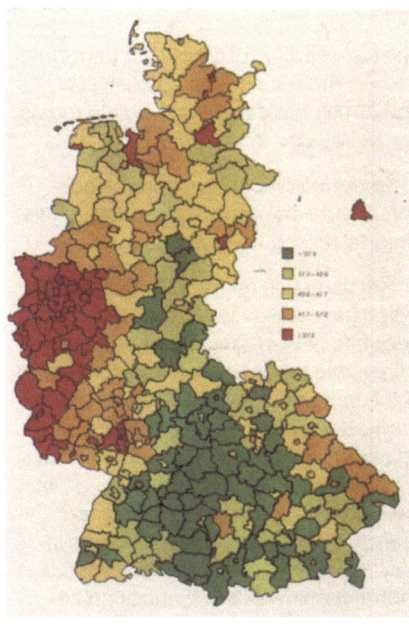

Rate of mortality from melanoma in men

## Secular Trends

The Cancer Atlas shows that, despite a relatively calm superficial picture of the overall cancer "landscape" (the total death rate has hardly altered), the development of individual tumor types is different: some are increasing, and some are decreasing.

In men in the period from 1952–1981, all the more frequent malignant neoplasias have increased apart from tumors of the esophagus, the stomach, connective tissue and bone. There is a major decline of gastric cancer (– 50%) as compared to an even greater rise of lung cancer (+ 118%). The four cancer localizations lungs, stomach, colon/rectum and prostate today account for almost 80% of all cancer deaths in men.

In women, there is a decline of esophageal, gastric, connective tissue and bone cancer as well as cancer of the corpus uteri. An increase is to be found particularly in tumors of the breast, the colon, the lungs as well as the pancreas. The most frequent causes of cancer death in women are cancers of the breast and the colon. In women, lung cancer still takes fifth place at the moment, but is showing an appreciable increase.

The five most frequent tumor types (breast cancer, large bowel cancer, stomach cancer, ovarian cancer and lung cancer) account for around 50% of all deaths from cancer in women.

The authors of the Cancer Atlas ascribe the decrease or increase of cancer mortality to an alteration of the localization-specific "supply" of carcinogenic factors. They attribute the (in some cases appreciable) geographical differences in the incidence of the different types of cancer largely to environmental factors. This entails the environment in the broadest sense. The term also comprises the social environment (occupation, social class), the individual lifestyle (smoking, nutrition) up to the environment of the still unborn child.

## Conclusions

The cancer atlas prompts the performance of more far-reaching analytical epidemiological studies. Two measures are necessary in this respect:

1. Epidemiological cancer registries should be established as rapidly as possible to record new disease cases.

2. The statistics on the cause of death, which have a high quality in the Federal Republic of Germany, must be made accessible to research. The background of the increase of cancer deaths can be clarified with the information provided by death certificates. Such studies have enabled substantial advances, e.g., in the field of occupational cancer research. These have led to progress in prevention (e.g., replacement of beta-naphthylamine as a vulcanization accelerator in the rubber industry or prohibiton of arsenic as an insecticide in viticulture). However, such research projects are not possible today without access to the death certificates of persons formerly employed in a risk area. Due to the increasingly stringent data protection regulations in the Federal Republic of Germany, unfortunately the epidemiologist is nowadays often refused access to death certificates.

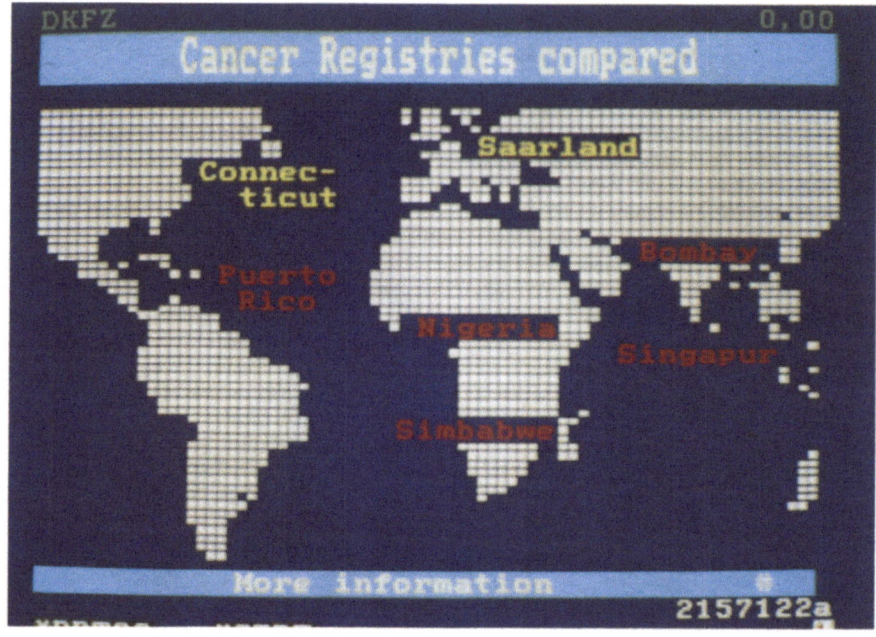

Fig. 81

## Criticism of the Cancer Atlas

The authors were surprised that the Cancer Atlas was the object of quite a overwhelming wave of journalistic attention even before its appearance on the book market. There were several television and radio programs, a title story in "Der Spiegel", an eight-page article in "Stern", a report in "Quick", and reports and articles in practically all West German daily papers. The exceptional publicity was supported in part by the fact that the Federal Minister of Research and Technology presented the book personally at a press conference in August 1984.

The first critical reactions came by return mail and before the critics concerned had seen the book, since it was not yet on the market. It may be observed that there has not been even remotely the amount of journalistic turbulence and criticism, quite missing the point of the book, in any other country on publication of the respective cancer atlas.

The rational and material criticism of the Cancer Atlas essentially concentrates on doubts as to the diagnostic validity of the official mortality statistics. This discussion is decades old, and pathologists and epidemiologists in particular have different views.

The validity of the diagnostic data on the death certificates has been disputed time and again by pathological anatomists. Of course, as is known by every epidemiologist, the diagnoses of the pathologists are more certain than those of clinicians. On the other hand, mere autopsy statistics cannot be used for epidemiological purposes, because they make statements on the basis of a highly selected material of about 8% of all deaths (mainly diagnostically difficult or unconfirmed cases), and these appraisals cannot be extrapolated to the 92% non-autopsied cases of death.

The often presented argument that the frequency of autopsies constitutes a direct measure for the quality of the official cause of death statistics in the different countries is invalid, not least since the autopsy results are not available at the time the death certificates are filled out and the latter are practically never amended.

Some misunderstandings are explained solely by the fact that the different objectives of death certification and autopsy report are not recognized.

In the statistics on the cause of death the immediate cause of death and, if appropriate, the underlying condition which led to this are included; on the other hand, the autopsy finding is intended to register all pathological findings present in the corpse. If the death certificate does not mention a tumor found on autopsy, this does not automatically entail an error in the issue of the death certificate. For example, a subclinical prostate carcinoma is a frequent autopsy finding in old men who have not died from cancer. It would be wrong to include such carcinomas in the cause of death statistics as immediate cause of death or as underlying condition. In some recent papers, pathologists from German institutes have considered it necessary to justify a higher rate of autopsy by the observation of a major discrepancy between clinical diagnoses and autopsy findings. Global

reference is made to differences of 50% and more between the clinical and pathological anatomical diagnoses.

However, as shown by experience, such global statements are of little use, since, on the one hand, the frequency of autopsy in different diseases and, on the other hand, the diagnostic validity in different groups of diagnose are very different. In particular, information on cancer on the death certificates is more reliable than that on some other groups of diagnoses, since practically almost every cancer patient has been examined radiologically and/or biopsied before his death (histological findings are available for about 70–80% of all cancer patients).

Any epidemiologist will admit that the data on the death certificates are not correct in an appreciable portion of cases. On the other hand, he may assume that the error frequency of the data in the north of the Federal Republic will not have another weight or follow another direction than in the south. He will be able to assume that the incorrectness of the data is randomly distributed. Thus, this does not disturb the comparability. If it is generally assumed that the clinician does not find so many cases of cancer and note them on the death certificates as the post mortem experts in the autopsy findings, this means that the data of the mortality statistics are merely minimal data which would have to be increased by a certain factor.

Thorough validation studies from home and abroad (e.g., from Heasman and Lipworth, Percy et al.) demonstrate the overall validity of the data on death certificates for the purposes of cancer epidemiology. In the 1973 WHO Copenhagen study (Medical Certifica-

tion of Causes of Death – Euro 4906), Koller observed for the Federal Republic that the "information available to the doctors issuing the death certificate is to be designated as good in 80%". Percy et al. from the Biometric Branch of the National Cancer Institute in Bethesda, USA found agreement between the data in the case documentation and on the death certificates in 82.7% of 48,826 cancer deaths. However, there were marked differences with regard to the different forms of cancer. Thus, colon cancer was mentioned more frequently on the death certificates, but rectal cancer was mentioned less frequently than on the medical records.

To summarize, with regard to the discussion on the reliability of post mortem certificates once more triggered off by the Cancer Atlas, it is to be stated that the critics of the Cancer Atlas have not provided new criteria or insights. So long as patent recipes for an improvement of the quality of mortality data are not in sight, the epidemiologist will have to live with the data available, even if these are doubtless not optimal.

The authors were also criticized in that an atlas of cancer morbidity (i.e. frequency of disease incidence) was said to be much more informative than an atlas of mortality. This is to be commented on as follows: first of all, only the diseases which lead to death are, of course, included in the statistics of cause of death. One thus obtains from the mortality data only information about those tumors which had a fatal outcome. Tumor types which lead to death will thus enter into in the statistics with a greater weighting than those with a relatively good curability. In the former, the mortality can be regarded as being representative of their incidence, and in the latter the mortality underestimates the incidence. This effect is the more pronounced the better the curability of a tumor. With malignancies, which rarely take a fatal course (e.g., certain skin tumors), mortality statistics provide practically no useful information on the frequency of occurrence.

A complete description of the current situation in a population requires two different data sources: firstly data on the morbidity (incidence = rate of occurrence of new disease and prevalence = number of existing cases) of the various cancer forms at defined times. (Such data are collected by so-called "cancer registries"; they are available only where there are well-functioning cancer registries); secondly, data on the mortality (cancer mortality) to be taken from the official mortality statistics of the individual countries. The two data sources provide supplementary information.

For certain decisions of health policy (e.g., the initiation of preventive measures, provision of beds, etc.), knowledge about incidence and prevalence is more important than that about mortality. In the case of a reduction in lethality with certain forms of cancer, due to improved therapy, mortality may fall despite an increase in the frequency of occurrence of the disease. In such a case, consideration of the mortality data alone would evoke a false impression of the economic and medical significance of the disease.

On the other hand, the mortality statistics are the essential instrument for obtaining information to evaluate the result of preventive measures in cancer control, even if cancer registries are available.

Both data sources (cancer registries as well as mortality statistics) are important for an efficient cancer epidemiology and should not be played off one against the other.

Apart from this, the criticism of the Cancer Atlas does not alter the fact that the official mortality statistics are the only regionally complete and internationally comparable data source available all over the world for epidemiological investigations.

It was further criticized that the Cancer Atlas only records the last domicile of the deceased person, which may be quite different from where he had spent most of his life and had been exposed to the most important environmental influences. The familiar example of Florida in the USA, where the highest rate of deaths from cancer is recorded (the "panhandle" phenomenon), shows that such "migratory movements" may play a role. The reason for this is that very many Americans retire to Florida. It was also found in Britain that a clinic for incurable cancer patients appreciably raised the mortality rate of the county concerned.

In the Federal Republic, the degree of mobility of the population is relatively small. It should be investigated first of all whether there also exist such "national senior citizens' homes" in this country. The clarification of the background of apparent "cancer nests" is one of the investigations which should be prompted by the Cancer Atlas.

The atlas is a reflection of the "cancer landscape", a product of descriptive epidemiology. It illustrates the situation, explains it, but does not appraise it. It is intended to give ideas and pointers for more far-reaching analytic studies. It should be used by people who can work with its data, be they scientists, doctors or persons responsible for health policy. However, it should not be used to produce public disquiet.

Of course, we would have been very pleased to present an atlas of cancer morbidity in the Federal Republic of Germany. However, the conditions for obtaining appropriate data (maintaining population-related cancer registries) do not as yet exist in the Federal Republic apart from Hamburg and the Saarland. If the public discussion triggered off by the Cancer Atlas has produced a further impulse in this direction, the authors' efforts would have been worthwhile.

Prof. Gustav Wagner
Epidemiology and Documentation
Institute of Documentation, Information and Statistics

Staff collaborating

Dr. Nikolaus Becker
Dr. Rainer Frentzel-Beyme

In collaboration with

Herbert Trojan
Department of Biophysics and Medical Radiophysics
Institute of Nuclear Medicine

Selected Publications

Heasman, M. A., Lipworth, L.: Accuracy of Certification of Death. London: H.M.S.O. (1968).

Howe, M.: National Atlas of Disease. Mortality in the United Kingdom. London: Nelson (1970).

Mason, T. J., McKay, F. W., Hoover, R., Fraumeni, J. F.: Atlas of Cancer Mortality for U.S. Countries: 1950–1969. DHEW Publication No. 75–780. Washington: U.S. Govt. Printing Office (1975).

Brooke, E. M.: Géographie de la Mortalité due au Cancer en Suisse 1969–1971. Lausanne: Dept. de l'Intérieur et de la Santé Publique (1976).

Day, N. E.: A New Measure of Age-Standardized Incidence – The Cumulative Rate. In J. Waterhouse, C. Muir, P. Correa, J. Powell (Eds): Cancer Incidence in Five Continents, Vol. III, pp. 443–445. Lyon: International Agency for Research on Cancer (1976).

Segi, M., Aoki, K.: Atlas of Cancer Mortality for Japan by cities and counties 1969–1971. Tokyo: Daiwa Health Foundation (1977).

Cislagh, C., DeCarli, A., Morosini, P., Puntoni, R.: Atlante della Mortalita per Tumori in Italia. Trienno 1970–1972. Roma: Lega Italiana per la lotta contra i Tumori (1978).

Chen, Kung-Pei, Wu, Hsin-Ying, Yeh, Ching-Chuan, Cheng, Yu-Jan: Color Atlas of Cancer Mortality by Administrative and Other Classified Districts in Taiwan Area: 1968–1976. Taipei: National Science Council (1979).

Frentzel-Beyme, R., Leutner, R., Wagner, G., Wiebelt, H.: Krebsatlas der Bundesrepublik Deutschland. Berlin-Heidelberg-New York: Springer (1979).

Centraal Bureau voor de Statistiek: Atlas of Cancer Mortality in the Netherlands 1969–1978. The Hague: Netherlands Central Bureau of Statistics (1980).

Minister of National Health and Welfare: Mortality Atlas of Canada. Vol. 1: Cancer. Hull/Québec: Canad. Gov. Publ. Centre (1980).

Chinese Institute of Medical Sciences: Atlas of Cancer Mortality in the People's Republic of China. Beijing: Chin. Acad. med. Sci., China Cartographic Publ. House (1981).

Percy, C., Stanek, E., Gloeckler, C.: Accuracy of cancer death certificates and its effect on cancer mortality statistics. Amer. J. publ. Hlth 71, 242–250 (1981).

Boyle, P.: Report on the Workshop on Mapping of Cancer, Lyon, 10–11 Dec. IARC International Technical Report No. 82/002 (1981).

Ministerie van Volksgezondheit en van het Gezin – Institut voor Hygiene en Epidemiologie: Atlas van de Kankermortaliteit in Belgie (1969–1976) – Atlas of Cancer Mortality in Belgium (1969–1976). Brussels (1983).

Becker, N., Frentzel-Beyme, R., Wagner, G.: Krebsatlas der Bundesrepublik Deutschland, 2. Aufl. – Atlas of Cancer Mortality in the Federal Republic of Germany, 2. edit. Berlin-Heidelberg-New York-Tokyo: Springer (1984).

Medical Research Council: Scientific Report No. 3. Maps and Cancer. Proceedings of a meeting held on 20th September 1983 at the MRC Environment Epidemiology Unit. Southampton: Southampton General Hospital (1984).

Bundesamt für Statistik (Hrsg.): Geografische Verteilung der Krebssterblichkeit in der Schweiz 1979–1981. Beiträge zur Schweizerischen Krebsstatistik Heft 119. Bern: Bundesamt für Statistik (1984).

Koller, S.: Studie über die Todesursachen auf den Todesbescheinigungen in der Bundesrepublik Deutschland, Mainz, ohne Jahr, sowie WHO Kopenhagen, Euro 4906.

Research Commitee on Geographical Distribution of Diseases: National Atlas of Major Disease Mortalities for Cities, Towns and Villages in Japan (1969–1978). Tokyo: Japan Health Promotion Foundation o.J.

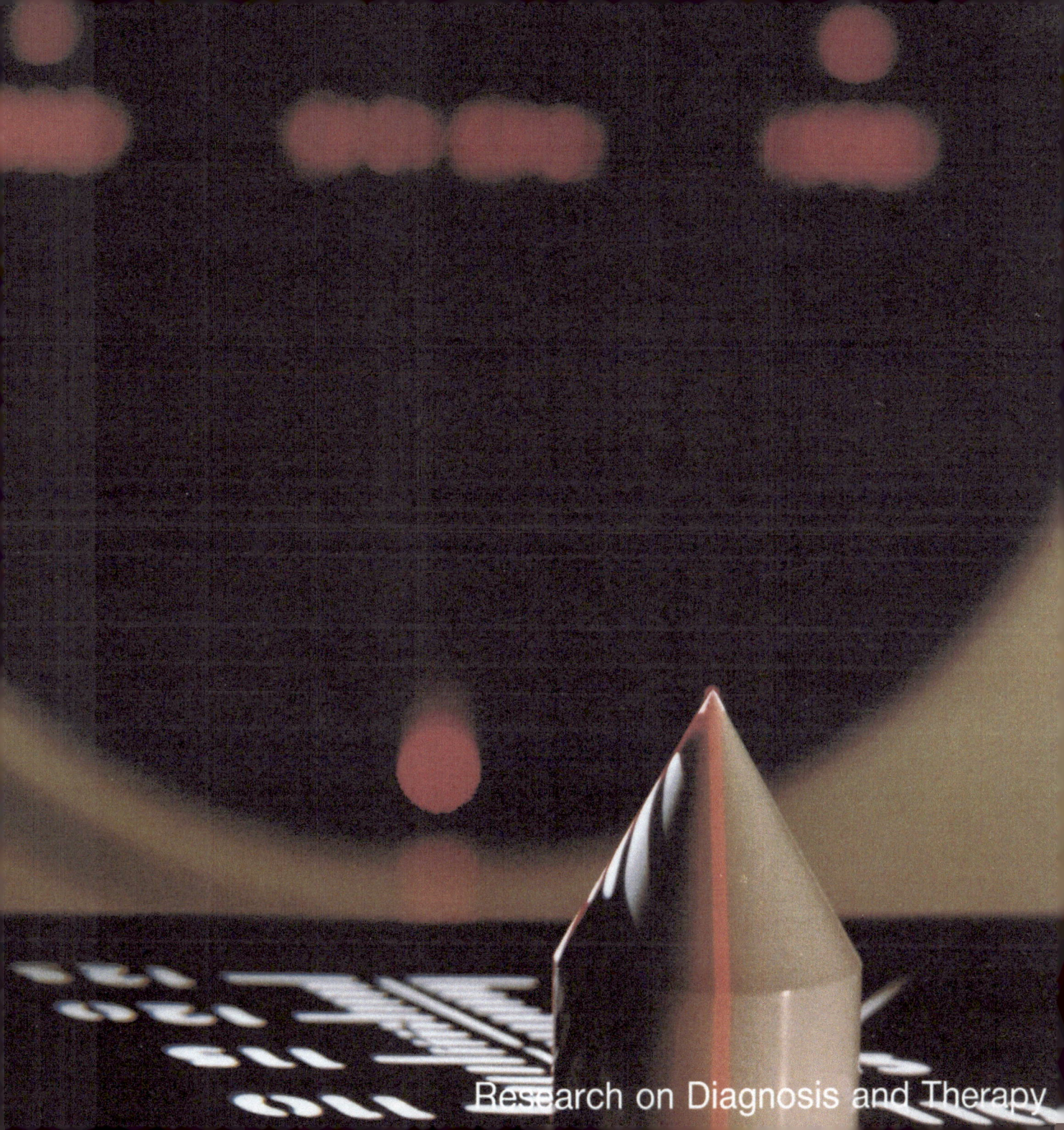

Research on Diagnosis and Therapy

# 5

## Research on Diagnosis and Therapy

In the battle against cancer, diagnosis has a crucial strategic significance. Diagnostic shortcomings will be difficult to counteract by therapy.

Tumor diagnostics has the following essential functions:

1. Detection of the tumor in as early a stage as possible
2. Determination of the size, localization, organ relation and extent of the tumor (staging)
3. Characterization of the tumor tissue on the basis of morphological, physiological and biochemical parameters
4. Control of the course of therapy
5. Diagnostic follow-up

The crucial first step in dealing with the individual disease is to obtain as early a diagnosis of the tumor as possible. The methods of investigation should only constitute a slight burden to the patients so that they can already be used on first suspicion. It is to be borne in mind that the tumor has generally been present in an asymptomatic phase for several years before it has grown to a certain size. As a rule, it has a size of more than 1 cm when it is discovered or gives rise to symptoms. This means that there are already several million tumor cells, even in the case of a relatively early diagnosis of a tumor.

If a tumor has been detected, the important subsequent diagnostic step is the determination of the tumor extension (staging). This is the decisive basis for the planning and management of therapy. To detect the size and anatomical situation of a tumor as well as its spreading in the body, various methods

Fig. 82

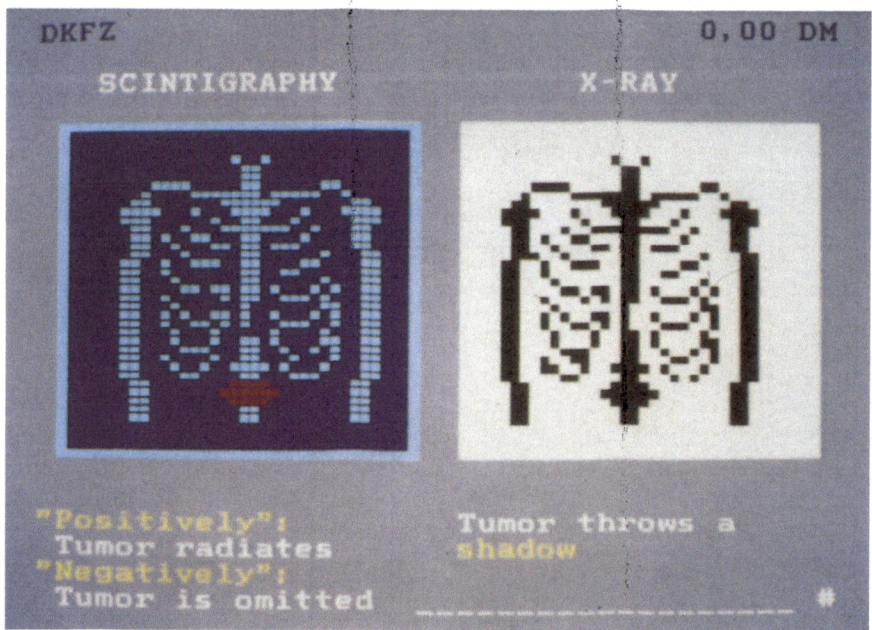

of investigation must be used depending on the tumor type. In particular, computer tomography has proved effective in this regard. As a rule, it is also the calculatory basis for planning modern radiotherapy.

A further diagnostic approach attempts to establish the special features of the respective tumor and its "inner life". On the one hand, macroscopic and, if appropriate, electron microscopic evaluation of the tissue of the tumor is employed for this purpose (grading). More recent approaches aim at detecting and quantifying physiological and biochemical parameters such as blood flow and metabolism both within the tumor and in the neighboring tissues which are not yet affected as well as in the metastases. Important information for the

planning and management of the therapy can be obtained from this data.

Monitoring of the course of therapy by means of modern diagnostic procedures makes a crucial contribution to optimization of treatment. The good or poor response of the tumor to therapy, which may for example result in an alteration of the treatment, can be detected more precisely and earlier than had been possible even about 15 years ago. After successful resection or regression of the tumor tissue, diagnostic surveillance or follow-up of the patient has as its objective early detection of local recurrence or metastases. It is understandable that noninvasive techniques are employed preferentially in follow-up.

For the diagnosis and evaluation of a tumor condition, there are in principle

various diagnostic methods:

1. Biochemical and immunological investigation of body fluids (blood, urine, effusions etc.)

2. Detection of tumor tissue with imaging techniques:
a) Radiodiagnostics
b) Endoscopy
c) Ultrasonography
d) Computer tomography
e) Nuclear magnetic resonance tomography
f) Scintigraphy including immuno-scintigraphy
g) Positron emission tomography

3. Detection of tumor cells (cytodiagnostics) in the sputum, smears or in puncture fluid

4. Pathohistological detection of tumor cell structures by biopsy from the suspicious tissues.

In recent years, diagnostic research at the German Cancer Research Center has been concerned with imaging techniques, in particular with ultrasonography, computer tomography and nuclear medical methods. In the field of cytodiagnostics, automatized cancer screening was made possible by means of "flow or impulse cytophotometry", which enables cells with atypical features to be sorted out in large samples for measurements. New image processing techniques have also been developed for the quantitative detection of histopathological alterations and used for solution of various diagnostic problems (cf. also articles in this volume).

Diagnostic research in coming years will also focus on the new methods for the evaluation of the functional activity and internal structure of tumors by noninvasive methods. Such investigations can be carried out today by means of nu-

Fig. 83

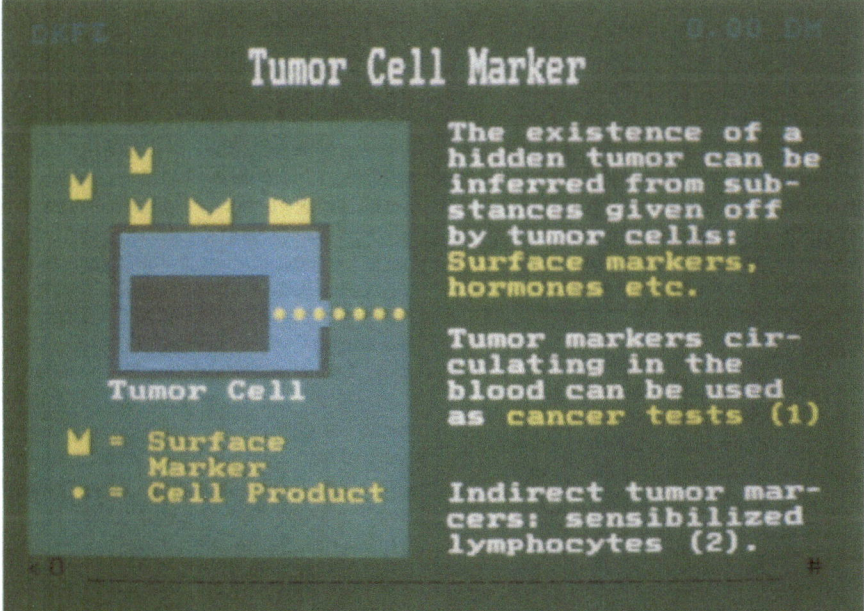

125

clear magnetic resonance tomography and positron emission tomography.

Nuclear magnetic resonance tomography is a technique in which regions of the body are imaged layer by layer in various directions so that their structures can be investigated. For this purpose, the patient is placed in a very strong magnetic field. Certain atomic nuclei which possess a rotatory impulse (spin) behave like tiny magnets oriented within the field. These nuclei can be excited by radiowaves of a frequency corresponding to their own precison frequency. They then emit high-frequency signals which contain extensive information on the state of the tissue concerned. However, it is necessary to decode these signals by means of modern data processing. In the application of high magnetic field intensities, this technique also enables insights into certain metabolic activities of the tissue.

In parallel to and in supplementation of these techniques, future investigations of tumor tissue will be carried out with positron emission tomography. This procedure allows the distribution of radioactively labelled organic substances in the body to be measured and visualized layer by layer. Radioactive labelling with an appropriate positron emitter does not alter the biological behavior of the molecule concerned. Above all, the quantity of the substance concerned can be measured in absolute terms, which is of crucial importance for the analysis of metabolic processes.

These two techniques are used for the diagnosis of the tumor, for staging, but above all for characterization of the tumor tissue in the living body and to check the course of therapy.

A further important approach in diagnostic research consists in the applica-

tion of molecular biological and immunological techniques. The primary objective is the detection of characteristic structures (antigens) on the tumor cells which allow delimitation from normal tissue in practicable test procedures. Today, hybridoma technology is used for this purpose. The corresponding monoclonal antibodies obtained with this technology can be used for diverse purposes. This technique has made it possible today to produce highly specific monoclonal antibodies. In the classical method of immunization of animals (by injection of a substance foreign to the animal, of an antigen), an antiserum can be obtained which contains the antibody. Attention has concentrated on antibody-producing cells or their precursors: lymphocytes from the spleen of immunized animals are fused with tumor cells of a corresponding type (myeloma cells) in the test tube. The hybrid cells formed contain important genetic features of both "parents": from the myeloma cell they have inherited the capacity to grow and to proliferate permanently in culture, and from the normal lymphocytes they have inherited the capacity to produce an antibody with a certain specificity. It is possible to clone hybrid cells producing such specific antibodies, i. e. to grow them in pure cultures so that the corresponding cell culture continuously produces one highly specific antibody.

Different tumor cell populations in a patient can be identified by means of immunohistochemical visualization of the antigen distribution in the tissue. Metastases can be assigned to the tumor of origin by detection of various proteins of the cytoskeleton (structural elements of the cell), i. e. it can be established whether a metastasis has derived, e. g., from hepatocytes or from connective

tissue. This identification enables specific screening for the tumor of origin, which is not known in many cases, and it makes a specific therapy of the tumor type possible.

Monoclonal antibodies against tumor-typical structures can also be used as vehicles for conveying radionuclides or other therapeutically active substances into the target tissue. Thus the indications for immunoscintigraphy, radioimmunotherapy and immunotherapy with cytostatic- or toxin (cell toxin)-conjugated antibodies are extended.

All these techniques have been developed in experimental models and must now be checked with regard to their clinical value.

These outline descriptions of diagnostic activities reveal the close interrelationship between diagnosis and therapy. This topic will be stressed in research in coming years.

## Therapeutic Research

The designation "cancer" does not refer to a uniform disease. On the contrary, it is a collective term for a large number of different tumors in various stages of development. In view of this diversity, it cannot be expected that all malignant tumors can be influenced or cured by one and the same therapeutic procedure. A fundamental difficulty of many therapeutic approaches is the fact that the tumor cell develops from a normal cell and hence exhibits very much fewer differences from the normal cell which can be utilized therapeutically than is the case, e. g., for bacteria.

There are various approaches to cancer treatment:

1. Surgical removal of the tumor tissue
2. Radiotherapy
3. Hyperthermia
4. Hormone therapy
5. Chemotherapy
6. Immunotherapy

Surgery and radiotherapy are employed for local treatment of a tumor. However, there are limits to surgical treatment and radiotherapy when the tumor has spread to one or more vitally important organs so that radical resection or elimination of the tumor is no longer possible in view of the concomitant damage to the healthy tissue. As far as can be evaluated so far, local hyperthermia can supplement radiotherapy in some tumors. Chemotherapy may be employed with some solid tumors when tumor metastases are already present. In malignant diseases of the hematopoietic tissue (leukemia), noteworthy successes could be achieved up to now with chemotherapy. Depending on the stage of the disease, primary malignant tumors of the lymph nodes can be favorably influenced by radiotherapy and/or chemotherapy. As a rule, hormone treatment is restricted to tumors of which the cells possess appropriate hormone receptors.

With regard to immunotherapy, an established technique cannot be offered today. There is hope that our constantly increasing knowledge of the natural and specific resistance in the body will lead to means of direct intervention in defence mechanisms, e. g., specific manipulation for the elimination of tumor cells or prevention of the development of metastases.

The future research activity of the German Cancer Research Center in the field of radiotherapy will pursue two new approaches with particular priority. The main objective is a complete elimination of the tumor whilst sparing the healthy surrounding tissue as far as possible. This can be achieved today by improving the planning of radiotherapy, especially by means of computer tomography and by use of electronic data processing.

One method is the stereotactic therapy of brain tumors. This procedure enables a target point in the brain to be reached with a deviation of less than 1 mm by means of a special puncture device. Via the cannula introduced, liquid or solid radioactive substances can be transported to specific points of the tumor. In this way, a largely selective irradiation of the tumor can be carried out from the inside. In connection with this approach to therapy, the therapeutic efficacy of local controlled hyperthermia in combination with radiotherapy is also being investigated.

A second therapeutic procedure is designated as convergence irradiation. The tumor is exposed to a crossfire from many directions from the outside. In this way, a very high dose is attained in the region of the tumor, whereas the exposure of the healthy tissue is relatively low. However, the question must be critically examined as to what advantages this technique has compared to conventional radiotherapy. Depending on the results and as far as technically possible, it will also be employed in other body regions apart from the skull. These radiotherapeutic programs are being carried through by the German Cancer Research Center in close collaboration with the Radiology Division, University of Heidelberg and the Neurosurgery Division, Center for Surgery at the University of Heidelberg.

Various tumor types have a different sensitivity to cytostatics. There may indeed be extraordinary individual differences within the same tumor type. In contrast to the sensitivity determinations (antibiogram) usual in bacterial disease, it has not been possible to predict adequately the possible influence which cytostatics have on tumor cells (tumor and metastases). A short-term in vitro test developed at the German Cancer Research Center enables the prediction of a tumor's resistance to certain anticancer drugs.

Besides the determination of resistance and investigations into cell kinetics of tumors and metastases (proliferating and nonproliferating portion of tumor cells, cell loss), the development and testing of new antineoplastic chemotherapeutics, clinically relevant tumor models, the reduction of detrimental side effects of the chemotherapeutics applied, the development of schemes for combination therapy as well as local regional chemotherapy are focal points of research in the field of chemotherapy. In some cases, these have been explored in cooperation with hospitals.

The antiviral and, where appropriate, antineoplastic action of xanthogenates which were initially investigated in cell cultures are also attaining increasing significance for research in animals.

The susceptibility of tumor cells and bone marrow cells to cytostatic drugs is tested in cell cultures to compare anti-tumor activity with undesired bone marrow toxicity.

The development and biological testing of new cytostatic drugs include experiments with triazenes, water-soluble nitrosourea derivatives and nitrosoureas linked to oligopeptides, alkyl-lysophospholipids and oxazaphosphorin metabolites. Besides the test of their efficacy in tumor models which are similar to human tumors, the pharmacokinetics and late toxicity (i. e. later development of cancer) of certain substances are investigated.

The reduction or abolition of toxicity by protective substances against the detrimental effects (i. e. nerve damage, bone marrow damage, carcinogenesis) of cytostatics used clinically is a focal point of research. For example, the later development of bladder cancer after treatment with cyclophosphamide has been prevented by a concurrent administration of Mesna (mercapto-ethane sulfonate).

The tumor models developed at the German Cancer Research Center can be applied under clinical conditions and enable the evaluation of cytostatic combinations of clinically used substances (excluding long-term toxicity).

In collaboration with the Surgical Hospital, University of Heidelberg, the treatment of hepatic metastases from colon cancer has been investigated by mere perfusion of the liver with anticancer drugs. These agents are introduced into the liver in a high dosage, and are less detrimental than orally or intervenously applied cytostatics, since the organ partially detoxifies the drug during its passage.

There is clinical collaboration with the University Division of Maxillofacial Surgery and the Tata Memorial Center in Bombay (India) in the field of ENT malignancies. The combination of clinically established cytostatics with uncleosides (autologous cell substances) to reduce the toxic side effects of the former, revealed a therapeutic advance in a pilot study. A control study is now being carried out.

In a clinical study of bronchial as well as ovarian carcinomas, cell kinetic parameters are measured by various methods in order to detect correlations of the cell type with the clinical course of the tumors.

Research in the field of immunotherapy is concentrated on a fundamental exploration and evaluation of the diverse possibilities of applying monoclonal antibodies in solid tumors, in tumors of the blood system and in bone marrow transplantation.

Interferon therapy may be classified under immunotherapy. It has recently helped to attain noteworthy results with some forms of cancer, especially hairy cell leukemia. At the German Cancer Research Center, fundamental research is being carried out on the mode of action of interferons (see the special contribution in this volume). Besides this, treatment protocols are scientifically tested in cooperation with hospitals. The mechanisms of the anti-tumor action of interferons are complex and have not been completely clarified. On the one hand, interferons combine the mode of action of a cytostatic with an immunostimulant substance; on the other hand, there are indications that tumor cells treated with interferon become less malignant, i. e. they partially lose the capacity for invasive growth. Therapy with the tumor necrosis factor (TNF) is likewise to be classified under immunotherapy. Like the interferons, TNF is a product of the body's own resistance and has shown therapeutic activity in a series of transplantation tumors in mice. At the German Cancer Research Center, the action of TNF on metastasizing and nonmetastasizing tumors is being investigated. In particular, various forms of application and combination of TNF with other immunologically active substances (lymphokins) are being tested. At the same time, the effect of TNF in virus-infected cells is studied, in addition to fundamental research on the biological mode of action of TNF. These investigations are concerned (inter alia) with the question as to why one tumor is sensitive and another insensitive to TNF. The action of TNF probably depends on the expression of the TNF receptor on the tumor cells. For this reason, the question is to be raised as to whether the sensitivity of tumors to TNF can be increased by specific measures to raise the TNF receptor expression on tumor cells.

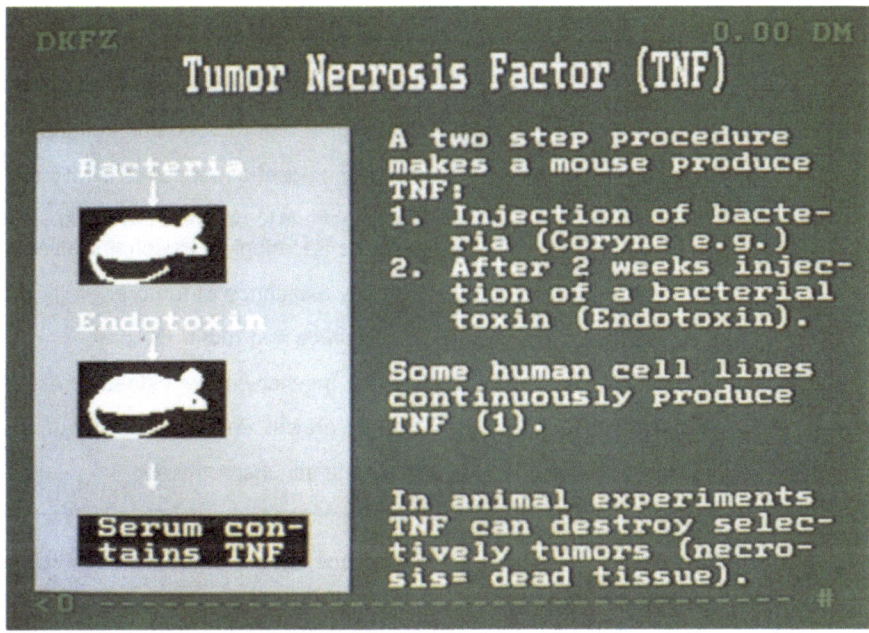

Fig. 84

## Research Activities focused on Diagnostic and Therapeutic Research

Monoclonal antibodies against tumor-associated antigens

Characterization of tumors with monoclonal antibodies: differentiation, progression, prognosis and localization in vivo

Nuclear magnetic resonance (NMR) tomography in cancer research (medical part)

Echographic diagnostics and computer echography in oncology

Computer tomography in oncological diagnostics, planning of therapy and follow-up

Nuclear medical diagnosis and therapy including positron tomography (PET) in oncology

Physics in oncological radiodiagnostics and NMR tomography

Physics in oncological nuclear medicine and positron tomography (PET)

Physics of radiotherapy

Development and application of computer-assisted techniques in oncological radiology

Development of techniques to visualize and label organic biomolecules

Development of radiopharmaceuticals for nuclear medical diagnosis and therapy

Nuclear magnetic resonance (NMR) for the investigation of tumor metabolism

Investigations to optimize the therapy of cancers in various stages in collaboration with the Radiological Hospital, University of Heidelberg

Therapy resistance of tumors

Cell kinetics and tumor therapy

Cellular mechanisms of cytostatic resistance

Cellular growth kinetics (MEDAC)

Experimental chemotherapy

Investigation of the effect of selected cytostatics on chemically induced leukemias

Chemotherapeutic characterization of new cytostatics

Development of new cytostatic nitrosourea derivatives

Improvement of the selectivity of antineoplastic chemotherapeutics

Investigation of the biochemical basis of the combination of antineoplastic chemotherapeutics with nucleosides

Improvement of the chemotherapy of carcinomas of the head and neck region

Antineoplastic effect of polyfunctional diterpenes

Biochemical basis of antineoplastic combination chemotherapy

Antiviral and antitumoral effect of xanthogenate derivatives

Interferon inducers and immunostimulants

Positron tomography for the investigation of tumor metabolism

Pathomorphological investigations on experimentally induced tumors

Pathomorphological diagnosis of experimentally induced cancer diseases

Information system of experimental oncopathology and registry of experimental tumors

Tumor cell enrichment by fluorescence-activated sorting (TEFAS)

Clinical cancer documentation (e. g., Study Group of German Tumor Centers (ADT), TNM field studies)

Development of the international cancer literature information system CANCERNET

Development of organization, documentation and electronic data processing techniques for the Tumor Center Heidelberg/Mannheim

Development and presentation of methods for producing and processing graphs and images

Statistical methods for clinical studies

Dosimetry for radiotherapy and calculation of integral dose in radiotherapy patients

Stereotactic brain tumor therapy (in collaboration with the Neurosurgical Division of the Surgical Hospital and the Radiological Hospital, University of Heidelberg)

Interferon gamma

Antiviral mechanisms of interferons

Immunoregulatory action of interferon gamma

Cellular immune defence mechanisms in metastasizing spontaneous tumors

## 5.1 Development of New Anticancer Drugs

by Gerhard Eisenbrand

Anticancer drugs are also termed cytostatics or cell poisons. They are drugs which are used for the chemical treatment of certain forms of cancer in "chemotherapy". Besides operations and radiotherapy, chemotherapy is the third major form of cancer therapy. As new activity principles have become available as a consequence of the worldwide search for substances with antitumor activity, chemotherapy has attained increasing importance.

Chemotherapy primarily affects cells in the process of division. The greatest problem of chemotherapy is that not only malignant neoplasms but also numerous healthy tissues in the body contain cells which are rapidly dividing, e. g., the skin, the intestinal mucosa, the bone marrow, the spleen. As a consequence, there are as a rule also numerous undesired side effects besides the desired effects on tumor tissue. Damage to the bone marrow is frequently so serious that it sets narrow limits to an aggressive antitumor therapy.

Besides inhibitors of cell division and cell metabolism, hormonally or antihormonally active substances, above all alkylating cytostatics, are used. Such compounds act by a chemical attack on the genetic material of the cell, the DNA (deoxyribonucleic acid). They do this in a basically similar manner to many chemical carcinogens and substances which alter the genetic material (mutagens) with the difference that most of

such cytostatically acting alkylating agents also alkylate bifunctionally, i. e. two complementary DNA strands are chemically crosslinked with each other. As a consequence of such crosslinks, the DNA strands no longer separate so that they can no longer be copied. It may be supposed that besides crosslinking, monofunctional alkylation, which also occurs, contributes less to the cytostatic action, but is on the contrary more likely to be responsible for undesired late effects, e. g., the generation of therapy-induced secondary tumors often years after primarily successful chemotherapy.

In animal models, 2-chloroethylnitrosoureas are amongst the most effective antineoplastically active compounds we know. However, clinical use of these substances which are highly active in experiments is greatly restricted owing to their massive side effects. It has, therefore, been attempted for many years to modify these compounds chemically in such a way that their high antineoplastic efficacy is maintained, but the side effects are reduced.

In our working group, we were able to produce a water-soluble analog of BCNU, a nitrosourea which is frequently employed clinically (BCNU). In contrast to other analogs with a good water-solubility, the new analog (HECNU) also shows a pronounced lipophilia, i. e. it accumulates in the lipid phase when partioned between the aqueous and lipid phase.

HECNU was tested preclinically on a very wide spectrum of experimental tumors. In the vast majority of about 30 tumor models in the mouse and 15 tumor models in the rat, it was at least

equally active or more active than reference compounds used clinically. In the therapy of tumors implanted into the brain, the substance was markedly superior to all reference substances. Since HECNU also showed good growth-inhibitory effects and sometimes also curative effects in human tumors transplanted into nude mice, it was logical to decide on a clinical trial. This applies all the more since HECNU had proved to be much less toxic and at the same time much less carcinogenic than BCNU after repeated administration in a long-term toxicity trial in the rat.

Results hitherto available from clinical studies on about 100 patients so far show that HECNU has an antitumor spectrum similar to that of other nitrosoureas in humans and appears to display a comparable antineoplastic efficacy. The efficacy in gastric carcinomas with a total response rate of 30% is to be emphasized; in colorectal carcinomas, a total response rate of 20% was observed. It is important that so far no effective chemotherapy has been available for these cancer conditions. The "response" to chemotherapy is not associated in principle with a significant prolongation of life; however, it indicates the fundamental effectiveness of the agent.

Three long-term partial remissions (i. e. reduction of tumor volume to less than 50% of the volume at start of therapy) in five patients with brain tumors treated so far are promising. A response was also observed in two out of four pancreatic carcinomas and lymphomas (non-Hodgkin) as well as in a few rarer tumor types. A comparison of the side effects of HECNU with those of other nitrosoureas reveals significantly reduced bone marrow toxicity and gastrointestinal toxicity (nausea, vomiting). A good venous tolerance and absence of alopecia due to therapy is to be emphasized.

The results show that even in a group of substances such as the nitrosoureas, which has been so intensively investigated, the ratio of antineoplastic to toxic action (i. e. the therapeutic range) can be markedly improved by relatively simple alterations in the molecular structure.

However, our structure-effect investigations on a large number of newly synthesized analogs subsequently showed that an apparently optimal value for the therapeutic range can only be exceeded to a small extent by this approach. We have, therefore, been concerned with finding suitable transport molecules for the nitrosourea group in order to attain specific transport to the tumor, sparing other sensitive tissues. Substances, which have an affinity to hormone receptors, appear to us to be especially promising. A series of human tumors contain receptors for hormones; for example, in breast cancers, receptors for estrogens, gestagens or androgenic hormones are frequently found. The content of hormone receptors in such tumors can be utilized in order to attain specific transport of cytostatically active groups to the tumor tissue by means of

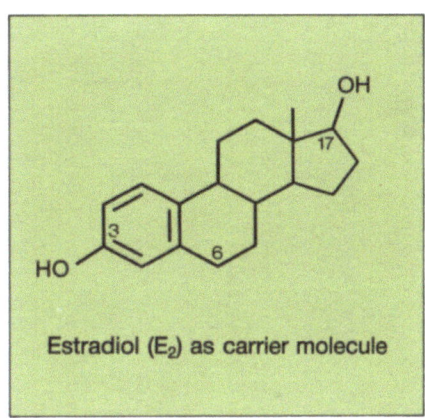

Estradiol ($E_2$) as carrier molecule

Fig. 85

carrier molecules with affinity to the receptors. The aim is to raise the concentration of the drug in the target tissue which simultaneously lowering the systemic toxicity (drug targeting). In principle, this idea is not new, but systematic structure-effect investigations on the most suitable kind of chemical bonding, the nature of carrier molecules and alkylating groups as well as the optimal linkage position are lacking.

We have commenced and intensively pursued such investigations. The results obtained so far can be illustrated by compounds in which the human sex hormone estradiol ($E_2$) takes over the function of the carrier molecule.

## Estradiol ($E_2$) as a Carrier Molecule

$E_2$ derivatives with a cytostatically active group in various positions of the carrier molecule.

To test the therapeutic concept described, experimental animal tumors are required which possess hormone receptors and correspond in their properties to human tumors. Such an experimental tumor is, for example, the chemically induced breast cancer of the rat. Testing the derivatives on this model showed that the 17-linked derivative is far superior to the other derivatives and also to the simple mixture of the hormone with the cytostatic agent, both with regard to reduced toxicity and with regard to its tumor-inhibitory action. The therapeutic superiority of the 17 derivative is also evident when compared to treatment with a clinically used antihormonal substance (tamoxifen) or to surgical removal of the ovaries (ovariectomy).

These encouraging experimental results caused us to intensify research on structure activity in this field. The work has been supported by mechanistic investigations with regard to receptor binding, receptor behavior under therapy, organ-specific DNA-DNA crosslinking and hormonal side effects. It is to be hoped that we will come closer to the objective of a tumor-specific therapy of tumors containing hormone receptors in the foreseeable future.

The research project is being supported by the Federal Ministry for Research and Technology within the project "Drug Development and Testing for Cancer Therapy".

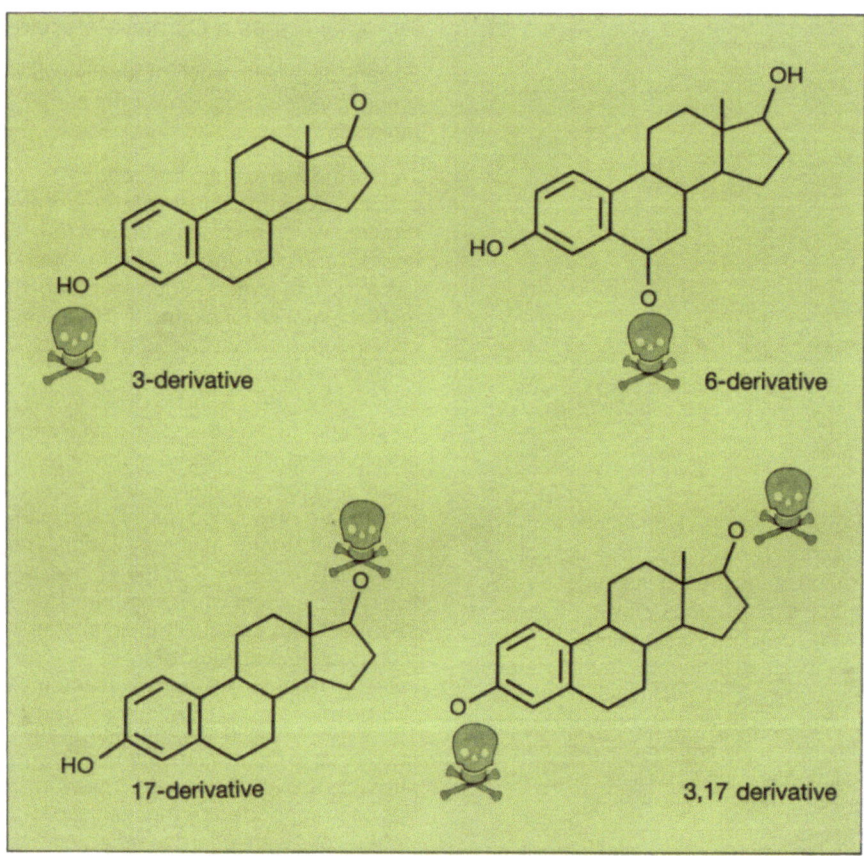

3-derivative

6-derivative

17-derivative

3,17 derivative

Fig. 86
E2 derivatives with cytostatically active group in
various positions of the carrier molecule

Prof. Gerhard Eisenbrand
Study Group Development of
Cytostatics,
Institute of Toxicology and
Chemotherapy,
German Cancer Research Center;
Food Chemistry and Environmental
Toxicology,
Faculty of Chemistry
University of Kaiserslautern

Staff collaborating

Study Group Development of
Cytostatics
Klaus Ehresmann
Karl Mühlbauer
Otto Zelezny

Food Chemistry and Environmental
Toxicology,
University of Kaiserslautern
Dr. Gabriele Heidt-Zapf
Maria Lorez
Joachim Schreiber
Wilhelm Stahl

In collaboration with

Dr. Martin Berger
Dr. Jean Floride
Dr. Thomas Henne
Department of Carcinogenesis and
Chemotherapy

Fig. 87
Chemical characterization of a freshly synthesized
cytostatic by means of nuclear magnetic resonance
spectroscopy

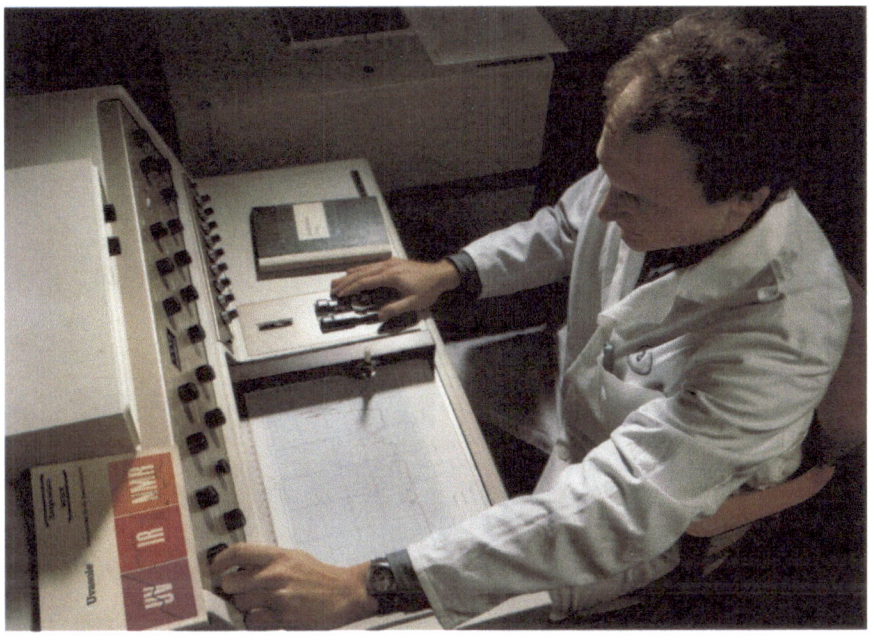

Priv.-Doz. Dr. Jens Zeller
Department of Perinatal Toxicology,
Institute of Toxicology and
Chemotherapy,
German Cancer Research Center

Priv.-Doz. Dr. Hans Heiner Fiebig and
coworkers,
University Medical School,
Albert Ludwig University of Freiburg

Members of the Screening & Pharmacology Group of the European Organization for Research on Tumor
Chemotherapy (EORTC)

Selected publications

Eisenbrand, G.: Anticancer nitrosoureas: investigations on antineoplastic, toxic and neoplastic activities. IARC Scientific Publ. No. 57, 695–708
(1984).

Eisenbrand, G.: Neue Entwicklungen auf dem Ge-
biet der Nitrosoharnstoffe. In: Beiträge zur Onkolo-
gie, Karger Verlag für Medizin und Naturwissen-
schaft, Basel, 18–35 (1984).

Zeller, W. J., Schreiber, J., Ho, A. D., Schmähl, D.,
Eisenbrand, G.: Cytostatic Activity of Steroid-Link-
ed Nitrosoureas. J. Cancer Res. clin. Oncol. 108,
164–168 (1984).

Berger, M. R., Floride, J., Schreiber, J., Schmähl,
D., Eisenbrand, G.: Evaluation of new estrogen-link-
ed 2-chloroethylnitrosoureas. J. Cancer Res. clin.
Oncol. 108, 148–153 (1984).

Bedford, P., Eisenbrand, G.: DNA-damage and repair in the bone-marrow of rats treated with four
chloroethyl nitrosoureas. Cancer Research 44,
514–518 (1984).

## 5.2 Cancer Chemotherapy – Biochemical Basis of Combination Effects

by Werner Kunz and Rüdiger Port

The development of cancer chemotherapy in the last 20 years has shown that advances are possible not only by the use of novel substances but also by a skilful combination of substances which have been known for a long time but of which each by itself has only shown unsatisfactory effects. The chemotherapeutic research activities of the department "Molecular Toxicology" of the Institute of Biochemistry aim at clarifying the biochemical basis of such favorable combination effects in the hope of thereby enabling a systematic further development of the schemes of combination therapy which have so far been drawn up on an empirical basis. The necessary experiments are being carried out together with the Department of Experimental Chemotherapy (Head: Prof. Hans Osswald) of the Institute of Toxicology and Chemotherapy. In this department, a scheme of combination therapy was developed on the basis of animal transplantation tumors which has proved to be exceedingly effective in humans in the treatment of malignant tumors of the oral cavity with a 30% cure by chemotherapy alone. However, the biochemical basis for the efficacy of this treatment is still largely unknown.

As an example for the work of the Department of Molecular Toxicology intended to enable a further systematic development of successful schemes of combination therapy, a study is described here which concerns the

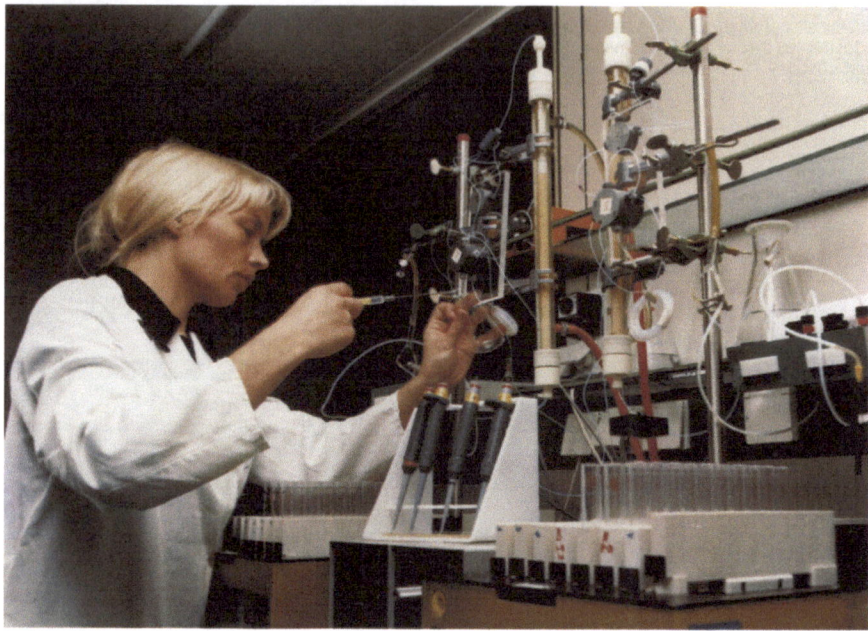

mechanism of interaction of the two anticancer drugs methotrexate and fluorouracil. These are two substances which inhibit the synthesis of nucleotides in the cell, i. e. of the building blocks for the nucleic acids bearing the genetic information. Clinically, the two substances are used in combination in the treatment of inoperable tumors of the breast, the ovaries and the gastrointestinal tract. A favorable interaction ("synergism") was observed when methotrexate was administered before fluorouracil. Experimental findings indicate that the effect is mutually attenuated when the chronological sequence of the two substances is reversed.

Fig. 88
Incorporation of radioactive fluoruracil in nucleic acid building blocks of cancer cells. Quantitative determination of the amount of the cytostatic agent incorporated

We investigated the question as to how the uptake and incorporation of fluorouracil into tumor cells is altered by pretreatment with methotrexate. The transplantable sarcoma 180 of the mouse in the ascites form was used as a tumor model. The investigations were conceived and carried out in collaboration with Professor Richard Herrmann (Medical Department, University of Heidelberg, since May 1985 Westend Clinic, Free University of Berlin), and Professor Hans Osswald.

Important results of the study are: the incorporation of fluorouracil into ribonucleic acid (a crucial step for the effect of the substance) is enhanced by pretreatment with methotrexate when the dose of methotrexate and the time interval between methotrexate and fluorouracil administration are correctly chosen. The desired effect was statistically significant only with the highest dose of methotrexate employed (150 mg/kg). In the lowest dose of methotrexate investigated (10 mg/kg), a moderate inhibition of fluorouracil incorporation was observed, i. e. the opposite of the desired effect. With regard to the time interval between methotrexate and fluorouracil administration, an interval of eight hours proved to be most favorable; with an interval, e. g., of four hours, the pretreatment was without effect.

Similar results were obtained with regard to the uptake of fluorouracil into the cell and with regard to the inhibition of thymidylate synthetase, an enzyme required for nucleic acid synthesis.

The results of the study make it understandable why the time intervals and dose conditions employed in the combination therapy of human tumors may be decisive for the result. A clinical study, in which a combination treatment with methotrexate and fluorouracil was applied in a seven-hour interval in patients with colon carcinoma, is in progress at present at the Department of Medicine, University of Heidelberg. The results obtained with methotrexate and fluorouracil in animal experiments were part of a study for which Richard Herrmann, Werner Kunz and Hans Osswald received the Farmitalia Carlo Erba Prize in 1985.

The present experimental studies on the synergism of methotrexate and fluorouracil are devoted to the question as to whether the time of day at which the substances are administered also influences their combination effect. First results indicate that this is the case.

Further studies in the department concerned a possible synergism between orotic acid (physiological nucleotide precursor) and fluorouracil. Precondition for the effect of fluorouracil is the conversion into phosphorylated metabolic products within the cell. This conversion is counteracted in various tissues by a more or less active mechanism by which, for example, in normal liver most of the fluorouracil which has entered the cell is rendered inactive. Orotic acid intensifies the protection of the normal cell against fluorouracil. Orotic acid is, on the other hand, only taken up by normal tissue. The therapeutic and toxic effect of fluorouracil decisively depends on its metabolism in the individual (malignant or normal) tissue. It would, therefore, be desirable to investigate its metabolism in the respective individual tumor before beginning treatment with fluorouracil. The development of methods for nuclear magnetic resonance spectroscopy of the metabolism of fluorouracil in the body appears at present to be the only feasible approach to obtaining information which may result in an improved application of fluorouracil without using radioactive substances and without surgical operations on the patient. Investigations on the metabolism of fluorouracil in humans with a high-resolution nuclear magnetic resonance instrument have recently been commenced in collaboration with the central study group on spectroscopy.

Prof. Werner Kunz
Dr. Rüdiger Port
Molecular Toxicology,
Institute of Biochemistry

Participating staff

Jürgen Reuter

In collaboration with

Prof. Hans Osswald
Experimental Chemotherapy,
Institute of Toxicology and
Chemotherapy

Prof. Richard Herrmann
Westend Clinic, Free University of Berlin

Margarete Ritter
Department of Medicine
University of Heidelberg

Selected publications

Herrmann, R., Kunz, W., Osswald, H., Ritter, M., Port, R.: The Effect of Methotrexate Pretreatment on 5-Fluorouracil Kinetics in Sarcoma 180 in vivo. European Journal of Cancer and Clinical Oncology 21, 753–758 (1985).

Port, R., Stein, W., Herrmann, R., Kunz, W., Osswald, H.: Modulation of 5-Fluorouracil Toxicity by Orotic Acid. Journal of Cancer Research and Clinical Oncology 109, A45 (1985).

## 5.3 Induction and Effect of Interferons and their Clinical Application

by Elke Storch and Holger Kirchner

Interferons are a group of autologous proteins which were originally discovered at the end of the 1950s on the basis of their antiviral properties. They are produced by cells in response to diverse stimuli. Their principle of action consists in their being bond to the membrane of the cells, converting them into a state of raised resistance within a few hours and thereby protecting them from viruses. Besides these antiviral properties, interferons evoke a whole series of further biological activities. They possess the capacity to inhibit cell growth both of normal and of cancer cells. They have a regulatory effect on a number of immune reactions in that they activate nonspecific defense cells such as macrophages and "natural killer cells", in that they modify antibody production by B lymphocytes and enhance the expression of certain surface antigens on the cells.

The expectations that interferons might be used therapeutically in virus infections and tumor diseases were based above all on their antiviral and growth-inhibitory properties. However, the small amounts of natural interferons isolated from human cell cultures at the beginning of the studies did not allow large-scale clinical testing. The situation has only improved since sufficient amounts of interferons could be produced by means of genetic engineering in recent years. The preparations, which are being tested all over the world today, are listed in Table 9. The only product li-

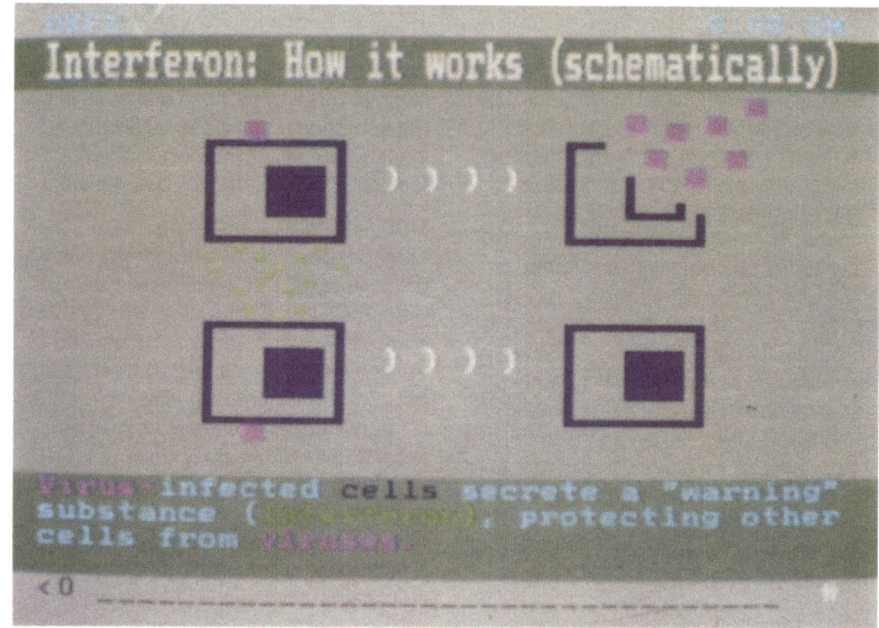

Fig. 89

cenced in the Federal Republic of Germany contains beta interferon isolated from human fibroblast cultures; however, further products are awaiting licencing.

Especially in view of this until very recently restricted availability, interferons have only been tested to a limited extent in clinical investigations. Differences in the results are based on the divergent selection, dosage and mode of application of the interferon preparations and in the often small and heterogenous patient groups. These studies clearly show that interferons lead to improvements, which can be rendered objective in some virus and tumor diseases, and

Tab. 9

| Interferon type | Production procedure |
| --- | --- |
| natural alpha | Induction of leukocyte cultures by viruses |
| natural alpha | Induction in lymphoblastoid cell cultures by viruses |
| alpha-1, alpha-2 | Genetic engineering |
| natural beta | Induction in fibroblasts by ds-RNA |
| beta | Genetic engineering |
| natural gamma | Induction in T cell lines by mitogens |
| gamma | Genetic engineering |

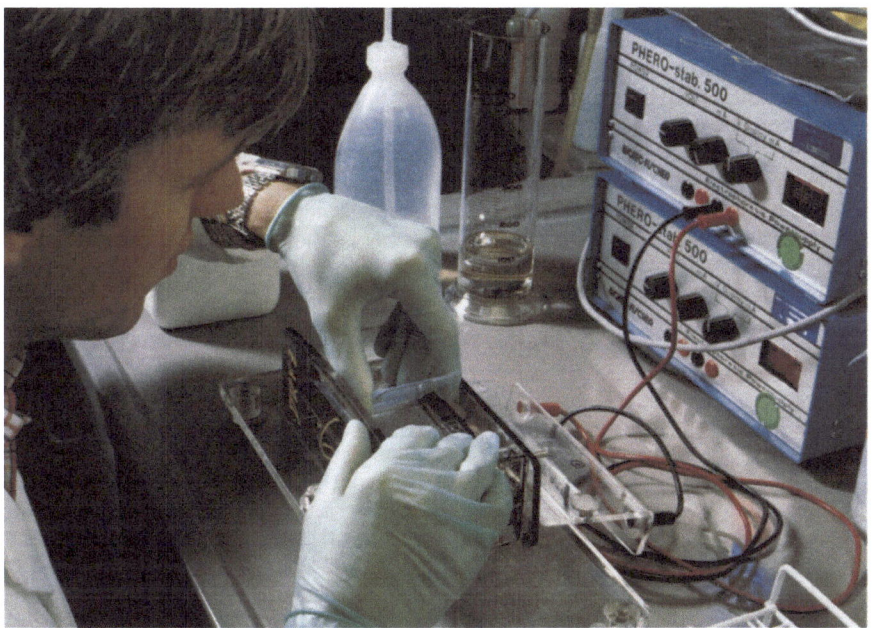

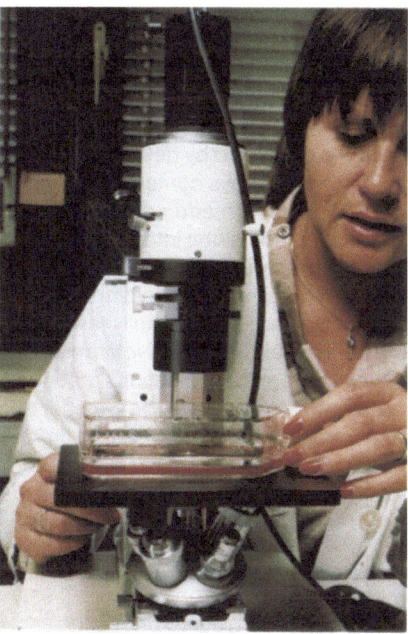

Fig. 90
Ribonucleic acid fragments from interferon-treated cells are separated in electrophoresis

Fig. 91
Here, it is tested whether cells grown in the culture flask are already dense enough to carry out investigations on interferon induction with them

that they should only be used in controlled clinical studies with quite specific indications.

Successful cures have been attained with interferons in viral diseases caused by viruses of the herpes group, as for example in herpes simplex keratitis (corneal inflammation), and in oral and genital herpes infections. High doses of interferon reduce the symptoms in shingles (caused by varicella zoster virus) and markedly accelerate healing. Very good results of interferon therapy have been reported in laryngeal papilloma. This disease is a benign laryngeal tumor caused by papilloma viruses. Its growth results in a major narrowing of the airways, necessitating frequent operations. In this tumor, interferon therapy delays the development of recurrences and thus raises the quality of life of the children affected. Interferon

treatment in encephalitis due to herpes virus is also promising. Interferon very probably does not constitute a cure-all against cold, since nasal sprays containing interferon can prevent a running nose, but the side effects of this local treatment are just as unpleasant as the disease symptoms themselves.

In cancer therapy, positive results of interferon treatment are to be recorded in some tumor forms which mostly occur rarely. On the other hand, the treatment appears to be ineffective in the numerically most important solidly growing tumors such as intestinal cancer, breast cancer and lung cancer. Multiple myeloma, chronic myeloid leukemia and Non-Hodgkin lymphomas appear to respond

to interferon therapy. Positive responses were also observed in bladder cancer, in kidney cancer and in Kaposi sarcoma. Appreciable improvements and high rates of healing were obtained above all in hairy cell leukemia. Treatment with interferon has thus proved successful in some viral and tumor diseases.

Interferons also display a series of side effects which are not to be neglected. Thus influenza-like symptoms occur, with fever, headaches, muscle pain and lassitude. Long-term therapy can lead above all to appreciable psychoneurological disorders. However, these side effects are reversible and regress after discontinuation of the drug.

Future therapeutic studies are intended to clarify an entire series of questions which are so far still open. Thus, a comparison of the individual interferon preparations has yet to be published. Interferons produced by genetic engineering methods always contain only a single subtype, e. g., interferon alpha 2, whereas natural alpha interferons are a mixture of various subtypes. There is no indication so far that these different interferons differ fundamentally in their antiviral and antiproliferative properties; however, there are indications that gamma interferon appears to be superior to other preparations with regard to its immunomodulatory properties. Detailed activity profiles of the different interferons have not yet been worked out so far.

Therapy with interferons also requires optimization with regard to dosage and mode of application. Thus, successful application of interferon with intravenous infusions in the treatment of shingles was reported at the International Interferon Congress which took place in Heidelberg in October 1984. Whether a long-term treatment with low doses is preferable to a high-dose short-term therapy in slowly progressing cancer is also under discussion.

Furthermore, it would be desirable if new knowledge on activity mechanisms would be utilized in therapy. Thus, better therapeutic results are to be expected from a combination of different interferon types, since experiments with cell cultures and animal experiments have both shown the synergistic effect of a simultaneous application of alpha or beta interferon with gamma interferon. In some cases, it has also proved to be advantageous to combine interferons with conventional drugs, e. g., cytostatics.

It is conceivable that, by means of genetic engineering, new interferon molecules may be produced which will show a therapeutic action with a reduction of side effects. At present, investigations are in progress on the conjugation of interferons with monoclonal antibodies so that interferons can be transported to specific target cells. It would also be important to know to what principles of activity the antitumoral effects of interferons are mainly attributable. It would likewise be important to know whether antiproliferative, immunomodulatory principles or effects on the differentiation of cells, such as are discussed especially in hairy-cell leukemia, are at the forefront. It is also important that interferons reduce the expression of oncogenes which are assumed to possess a regulatory role in cell growth and in the transition from the normal to the transformed state.

Since the optimization of a therapy with interferons is also likely to require a long time, the development of therapies with interferon inducers, i. e. with agents which induce the formation of interferons in the body itself, constitutes a rational alternative. Positive results of an adjuvant therapy with synthetic poly-nucleotides (polyA, polyU, polyI-polyC-lysine) have been described in tumor patients who had previously been treated surgically. The limitation of this form of therapy is based inter alia on the toxicity of these substances, and its advantage consists in that relatively high concentrations of interferons can act directly on the target cells at the site of formation.

In our study group, we are investigating low molecular weight substances (including acridine derivatives) as to their capacity to induce interferons. We are also studying mechanisms which influence this interferon response both in the body and in cell cultures. The objective of these investigations is to attain a high interferon response, keeping toxic side effects as low as possible. Thus, the interferon response to low amounts of 10-carboxymethyl-9-acridanone (CMA), for example in cell cultures, can be increased by more than 100 times by simultaneous administration of anti-inflammatory substances such as indomethacin. In the animal, the pretreatment with the immunomodulator Corynebacterium parvum has proved to be especially successful, above all locally in enhancing the interferon response to inducers. This raised interferon formation correlates with an enhanced protection of mice infected with herpes simplex virus which otherwise has a fatal course (Fig. 92). We are now testing this antivirally active double stimulation protocol (administration of Corynebacterium parvum and interferon inducers) for its effectiveness in mouse tumor models.

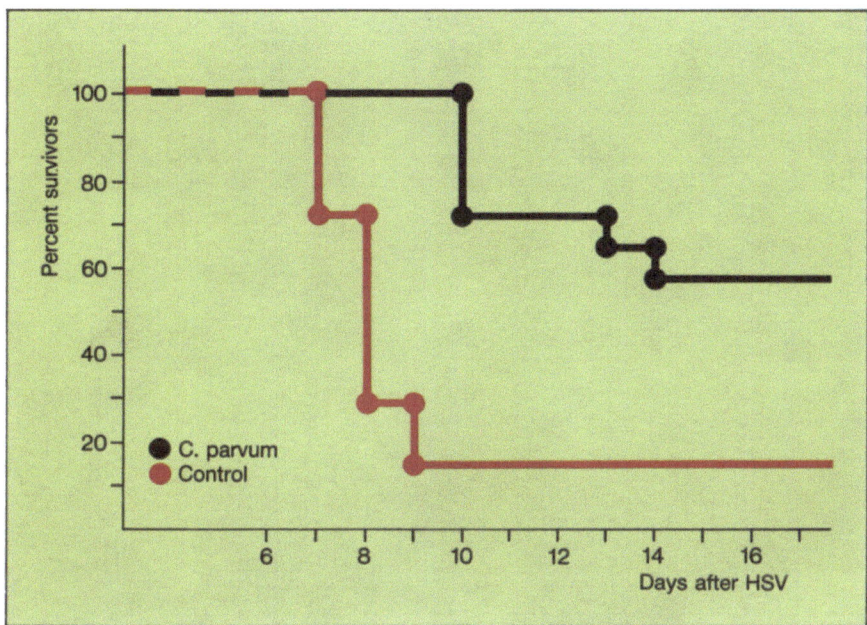

Fig. 92
The interferon inducer poly I-C does not protect mice especially well against a herpes simplex infection. However, if the animals are treated with C. parvum before treatment with poly I-C, the nonspecific defence is stimulated, and a higher percentage of the animals survives the otherwise fatal virus infection

antiproliferative effect of the interferons. This would contribute to a better understanding of the still fully unexplained phenomenon of physiological growth control of cells.

Dr. Elke Storch
Prof. Holger Kirchner
Tumor Virus Immunology,
Institute of Virus Research

Participating staff

Dr. Helmut Jakobson
Dr. Ingrid Opitz-Domke

Selected Publications

Jacobsen, H., Krause, D., Friedman, R. M., Silverman, R. H.: Induction of ppp(A2'p)$_n$ A-dependent RNase in murine JLS-V9R cells during growth inhibition. Proc. Natl. Acad. Sci. USA 80, 4954–4958 (1983).

Storch, E., Baumgartl, D., Kirchner, H.: Protection by polyI : polyC against infection with herpes simplex virus in mice pretreated with Corynebacterium parvum. Nat. Immun. Cell Growth Regul. 3, 134–142 (1984).

Brücher, J., Domke, I., Schröder, C. H., Kirchner, H.: Experimental infection of inbred mice with HSV, VI. Effect of IFN on in vitro virus replication in macrophages. Arch. Virol 82, 83–93 (1984).

Kirchner, H., Giebler, D., Keyssner, K., Nicklas, W.: Lymphoproliferation induced in mouse spleen cells by mycoplasma arthritidis mitogen. Scand. J. Immunol. 20, 133–139 (1984).

The molecular mechanism of the antiviral effect of interferons depends on the virus investigated and has so far been clarified only for a few viruses. It is unknown how interferon inhibits the proliferation of herpes simplex virus. In our department, this is investigated in macrophages. This model is especially interesting, as unspecific defense cells (macrophages) in the body can destroy viruses. In addition, the inhibition of herpes simplex virus replication in these cells due to interferon is very pronounced. In this way, it becomes possible to investigate molecular parameters in the viral replication cycle. Since application of interferons against herpes infections has also proved its effectiveness clinically, it is important to clarify the mechanism of the antiviral effect.

One of the focuses of research interest in our department is the characterization of the enzyme systems responsible for the effects of interferon. On the one hand, we are attempting to analyse more closely the role of already known enzyme activities (e. g., 2'–5'-oligoadenylate system) associated with the interferon response and in particular to elucidate their involvement in normal processes of the cells such as growth and differentiation. On the other hand, we are concerned with defining further molecular systems which have been unknown so far but the existence of which is to be postulated in view of the broad activity of the interferons (antiviral, antiproliferative, and immunomodulatory). In order to achieve this objective, we used the technique of gene cloning. It would be of particular interest to elucidate the mechanisms involved in the

## 5.4 Monoclonal Antibodies – New Approaches in Cancer Research

by Günter Hämmerling

Almost nine years have now passed since Köhler and Milstein described the production of monoclonal antibodies. Since then, a great deal of publicity and euphoria have been devoted to the topic of monoclonal antibodies in the press, with headlines such as "Breakthrough in cancer research", "Magic bullet against cancer", etc. Articles began as follows: "Imagine a new method of cancer treatment which is based on the principle of guided weapons. A small submicroscopic missile with an automatic search head is injected into the body, where it specifically searches out the cancer cells and destroys them, whereas normal healthy tissue is not affected. Such a powerful anti-cancer weapon does not yet exist, but everything indicates that it will be available in the near future". This is a quotation from the Wallstreet Journal of 1981, a newspaper which is otherwise very sober and cautious. It is undisputed that today monoclonal antibodies have gained entry into innumerable fields of biology and medicine which are no longer conceivable without them. This applies both to research and to industry. However, what has remained of optimistic formulations such as "magic bullet" and "breakthrough in cancer research"? Before presenting a survey of the current situation, I should like to recapitulate briefly what monoclonal antibodies are and what they are able to do.

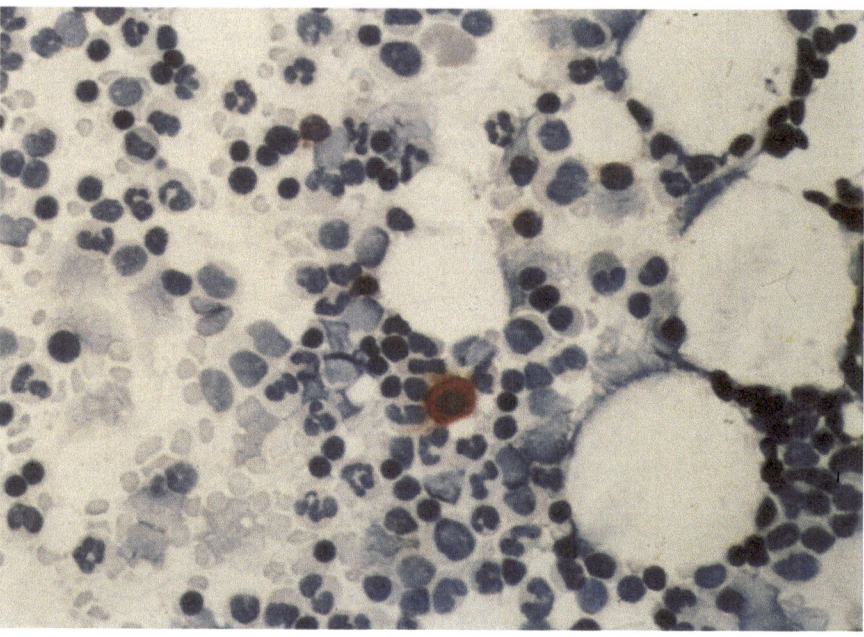

Antibodies are the natural weapons of defence of the body against disease organisms such as viruses and bacteria. Humans and animals are able to produce about ten million different antibodies. These fit like a key in a lock to recognize structures on foreign substances called antigens, e. g., micro organisms or vaccines. Since a foreign substance usually possesses many different recognition structures for antibodies, in general a confusing mixture of antibodies is obtained by the vaccination of an animal. Such a mixture of antibodies is sufficient for many medical and biological purposes. However, for very many other applications antibodies are required which are directed only against this single specific recognition structure. This problem was solved in an elegant way by Köhler and Milstein in Cambridge. Antibodies are produced by white blood cells which are very short-

Fig. 93
Detection of a single tumor cell in the bone marrow. Smear of a patient with a malignant lymphoma (cancer of the lymph glands). The tumor cell was stained red with a monoclonal antibody and with an enzyme reaction. The infiltration of the bone marrow shows a generalized stage of disease

lived. The trick of Köhler and Milstein was to immortalize the blood cell which produces a desired antibody by hybridizing it with a tumor cell in the test tube. These mixed cells (hybrids) received the desired properties from each of the two partners: from the tumor cell they received the capacity for unlimited proliferation, and from the blood cell the capacity for production of the desired antibody. All progeny of this mixed cell are identical (i. e. they are a clone) and always produce the same antibody which is therefore called "monoclonal antibody". They can grow forever, in suitable nutrient media, where they produce large amounts of the antibody. In conclusion, monoclonal antibodies are highly specific reagents suitable for the identification and measurement of almost any molecule occurring in nature or synthesized by chemists.

One of the major problems in the diagnosis of cancer is to distinguish normal tumor tissue as well as the precise classification of the tumor. So far, the various kinds of cancer have been classified by the somewhat different shape of the cancer cells under the microscope. However, such a diagnosis was often inconclusive or not possible at all. Monoclonal antibodies against certain structures in the tumor cells are now already being used as quasi-irreplaceable aids. To mention some examples from our own studies: under the collective term "leukemia and lymphomas", various kinds of cancer of white blood cells are subsumed. Some of them are exceedingly malignant and must be treated very aggressively, resulting in corresponding by serious side effects for the patients, whereas others can be given relatively mild treatment. It is frequently

not possible to distinguish these cancer types on the basis of their shape alone. Together with Dr. Bernd Dörken and Prof. Werner Hunstein from the Heidelberg Policlinic, we are working with Dr. Gerhard Moldenhauer in the German Cancer Research Center on a series of monoclonal antibodies with which the different classes of leukemias and lymphomas can be identified relatively simply. For example, we have developed monoclonal antibodies with which the malignant form of acute lymphoblastic leukemia can be distinguished from the less malignant form, which was not possible so far on the basis of purely morphological criteria. Although these antibodies are so far purely research reagents, they are already frequently used in Heidelberg for routine diagnosis, and therapy is carried out in accordance with the result. The antibodies also allow

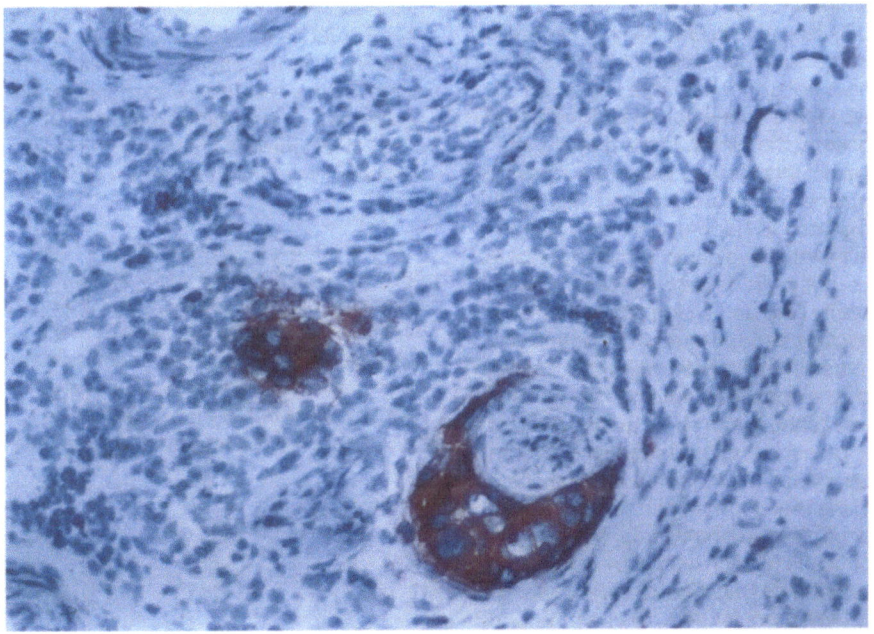

Fig. 94
Tumor cells stained with monoclonal antibodies have settled along a nerve tract

the extent of the cancer disease to be determined. If, for example, lymphoma cells are found in the bone marrow, then the disease is already generalized, and it must be therapied aggressively. In Fig. 93, we see that a single tumor cell among many thousand normal bone marrow cells can be rendered visible with a monoclonal antibody labelled with a red dye. This one cell could never be discovered without labelling the antibody. Such antibodies can likewise be used to check whether a therapy has been successful, i. e. whether the tumor cells have disappeared from the bone marrow.

Another example is the retrospective investigation of a surgically removed colon tumor with monoclonal antibodies developed by Dr. Frank Momburg and Dr. Gerhard Moldenhauer in the German Cancer Research Center. These investigations are carried out in a combined project with Prof. Peter Schlag from the Surgical Hospital and Dr. Peter Müller from the Institute of Pathology, University of Heidelberg. It is seen in Fig. 94 that very few of the tumor cells stained red here with antibodies have already settled on a nerve cord. Experience shows that this is a prognostically unfavorable sign so that these patients must receive more intensive chemotherapy. Without the stained antibodies, one would not have been able to discover these small metastases on the nerve cord.

A further example is a patient displaying swollen lymph nodes. An investigation of the lymph node with monoclonal antibodies carried out by Prof. Werner Franke in the German Cancer Research Center revealed that some epithelial cells were found in the lymph nodes. These derive from other organs of the body, since such cells do not normally

occur in lymph nodes; the diagnosis was as follows: the cells in the lymph nodes are tiny metastases of a carcinoma, i. e. the patient must have a tumor. This diagnosis was indeed confirmed by the discovery of a gastric cancer. Without the monoclonal antibodies, the tiny metastases in the lymph node would never have been detected.

These few examples are intended to illustrate the enormous diagnostic potential of monoclonal antibodies. The strength of the antibodies consists especially in the visualization of a small number of tumor cells and in the classification of tumors.

What is the situation with regard to monoclonal antibodies in therapy? Just as antibodies can destroy bacteria, they also have the capacity to destroy tumor tissue. Some patients have already been treated successfully with monoclonal antibodies against tumor cells, in the USA and also in Germany. The problem with this kind of treatment is that we have so far been unable to predict whether the injection of antibodies will destroy the tumor. In the majority of cases, this therapy was not successful, but the successes attained may be designated as hopeful. In my view, however, intensive basic immunological research must be carried out in order to clarify how and which antibodies can destroy tumor tissues. The notion of tumor-specific antibodies charged with cell poisons themselves finding their way to the tumor like a guided weapon and destroying it, as mentioned at the beginning in the quotations from the Wallstreet Journal, has so far not yet been put into practice. By the way, the principle of such a therapy was developed by Paul Ehrlich, who already spoke of poisoned arrows at the begin-

ning of the century, meaning antibodies charged with cell poisons. There have been some hopeful approaches in animal studies, but a great deal of research and development work must still be invested here before this procedure can be applied in humans.

The therapeutic application of monoclonal antibodies appears to be more hopeful in autologous bone marrow transplantation. Tumor tissue can be destroyed by irradiation and chemotherapy. However, normal tissue is also impaired. The cells of the hematopoietic system in the bone marrow, which are vital to life, are especially sensitive to irradiation and chemotherapy. In autologous bone marrow transplantation, bone marrow is removed from the patient before irradiation and reinjected again after radiotherapy so that the hematopoietic system can regenerate. However, since tumor cells are also present in the bone marrow, these must be removed before the latter is returned to the patient. This can be achieved in a test tube with monoclonal antibodies, a procedure which has already been carried out successfully several times in various countries of the world.

To summarize, the following appraisal can be made as to the value of monoclonal antibodies in cancer research: They are exceedingly useful and will soon be indispensable in cancer diagnosis. However, a great deal of research and development work will be necessary before reliable therapeutic application.

As a scientist engaged in cancer research, one is constrained to applying the information obtained from basic research. However, to achieve this appropriate financing and cooperation with clinicians is necessary. This cooperation is greatly promoted in Heidelberg by the facilities of the Heidelberg/Mannheim Tumor Center. Clinicians and basic researchers are brought together in the Tumor Center. Here I should like to mention expressly that the fruitful and gratifying cooperation with colleagues from the hospitals described by a few examples is financed almost exclusively by donation funds of the German Cancer Research Center by the German Research Association (DFG) and, above all, by project funds made available via the Tumor Center, i. e. from the Federal Ministry of Research and Technology and from the Ministry of Science and Arts of the Land Baden-Württemberg.

In the context of monoclonal antibodies, I have emphasized the application-oriented aspects of cancer research. However, cancer research cannot and shall not be exclusively application-oriented. In my opinion, cancer research, which is restricted to the investigation of cancer cells, will fail. In order to be able to cure cancer, one must understand the function of normal cells and of the healthy body. The dilemma in promoting research is to establish where cancer research begins and where it ends. Many of the major breakthroughs, which are important for our understanding of the neoplastic cell, do not originate directly from cancer research, but from general basic research. When Köhler and Milstein first developed monoclonal antibodies in 1975, they were not thinking of cancer diagnosis or therapy. On the contrary, they were pursuing the very theoretical and abstract question as to how the immune system can produce ten million different antibodies. As a byproduct, they developed a novel, revolutionary technology which is of central importance in cancer research even now.

Prof. Günter Hämmerling
Somatic Genetics,
Institute of Immunology and Genetics

Selected publications

Moldenhauer, G., Dörken, B., Pezzutto, A., Schwartz, R., Knops, J., Hämmerling, G. J.: Monitoring of a human B cell lymphoma with monoclonal anti-idiotype antibodies. In: Protides of the Biological Fluids. Ed. H. Peeters, Vol. 32, Pergamon Press, 863–866 (1985).

Dörken, B., Schwartz, R., Moldenhauer, G., Pezzutto, A., Hämmerling, G. J., Hunstein, W.: Monoclonal Antibody (HD 39) reactive with a human B lymphocyte-specific antigen expressed on late stages of B cell maturation. In: Protides of the Biological Fluids. Ed. H. Peeter, Vol. 32, Pergamon Press, 867–870 (1985).

Moldenhauer, G., Dörken, B., Schwartz, R. Pezzutto, A., Hämmerling, G. J.: Characterization of a human B lymphocyte-specific antigen defined by monoclonal antibodies HD 6 and HD 39. In: Leukocyte Typing II, Vol. 2, Eds. Reinherz, Haynes, Nadler, Bernstein; Springer-Verlag (1985).

Momburg, F., Moldenhauer, G., Möller, P., Hämmerling, G. J.: A new epithelium-specific antigen defined by monoclonal antibody 1 HT 125. Cancer Res. Clin. Oncol. 109: A 35 (1985).

## 5.5 Diagnosis and Therapy of Melanomas – Application of Antibodies

by Siegfried Matzku and Wolfgang Tilgen

The technique of hybridization developed by Köhler and Milstein in 1975 has enabled the production of highly specific monoclonal antibodies. By the classical method of immunization of animals (by injection of a substance foreign to the animal, an antigen), an antiserum containing antibodies can be obtained. In the new technique, interest was concentrated initially on the antibody-producing cells or their precursors. Lymphocytes from the spleen of immunized animals are hybridized with tumor cells of a corresponding type (myeloma cells) in the test tube. The hybrid cells formed received important genetic characteristics from both "parents": from the myeloma cell they received the ability to grow permanently and to proliferate in culture, and from normal lymphocytes they received the capacity to produce an antibody of definite specificity. It is possible to clone such specific antibody-producing hybrid cells (i. e. to grow them in pure culture) so that the corresponding cell culture continuously produces a quite definite, highly specific antibody. The hybrid cells can be stored for as long as required in liquid nitrogen; they can be reactivated as needed. In contrast to such monoclonal antibodies, which only react with quite definite antigen determinants, antisera are always mixtures of antibodies. It is hence possible to better define subtle differences in structure by means of monoclonal antibodies.

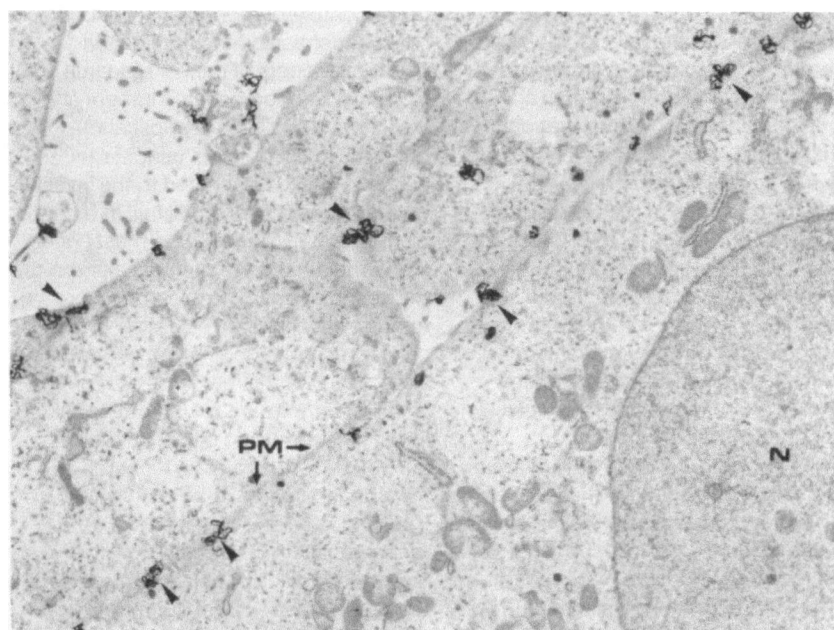

Fig. 95 a, b, c
Autoradiography of ultrathin sections of melanoma cells. Thirty minutes after addition of labeled antibody M 2.9.4, decay tracks are found at the cell membrane only. After two hours the antibody has entered the cell. Now decay tracks are found in the interior, in close association with vesicular structures

We want to devote ourselves to the possibilities and problems involved in the diagnostics and therapy of solid tumors. A skin cancer, malignant melanoma, is representative for this group of tumors, since two particular conditions for comprehensive experimental studies are fulfilled in this tumor type:
1. Availability of melanoma cells in culture and as transplant in the athymic nude mouse;
2. Knowledge of the maturation sequence of melanocytes as the "normal" equivalent of melanoma cells.

We will first describe the general problems in using monoclonal antibodies in solid tumors. We will then discuss our concrete approaches in the melanoma system. The problems are outlined by the following questions:

- What does the monoclonal antibody actually recognize (problem of specificity)?
- How is a sufficiently large amount of antibody introduced into solid tumor tissue?
- What functional principle is therapeutically successful?

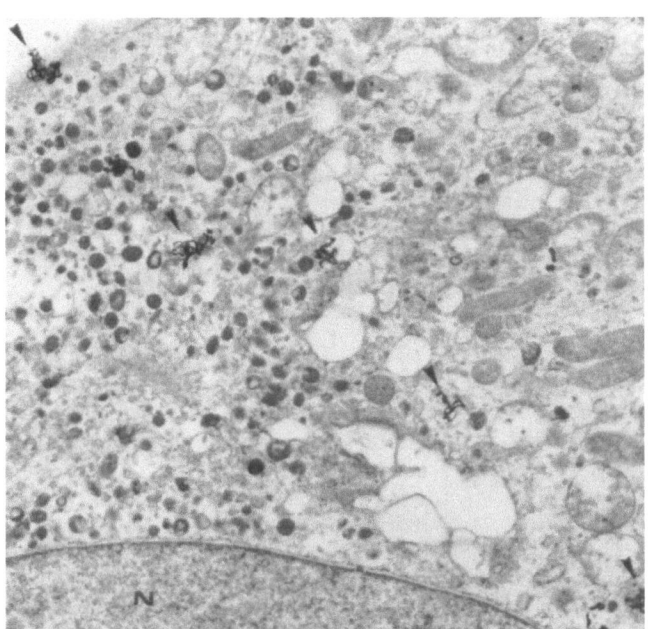 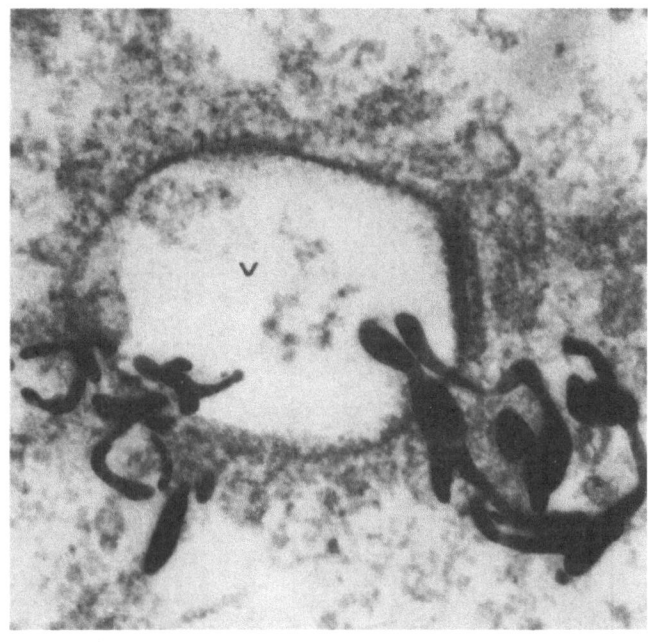

## What does the Monoclonal Antibody Actually Recognize?

Today agreement exists to a large extent that "tumor-specific" structures can be discovered neither with conventional antisera nor with monoclonal antibodies. The various study groups have, on the contrary, suggested autologous substances as a feature for the classification of tumor cells (i. e. tumor "markers"). However, these substances occur in an irregular arrangement, in unusual amounts, at unusual sites or at an unusual time in the development of the individual. Each of the tumor markers described can thus be found in a different place or at a different time in the healthy body. However, antibodies against such markers can nevertheless be used for diagnosis and therapy if the corresponding antigen (= marker) occurs in a relatively large amount on tumor cells or if antigen-positive normal tissue is shielded by a barrier which cannot be penetrated. An impressive example of such a barrier is present in the brain: due to the blood-brain barrier, structures within the tissue of the brain which bear a certain antigen are practically inaccessible for the antibodies against this antigen circulating in the body.

These problems are less serious in the diagnostic application of monoclonal antibodies in cell culture (in vitro). Furthermore, decisive advances in the understanding of the heterogeneity, the diversity of tumors could already be achieved with the methods of immunohistology. We know today that the appearance of a specific kind of tumor cell can vary from individual to individual and, within one patient, from the primary tumor to the metastasis, and indeed within a single tumor nodule. If it is known which of the different known antigens is present in sufficient amounts in an individual tumor, it can be predicted what monoclonal antibody gives rise to the expectation of maximum accumulation in the tumor tissue and thus high contrast in the scintigraphic representation.

A further important criterion is the stability of antigen expression. The antibody should be directed against an antigen which is not shedded and then appears in a soluble form in the circulation. Furthermore, the antigen should not be altered after binding by the antibody, i. e. it should not disappear from the cell surface.

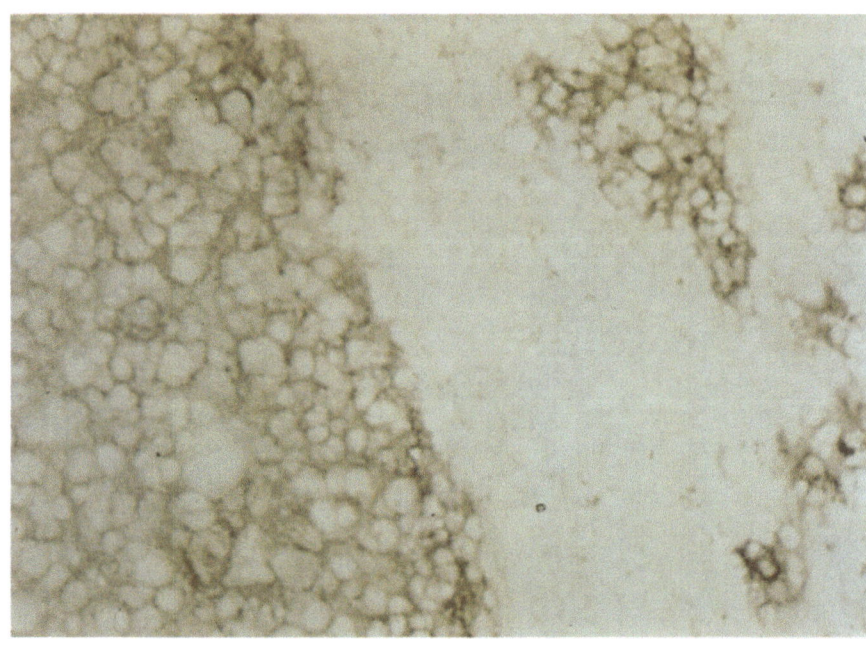

Fig. 96
Histological section through a metastasis of a malignant melanoma. Normal liver tissue (right side) is not stained, while melanoma tissue binds antibody R24 and is stained by a peroxidase-mediated reaction

From these criteria, we obtained the following answer to the question as to what the antibody actually recognizes: It should be effective against an antigen that is present in large amounts on (if possible) all tumor cells which have a free connection with the vascular system, but not on normal cells; the antigen should be stably anchored in the cell membrane.

## How can a Sufficiently Large Amount of Antibody be Introduced into Solid Tumor Tissue?

Molecules of the size of immunoglobulins (i. e. more than 150,000 Daltons) can leave the intravascular space only very slowly or not at all, since the blood vessels are lined with endothelial cells and the basal membrane which do not allow passage of molecules of this size (permeability barrier). Transport processes take place through pores (sieve effect). In the tumor vessels, the lining is mostly fragmentary or entirely lacking. The barrier is interrupted and the tumor tissue is preferentially accessible. Nevertheless, the diffusion or channeling through of large molecules up to the tumor cells situated farther away from the vessels is a slow process.

Efforts to raise antibody transport into solid tissue are concentrated on two points: on the one hand, it is observed that tumor vessels and normal vessels react differently to regulatory signals (e. g., for dilatation or constriction) so that a specifically increased blood flow in the tumor can be attained by pharmacological intervention, and the permeability of the barrier is raised. The practical value of this approach has still to be proved, however. On the other hand, it is attempted to facilitate the transport within the tissue, e. g., by reducing the size of the antibody molecules. Indeed, it was observed that enzymatically fragmented antibodies which still contain the antigen binding site (Fab and F(ab')₂ fragments), show a very much greater accumulation in tumor tissue.

A further consequence of enzymatic size reduction is the more rapid elimination of these antibody fragments from the intravascular space. What is not bound disappears rapidly from the blood. From this there results high contrast, a useful element in radioimmuno localization, but not a large absolute amount of antibody in the tumor under all circumstances.

Fig. 97
Immunoscintigram of a nude mouse with a melanoma transplant three days after injection of radioiodinated antibody M 2.7.6. The radioactive antibody is accumulated in the tumor node (left side). The head of the mouse is on top of the scintigram

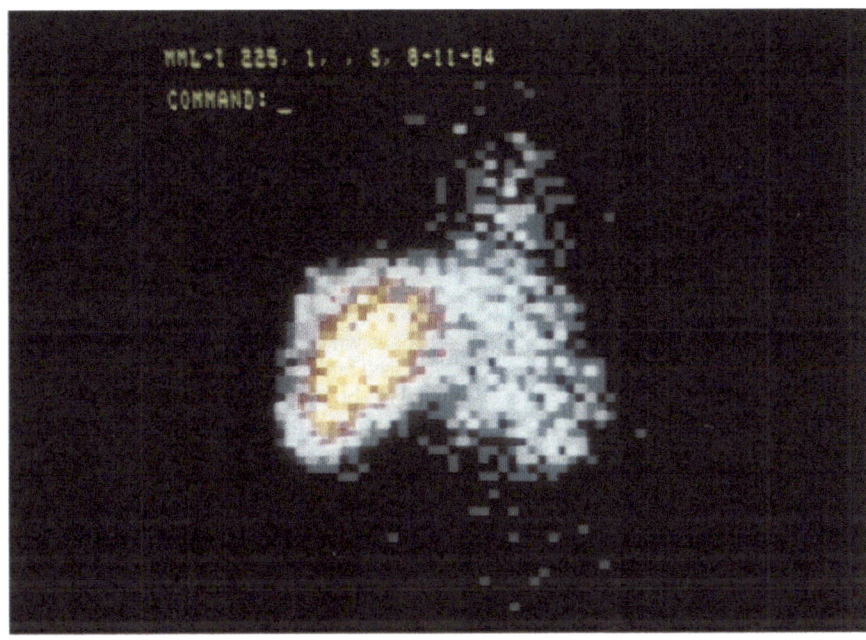

## What Functional Principle is Therapeutically Successful?

If a suitable antibody has been found and one knows how to attain a high concentration in the solid tumor tissue, the question arises as to the adequate functional principle for therapy. Antibodies can destroy tumor cells directly in interaction with other components of autologous resistance (e. g., with complement or killer cells bearing Fc receptors). This direct antibody effect has the advantage that material not directly bound to the tumor (i. e. the major part of the injected dose) does not create dramatic damage in the healthy body. It is known that the various mechanisms of direct antibody action depend on the subclass (isotype) of the antibody. However, it has not yet been clarified unequivocally which of the mechanisms described in vitro is also active in vivo (i. e.

in the patient). Furthermore, it is unclear what consequences arise due to the occurrence of autologous antibodies against the monoclonal antibodies used: so far, experiments with both positive and negative effects have been reported on.

In the indirect antibody action, the antibody is used as a vehicle which is intended to transport a nonspecific toxic principle to the site of action. A distinction must be made between toxic agents, which only have to reach the vicinity of the tumor cell in order to manifest their activity (e. g. radionuclides), toxic agents which have to reach the cell membrane (certain enzymes) and toxic agents which must reach a certain site of action in the interior of the cell (e. g., toxins of the ricin type). In the latter case, the antibody-conjugated toxin is exposed to the very destructive medium

of lysosomal vesicles during the process of transport into the cell. This makes the therapeutic action doubtful, although in principle only a few toxin molecules in the cell are sufficient for its destruction. Experimental tumor research is, therefore, investigating means of "packaging" the toxic principle in such a way that it can survive the process of transport into the cell without damage. At all events, antibody-conjugated active substance combinations which are not bound to tumor cells are degraded elsewhere in the body and are thus a burden to the cancer patient. For the practical evaluation of therapeutic effectiveness, only in vivo models are suitable, since the problem of accumulation in solid tissue and degradation of non-bound antibodies cannot be simulated in cell cultures.

## Experimental and Clinical Approaches in Malignant Melanoma

The production of monoclonal antibodies specific for melanoma cells has led to the discovery of various identical markers in the last five years, i. e. certain surface structures are "immunodominant". In our estimation, from the large number of known "published" antibodies, four are of major significance, since practical (clinical) results have already been attained using these antibodies.

It is only consistent with this that these antibodies are also the focus of our interest and the subject of various cooperative projects. The antibody 225.285 (Dr. Soldano Ferrone, New York) is effective against the "high molecular weight melanoma antigen" and can be used for the immunoscintigraphic localization of melanoma metastases. The antibody R 24 (Dr. Wolfgang G. Dippold, University of Mainz) can be used for immunotherapeutic purposes, above all because it exerts an antitumoral action even without conjugation with toxic molecules. The antibody 96.5 (Dr. Karl Erik and Dr. Ingegert Hellström, University of Seattle) as well as L 10 and O 12 (Dr. Wolfgang G. Dippold, University of Mainz) are effective against different areas of the "p 97" molecule on melanoma cells. With regard to 96.5, experience already exists both of diagnostic and therapeutic applicability. There are strong indications in this direction for the other two antibodies.

However, these antibodies do not yet completely meet the demands described. The search for new preparations with a better spectrum of properties hence continues to occupy a large part of our research activities. Furthermore, the question of antigen modulation in the sense of the disappearance of the antigen from the cell surface after antibody binding or transport of antigen-antibody complexes into the interior of the cells is gaining increasing significance.

In order to reduce animal experiments as much as possible, we have developed test techniques for both purposes which allow a far-reaching appraisal of the applicability of an antibody in vivo on the basis of data obtained with cell cultures. It has been shown that the most important parameters in this connection are the amount of antigen on different melanoma types, the binding strength of the antibody conjugated, for example, with radionuclide and the dynamics of antibody binding and detachment in various metabolic situations of the tumor cell.

A further focal point is the exploration of the therapeutic principles effective in vivo as well as the appropriate administration protocols. Here, animal experiments with melanoma transplants in nude mice are indispensable, since for fundamental reasons certain physiological and pharmacodynamic correlations are not evident in cell culture systems. However, even melanoma transplants in the nude mouse do not yet allow any definitive appraisal. In this model, for example, the effects of small amounts of antigen in normal tissues on the accumulation of antibody in tumor tissue cannot be investigated, since the mouse does not have such antigens.

The influence of this factor can consequently only be investigated in tumor patients. However, an important restriction is to be considered even here: for ethical reasons, clinical studies with novel drugs must only include patients with far advanced tumor conditions. The result of therapy is often measured in terms of alterations in volume of large tumor nodules. However, the question may be posed as to whether antibodies are the agent of choice for the reduction of large tumor masses as such or as vehicles for toxic substances. It is, on the contrary, logical to design a systemic therapy of disseminated tumor cells with antibodies after surgical removal of the tumor mass or reduction of its size. Such applications cannot be checked in clinical studies. Here, once again animal experiments are necessary to investigate this problem.

This project is being supported and carried out in the context of the special research field 136 "Cancer Research" (Sonderforschungsbereich 136).

Dr. habil. Siegfried Matzku
Radiochemistry, Radiopharmacology,
Institute of Nuclear Medicine

Dr. Wolfgang Tilgen, leading physician,
Dermatological Hospital, University of
Heidelberg


In collaboration with

Eva Bettina Bröcker
Josef Brüggen
Clemens Sorg
University of Münster

Dr. Wolfgang G. Dippold
I. Medical Division,
Johannes-Gutenberg-University Mainz

Dr. Soldano Ferrone
Department of Microbiology,
Walhalla, New York, USA

Dr. Karl Erik and
Dr. Ingegert Hellström
University of Seattle, USA

Selected publications

Dippold, W. G., Lloyd, K. O., Li, L. T. C., Ikeda, H., Oettgen, H. F., Old, L. J.: Cell surface antigens of human malignant melanoma: Definition of six antigenic systems with mouse monoclonal antibodies. Proc. Natl. Acad. Sci. USA 77, 6114–6118 (1980).

Garrigues, H. J., Tilgen, W., Hellström, I., Franke, W., Hellström, K. E.: Detection of a human melanoma-associated antigen, p97, in histological sections of primary human melanomas. Int. J. Cancer 29, 511–519 (1982).

Wilson, B. S., Ruberto, G., Ferrone, S.: Immunochemical characterization of a human high molecular weight-melanoma associated antigen identified with monoclonal antibodies. Cancer Immunol. Immunother. 14, 196–201 (1983).

Suter, L., Bröcker, E.-B., Brüggen, J., Ruiter, D. J., Sorg, C.: Heterogenecity of primary and metastatic human malignant melanoma as detected with monoclonal antibodies in cryostat sections of biopsies. Cancer Immunol. Immunother. 16, 53–58 (1983).

Matzku, S., Tilgen, W.: Experimentelle Grundlagen der Radioimmundiagnostik und -therapie humaner Melanome mit monoklonalen Antikörpern. Dermatol. und Nuklearmed., Hrsg. Holzmann, Altmeyer, Hör, Hahn; Springer-Verlag Berlin, Heidelberg, 137–147 (1985).

## 5.6 New Criteria for Prognosis in Lung Cancer

by Manfred Volm

Lung cancer is the most frequent cancer in men and takes fifth place all over the world in women. It is among the cancer types with an exceedingly unfavorable prognosis. Only about 10% of all patients live for more than five years after the diagnosis of their disease.

The prognosis of patients with lung cancer is largely determined by histologic diagnosis and tumor stage. The majority of lung carcinomas are classified histologically into four types: small cell lung carcinomas, epidermoid cell carcinomas, adenocarcinomas and large cell carcinomas. Histologic features, ultrastructure, clinical course and response to therapy indicate that the small cell carcinoma is a separate entitiy. The non-small cell carcinoma represents a mixed group of tumors with distinct but overlapping histologic properties, clinical course and biological behavior. Therefore, most treatment protocols combine these tumors in a single group. It should, however, be possible to further improve the treatment of non-small cell lung carcinomas if additional discriminatory factors could be better defined. Such discriminatory factors seem to be DNA abnormality and growth kinetics.

In the study carried out at our department, together with the Chest Hospital in Heidelberg-Rohrbach, 240 patients with non-small cell tumors of the lung were investigated with various biochemical and physical methods in the hope of finding new criteria for a prognosis of the disease.

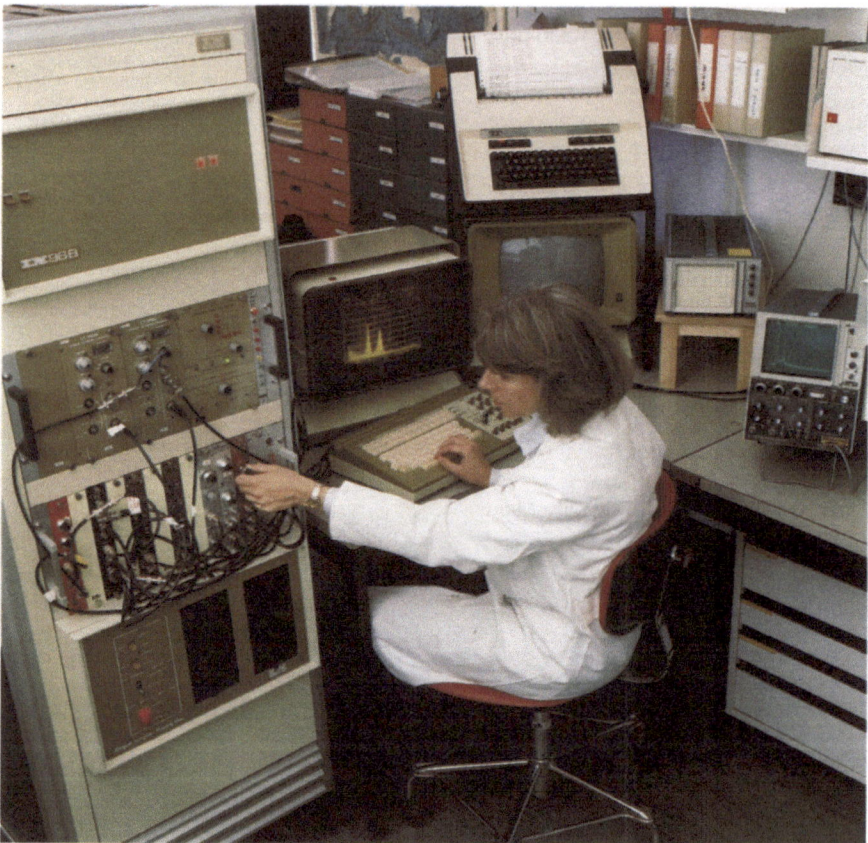

Fig. 98
Measurement of the genetic substance and the growth behavior in human lung tumors to determine the prognosis of the disease

For example, the amount of nucleic acids (DNA) in the cell nuclei was determined by means of flow cytophotometry and specific staining with fluorescent dyes (Fig. 99). The technique allows investigation of several hundred cells per second and provides information on 20,000–50,000 cell nuclei of the investigated tumor. The amount of DNA constitutes a measure for the evaluation of the normality of the cells. Normal cells possess a double (diploid) chromosome set; tumors frequently show deviations.

Our study has shown that the DNA content of lung tumors is prognostically significant for the survival time of the patients. Patients with diploid tumors live longer than patients with abnormal (aneuploid) tumors (Fig. 100).

By means of flow cytophotometry, it can likewise be established whether and to what extent the cells of a tumor proliferate. This can be determined by means of cell cycle analysis. It provides information on how many of the investigated cells are in the different phases of the cell cycle at a certain time on the basis of their DNA amount. Each tumor has a certain proportion of resting and growing cells. Growing cells double their DNA amount in the synthesis phase (S phase), pass through an intermediate stage ($G_2$ phase) and divide in mitosis (M phase).

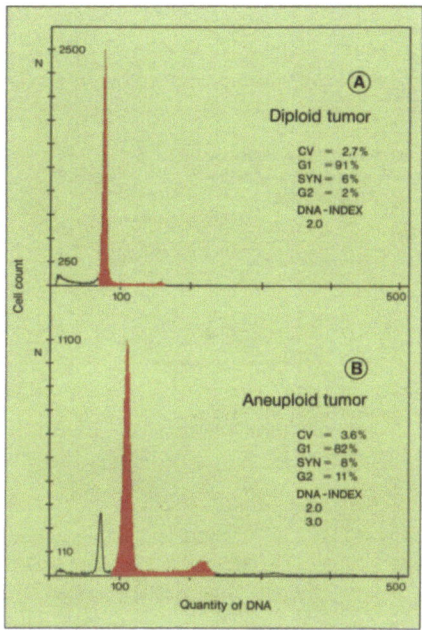

Fig. 99
Frequency of cells with different amounts of DNA

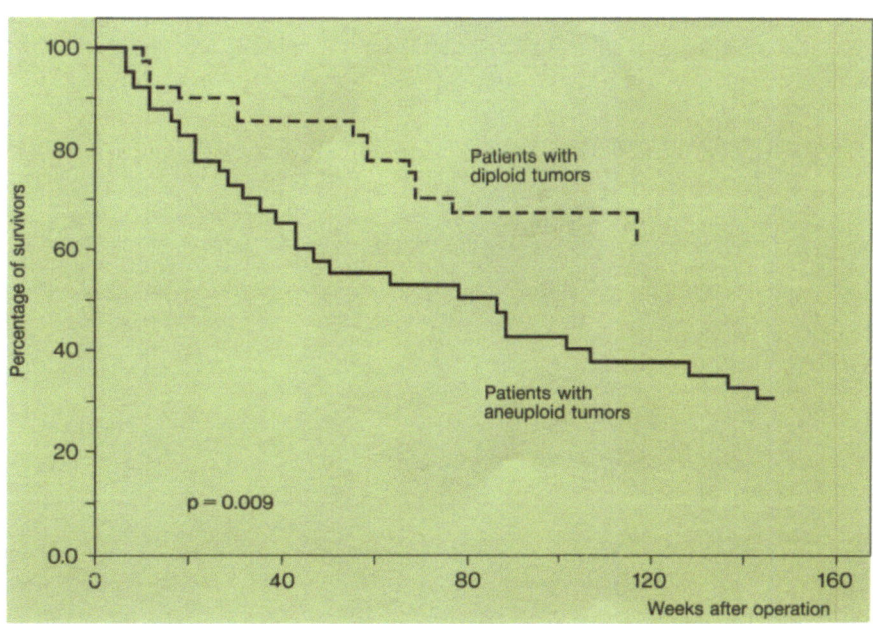

Fig. 100
Survival times of patients broken down according to the amount of DNA in their tumors

153

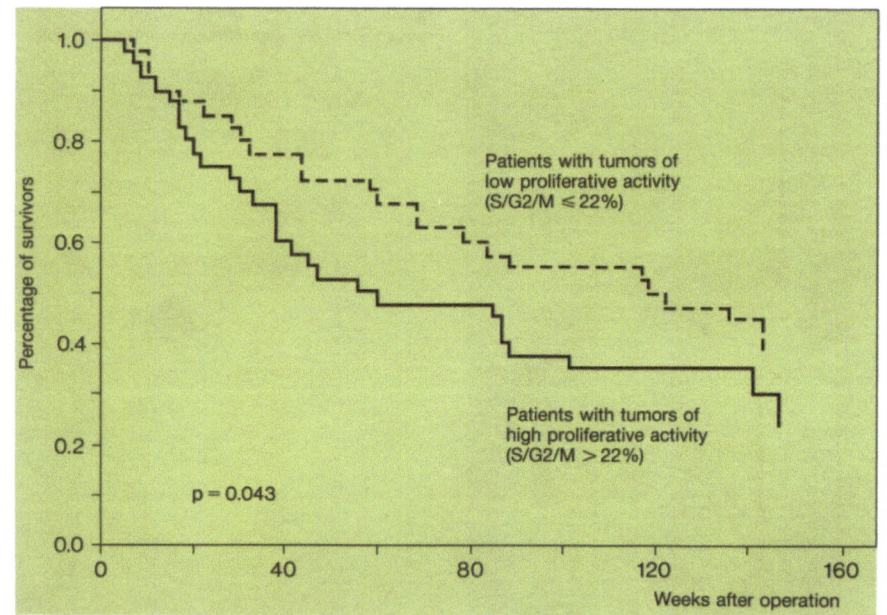

Fig. 101
Survival times of patients broken down according to the growth state of the tumors

Fig. 102

In the study, tumors with a high proportion of cells in the S and $G_2/M$ phase showed a more intense growth (high proliferative activity). The high proliferative activity also had prognostic significance for the survival time of patients with lung tumors. Patients with tumors of low proliferative activity live longer than patients with tumors of high proliferative activity (Fig. 101).

Prof. Manfred Volm
Cell Biology,
Institute of Experimental Pathology

Scientists participating

Dr. Jürgen Mattern
Dr. Jaroslav Sonka
Dr. Klaus Wayss

In collaboration with

Prof. Peter Drings
Prof. Ingolf Vogt-Moykopf
Chest Hospital
Heidelberg-Rohrbach

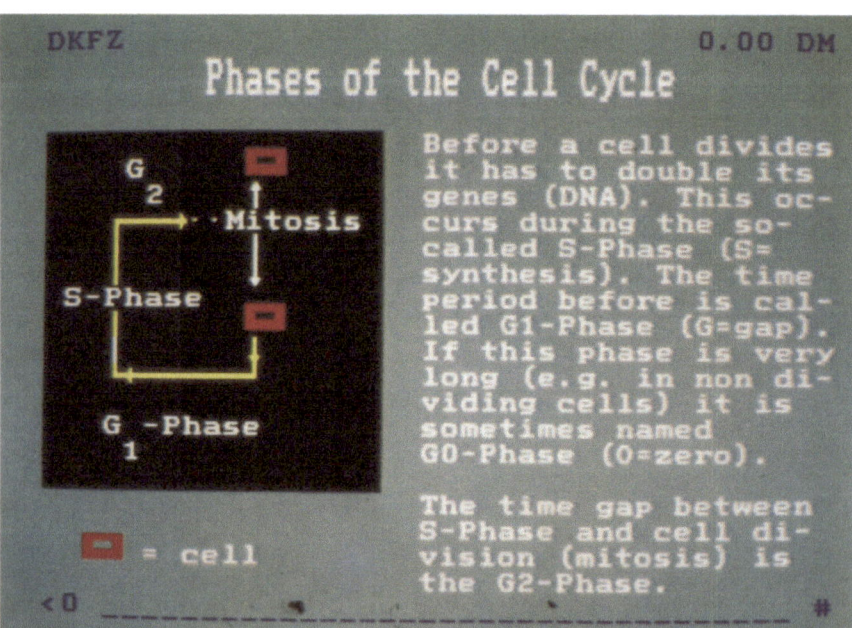

DKFZ                                    0.00 DM

## Phases of the Cell Cycle

G2

Mitosis

S-Phase

G1-Phase

= cell

Before a cell divides it has to double its genes (DNA). This occurs during the so-called S-Phase (S=synthesis). The time period before is called G1-Phase (G=gap). If this phase is very long (e.g. in non dividing cells) it is sometimes named G0-Phase (0=zero).

The time gap between S-Phase and cell division (mitosis) is the G2-Phase.

Selected publications

Volm, M., Mattern, J., Sonka, J., Wayss, K., Drings, P., Vogt-Moykopf, I.: Prognostische Bedeutung von Ploidie und proliferativer Aktivität bei nicht-kleinzelligen Bronchialkarzinomen. Tumor Diagnostik und Therapie 6, 8–13 (1985).

Volm, M., Drings, P., Mattern, J., Sonka, J., Vogt-Moykopf, I., Wayss, K.: Prognostic significance of DNA patterns and resistance-predictive tests in non-small cell lung carcinom. Cancer 56, 1396–1403 (1985).

Volm, M., Mattern, J., Sonka, J., Vogt-Schaden, M., Wayss, K.: DNA distribution in non-small cell lung carcinomas and its relationship to clinical behavior. Cytometry 6 (1985).

## 5.7 Radiosurgery in the Brain – a Special External Irradiation with a Linear Accelerator

by Günther Hartmann and Volker Sturm

The treatment of malignant tumors with ionizing radiation (briefly termed radiotherapy) occupies an important place in many therapeutical concepts. However, by its nature it is a local treatment, i. e. a curative effect is aimed at and expected only in the body region receiving pinpointed treatment. The physician's job is to attain as even as possible a distribution of the dose of radiation in the foreseen target volume, sparing the healthy surrounding tissue as much as possible.

In recent years, the development in the field of radiation equipment and radiation planning has steadily progressed and has been employed in practical radiotherapy. These developments make a major contribution to an improvement of the healing figures in certain local tumors. One of these developments will be described below.

### Stereotactic Convergent Irradiation

The stereotactic convergent beam irradiation developed at the German Cancer Research Center and applied in patients constitutes a very specific form of radiotherapy in which the aspect of local treatment is especially pronounced (Fig. 103). The goal of this technique is to attain such a high concentration of the radiation dose in small volumes in the brain that the destructive effect of the irradiation can be used, so to speak, like a surgical instrument (= radiosurgery). Especially in deep tumors and angiomas in the brain, which are not accessible to any operation and which are small and well-circumscribed, this may be the sole possible method of treatment.

Since 1979, the research project "Interstitial Tumor Brain Therapy" is being carried out at the Institute of Nuclear Medicine in close collaboration with the Neurosurgery Division at the Surgical Hospital, University of Heidelberg (Project Heads: Prof. Volker Sturm, Prof. Walter J. Lorenz). Here, extensive experience has been obtained in the treatment of inoperable tumors by means of interstitial or intracavitary tumor irradiation. In this method, radioactive substances are introduced stereotactically, i. e. specifically through an injection channel into the tumor to be irradiated.

Within this research project, the technique of external stereotactic irradiation using a linear accelerator has now been worked out as an alternative to irradiation from the inside. The objective was to obtain a technique of radiosurgery with which a precisely localized and sharply delimited dose distribution similar to that of an internal irradiation can be attained.

The model for this new technique of irradiation was the convergent beam irradiation developed by Lars Leksell et al. (1951) at the Karolinska Institute in Stockholm. In this technique, a large number of radioactive sources are used. The radiation from the individual sources arranged hemispherically is collimated to narrow radiation beams and focused on a single point in the brain. Since the radiation dose is thus concentrated in such an extreme manner on a small volume of tissue, the entire radiation dose to be used can be administered in a single treatment of about one hour's duration. In contrast to this, the foreseen total dose is administered in 20 or 30 fractions within a period of several weeks in a conventional radiation treatment. For the new type of treatment, the designation "stereotactic single dose irradiation" is also used.

The irradiation equipment by Lars Leksell specifically for radiosurgery uses 179 single cobalt 60 radiation sources. The equivalent is elaborate and expensive (price: about 6 million DM) because of the problems of screening and collimation connected with it. It is simpler to use the movement irradiation (movement of the irradiation source during the radiotherapy) available with a modern accelerator in combination with the rotation of the patient table for the stereotactic single dose irradiation. This technique of radiotherapy was put into practice for brain tumors in the linear accelerator equipment Mevatron 77 at the German Cancer Research Center.

Fig. 104

Fig. 103
A special radiotherapy developed in the German Cancer Research Center (convergence irradation) under test for vascular malformations in the brain and for certain brain tumors

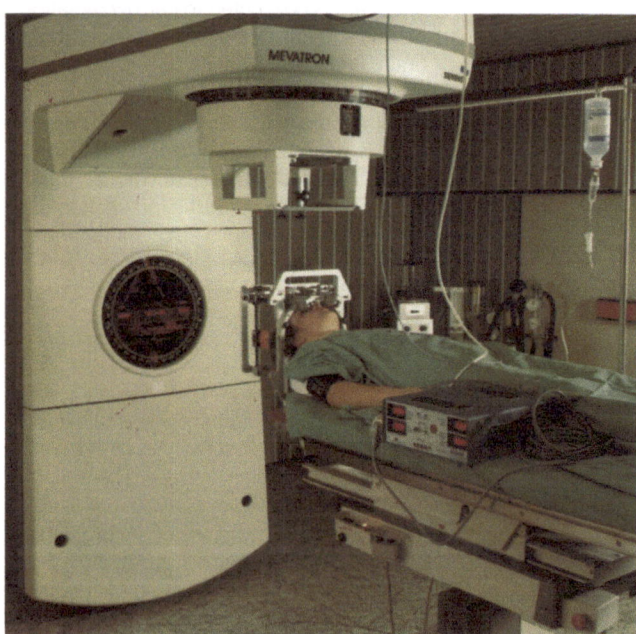

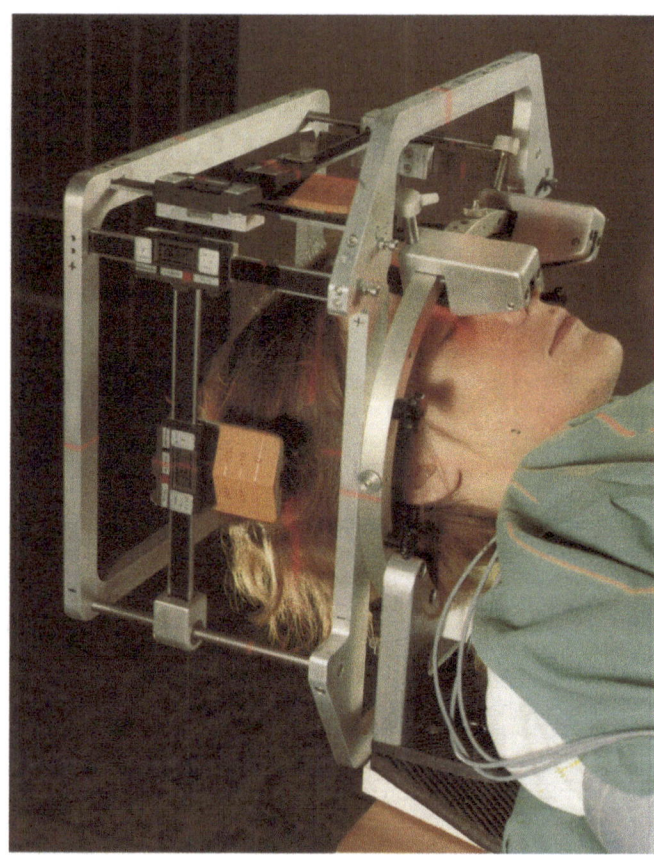

## Localization and Irradiation Technique

The basis for establishing the target of irradiation are the methods already developed and employed up to now at the Institute of Nuclear Medicine: a coordination matrix, in which every point in the brain is unequivocally allocated a position and thus made accessible to stereotactic operations with high precision, is defined by using computer tomographic data and computer programs. The base lines of the coordination matrix are represented by the stereotactic base ring fixed on the patient's head. Precondition for an external stereotactic irradiation is that the volume to be irradiated is placed exactly at the intersection point of the rays from various directions during the movement irradiation.

The high accuracy of aim required is attained by the use of a neurosurgical stereotactic technique. Figure 104 shows the principle of this technique. A base ring (modified Riechert-Mundinger system) is screwed firmly on the skull bone by means of four adjustable pins.

This is carried out under local anesthesia. This ring then constitutes a fixed reference system in which each point in the brain is unequivocally allocated a position and is thus accessible to sterotactic irradiation techniques with high precision. In the figure, the base ring is to be seen together with the positioning system. With this arrangement, the designated target point in the brain can be adjusted exactly at the intersection point of the beams produced with the linear accelerator.

The convergent beam irradiation is carried out by superposition of several movement irradiations, which are distributed over the entire upper half of the cranium. All radiation directions cross in the designated target point. Fig. 106 shows a schematic representation of this irradiation technique.

## Application

The first patient treated in the German Cancer Research Center suffered from an inoperable angioma. Since that time, about 70 further patients with angiomas or other tumor conditions in the brain have been treated. In a prospective study, the possibilities of the treatment of brain metastases and malignant gliomas are investigated. All cases involve patients in whom healing is not possible by open surgery due to the unfavorable position of the tumor. The technique, which is still elaborate today, requires the collaboration of physicians, physicists engineers and technical assistants. The results available so far justify the hope that the method of irradiation presented here is suitable for curing certain brain tumors.

Dr. Günther H. Hartmann
Central Radiation Protection and
Dosimetry Division
Department of Biophysics and Medical
Radiation Physics
Institute of Nuclear Medicine

Prof. Volker Sturm
Neurosurgery at the Surgical Hospital,
University of Heidelberg

Participating staff

Dipl. phys. Robert Boesecke
Dr. Karl-Heinz Höver
Prof. Walter J. Lorenz
Eng. Otto Pastyr
Dr. Wolfgang Schlegel
Dr. Gerd Wolber

In collaboration with

Dr. Bernd Kober
Radiological Hospital
University of Heidelberg

Selected publications

Sturm, V., Pastyr, O., Schlegel, W., Scharfenberg, H., Zabel, H.-J., Netzeband, G., Schabbert, S., Berberich, W.: Stereotactic computer tomography with a modified Riechert-Mundinger device as the basis for integrated stereotactic neuroradiological investigations. Acta Neurochir. 68, 11–17 (1983).

Hartmann, G. H., Schlegel, W., Sturm, V., Kober, B., Lorenz, W. J.: Cerebral radiation surgery using moving field irradiation at a linear accelerator facility. Int. J. Rad. Oncol. Biol. Phys. 11, 1185–1192 (1985).

Fig. 105
The precise position of the midpoint of irradation is checked with laser beams

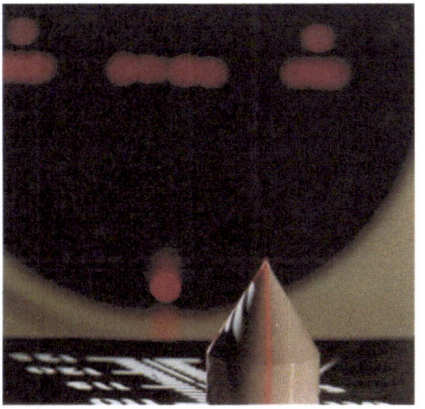

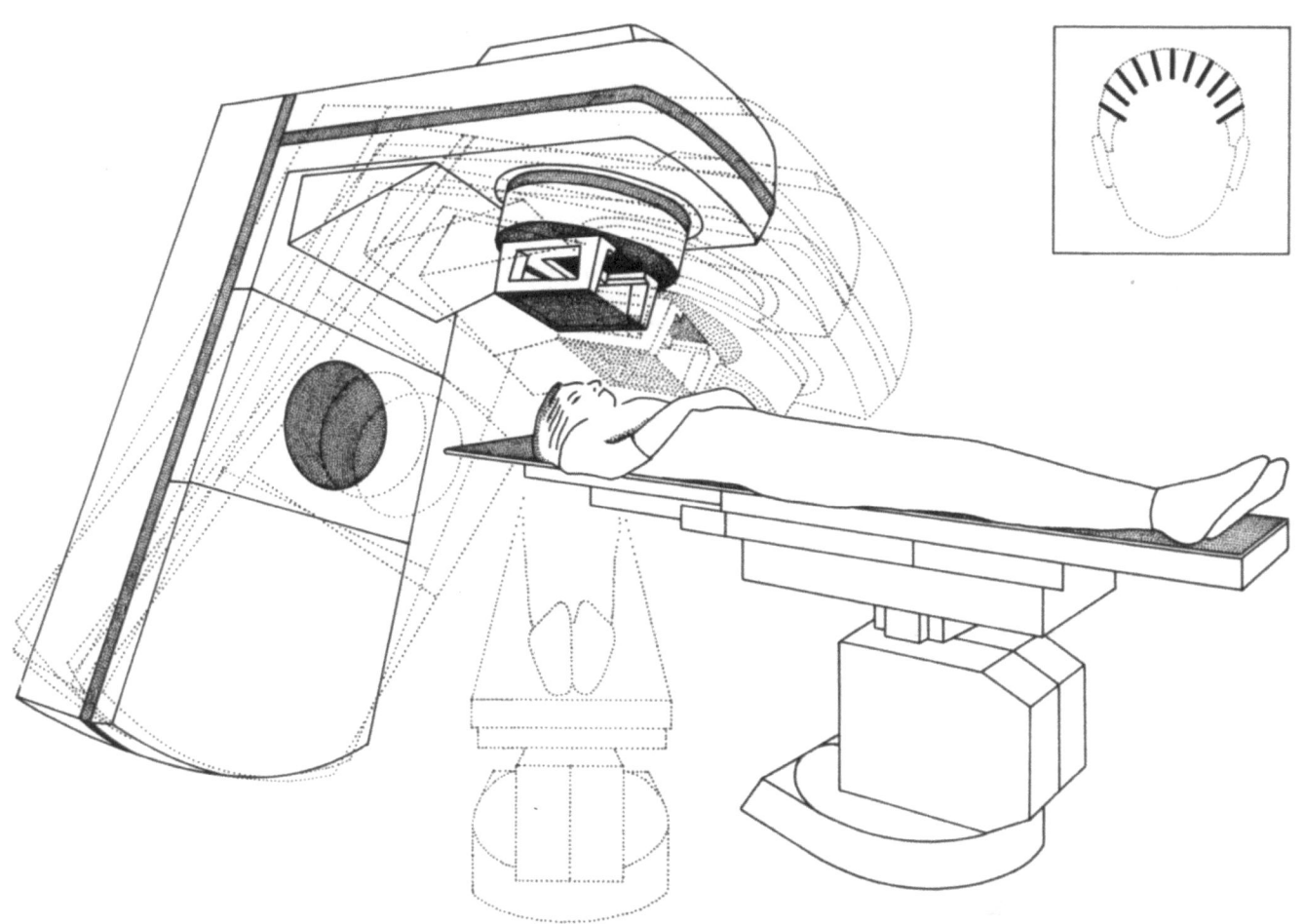

Fig. 106
Schematic representation of the irradiation technique. In the figure at the right at the top, the regions into which the beams penetrate, are labelled black

## 5.8 Spatial Image Representation – Support of Therapy Planning

by Wolfgang Schlegel and Bernhard Bauer

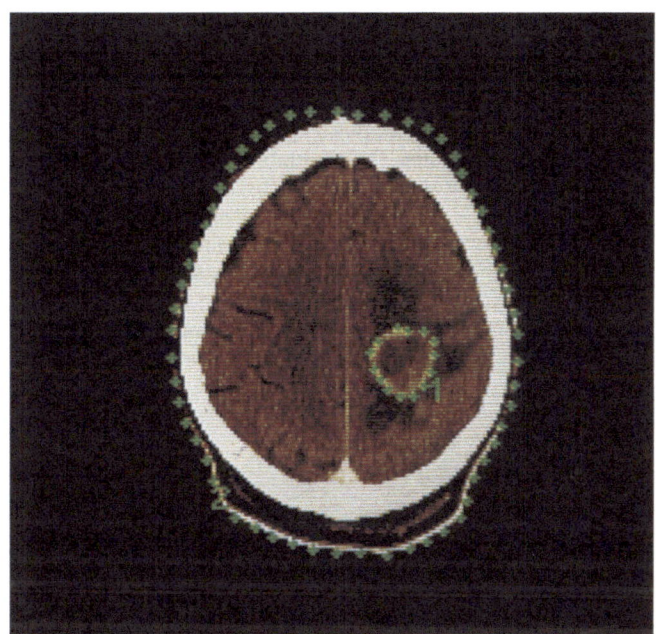

Fig. 107

Modern imaging techniques in medicine have brought about a decisive change in medical diagnosis within a short time: the physician no longer depends on the two-dimensional shadow picture of the X-ray alone, but can obtain three-dimensional anatomical information on the patient with the aid of the computer and appropriate measurement systems. This three-dimensional information is available in the computer memory as an abundance of numbers of which each represents one point in the picture initially invisible for man. If one wanted to put on paper the numbers, from which the three-dimensional image of a body region of about 30 cm long is composed, about 5,000 typewritten pages would be necessary!

The enormous flood of information of a three-dimensional image cannot be summarized in a single spatial representation. Hence, one requires sectional representation: from the three-dimensional picture data of the patient, a layer is "cut out" in the longitudinal transverse direction and presented as a two-dimensional picture (Fig. 107). In this way, the problem of the representation of a spatial picture is reduced to the production of a series of two-dimensional tomograms. This mode of presentation has the advantage that none of the information contained in the overall picture is lost, the recognizability of the data in the individual sections is very high, and anatomical structures and

pathological alterations in organs and in the tissue can thus be well evaluated. However, the conceptional capacity of a human being is, as a rule, overtaxed if the organs and structures presented in a series of tomograms are to be exactly located in space. However, for the therapist it is important to know how the spatial position of organs, body structures and pathological tissue changes in relation to each other: properties such as form, volume and distances from neighbouring organs are decisive for the therapeutic procedure, e. g., in radiotherapy or surgery. Although this information, which is important for the planning of therapy, is contained in image data, which are obtained with a computer tomograph, they cannot be directly perceived via the sectional presentation.

A spatial presentation of the position and form of organ surfaces can be attained with the method of "computer-aided design" (CAD). CAD computer programs were first developed for body work and machine building as well as for the production of cartoon films. Our group has adopted such a program which is now available on the market. We have altered and extended it in such a way that it can now also be used for the presentation of body surfaces and organs.

The reconstruction and presentation of body and organ surfaces with this method are shown in Fig. 107 to 110.

To produce a three-dimensional image, three processing steps are necessary: first of all, the contours of the surfaces to be presented must be labelled in the CT images (Fig. 107). In the second step, the contours are then linked to each other in such a way that a large number of individual surface elements arises. In this way, a wire frame model of the entire surface is obtained. Represented as a line drawing (Fig. 108), this already gives a spatial impression. In order to render a closed surface visible, the individual surface elements are then

stained in the third step (Fig. 108). In order to obtain a differentiated mode of consideration, we designate the different organs with different colors. The spatial images of the organs obtained in this way can be examined from all sides on the screen.

Fig. 108

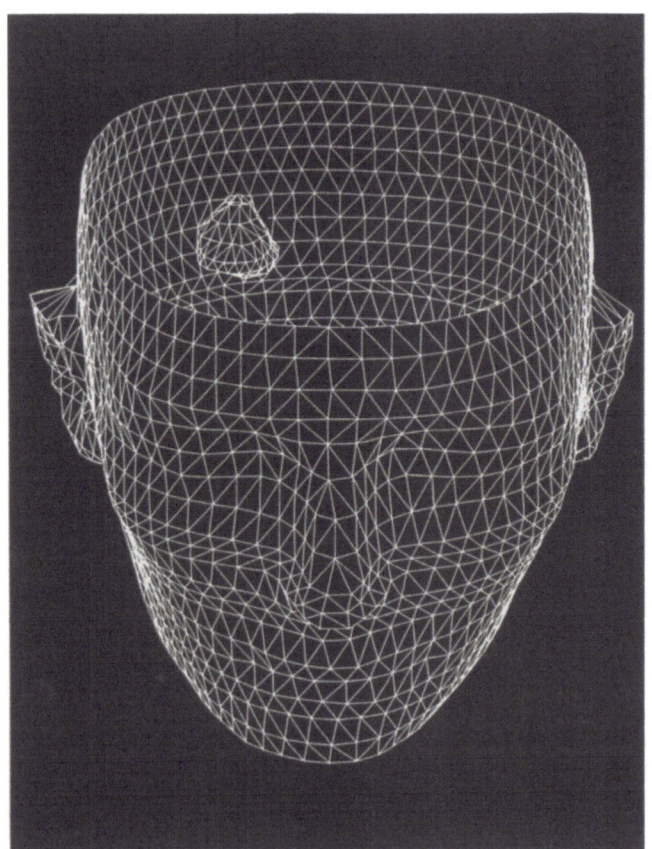

Fig. 109

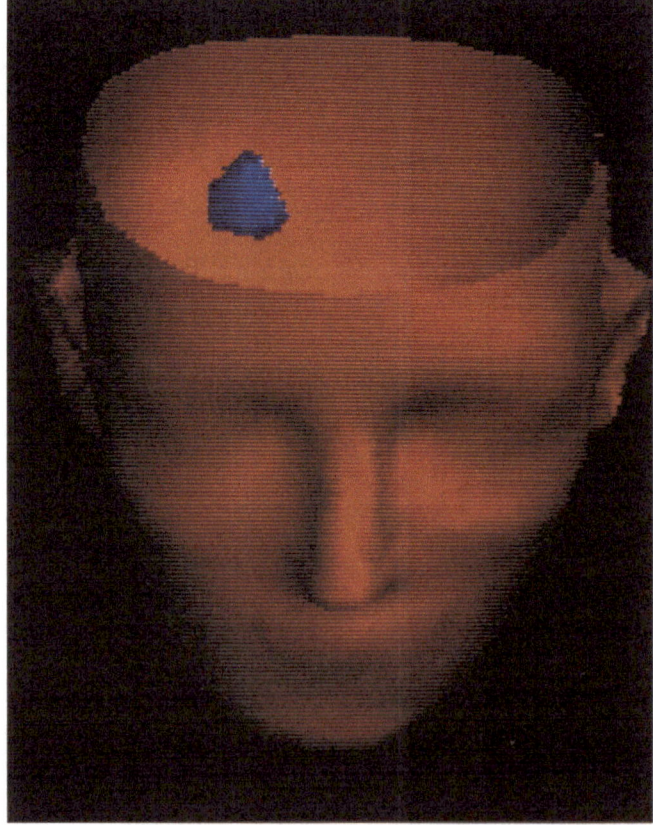

This technique has been employed so far in the planning of radiotherapy and of neurosurgical operations. In Fig. 110, a computer tomographic transverse picture of a patient with a bronchial tumor is shown first of all as an example for the application in planning radiotherapy. In the picture, the contours of the area to be treated are displayed; this area comprises the tumor itself and the adjacent mediastinal tissue. The spinal canal is likewise characterized as especially radiosensitive and hence to be spared. In this way, the treatment area and the spinal cord are drawn in all tomograms of this patient.

Furthermore, the spatial distribution of the radiation dose to be applied as calculated by the computer is shown in Fig. 110. The therapeutically active region (the "80% isodose" line) encloses the treatment region. The tissue to be treated is thus given a dose of radiation adequate to destroying the tumor. The outer range of activity (the 50% isodose line) delimits the tolerance region for the radiosensitive nervous tissue of the spinal cord. In this tomogram, the spinal cord is outside the critical region.

Fig. 111 now shows the three-dimensional presentation of the treatment area (red), the spinal cord (blue), the therapeutically active dose range (80% isodose lines). Fig. 112 shows the same body structures with a characterization of the spinal cord tolerance dose (50% isodose lines) for a conventional method of radiation treatment. In these two three-dimensional presentations, two deficiencies in planning can be discovered which could not be seen in the two-dimensional plan (Fig. 110):

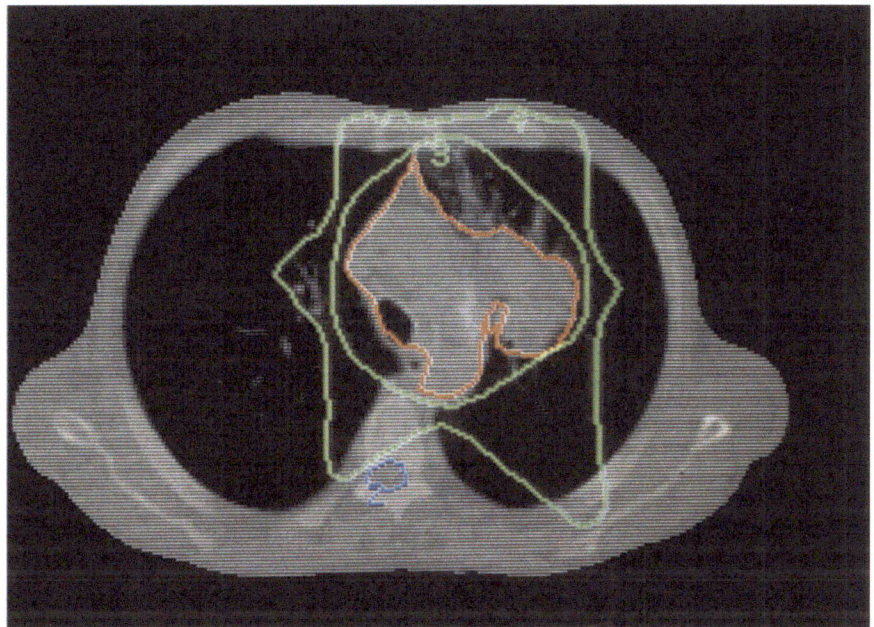

Fig. 110

- In certain areas of the treatment volumes, the therapeutically required dose is not completely reached (Fig. 111).
- In certain regions of the spinal cord, the tolerated dose is exceeded (Fig. 112).

Exceeding the therapeutically required dose can trigger off the development of a new tumor after completion of radiotherapy. On the other hand, exceeding the tolerated dose can elicit side effects which are a burden to the patient.

If these dangers can be recognized from the spatial presentation, it is possible to revise the originally planned mode of treatment once more: the treatment conditions are "optimized" with the aid of the computer.

After conclusion of the optimization process, the therapeutic dose is now shown adapted to the treatment volume in an ideal way (Fig. 113), and the danger of damage to the spinal cord is very largely precluded (Fig. 114).

This example shows the significance of three-dimensional calculations and representations in the planning of therapy: underdosages in the treatment region and overdosage in the critical regions can be avoided better than was previously the case.

By use of modern computer technology, one has thus come closer to the objective aimed at in cancer therapy, namely to improve the chances of healing and to reduce the side effects.

Dr. Wolfgang Schlegel
Bernhard Bauer
Biophysics and Medical
Radiation Physics,
Institute of Nuclear Medicine

Participating scientists

Dipl. Ing. Josef Doll
Prof. Dr. Walter J. Lorenz
Dipl. Inf. med. Timm Werner

Dr. Bernd Kober
Radiological Hospital, University of
Heidelberg

Prof. Volker Sturm
Department of Neurosurgery,
Surgical Hospital, University of Heidelberg

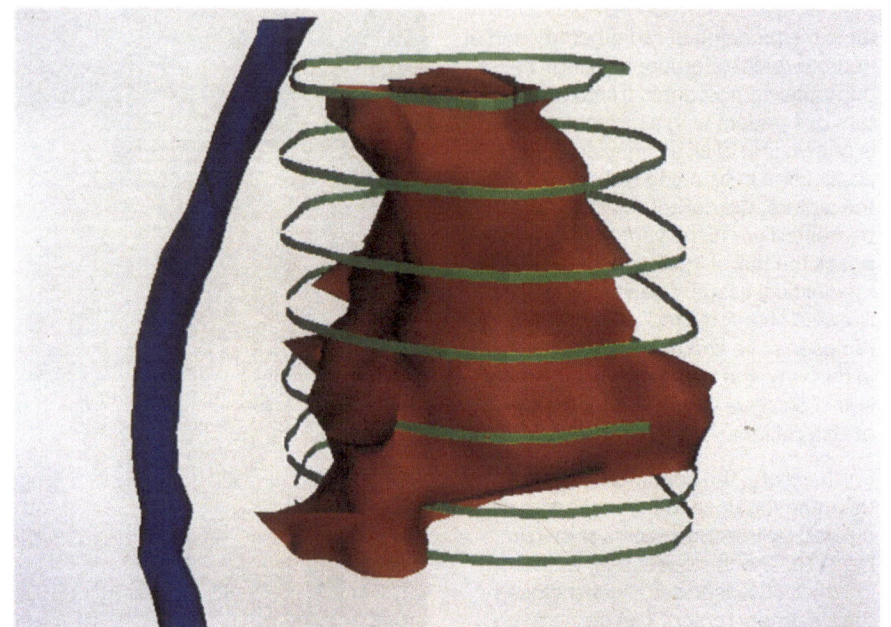

Fig. 111      Fig. 112

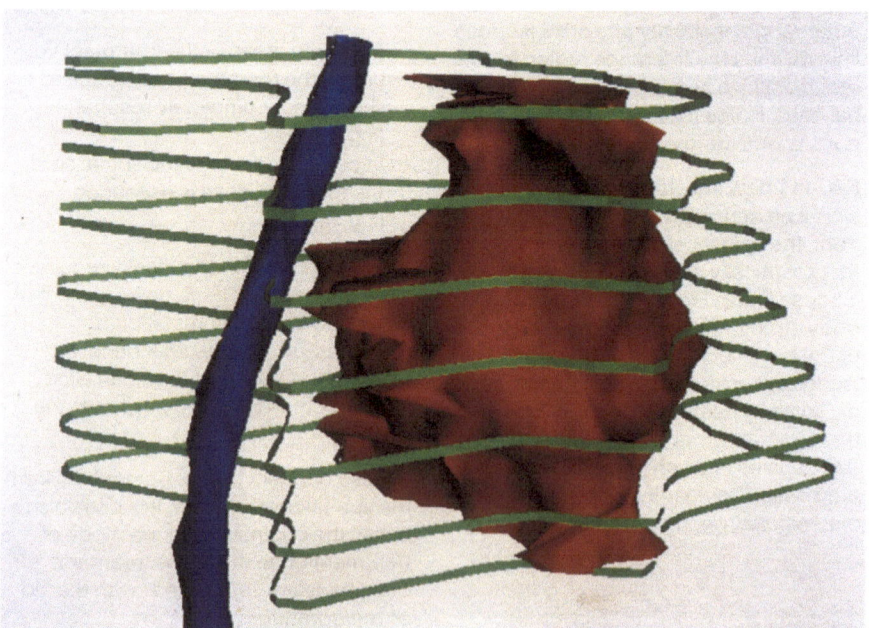

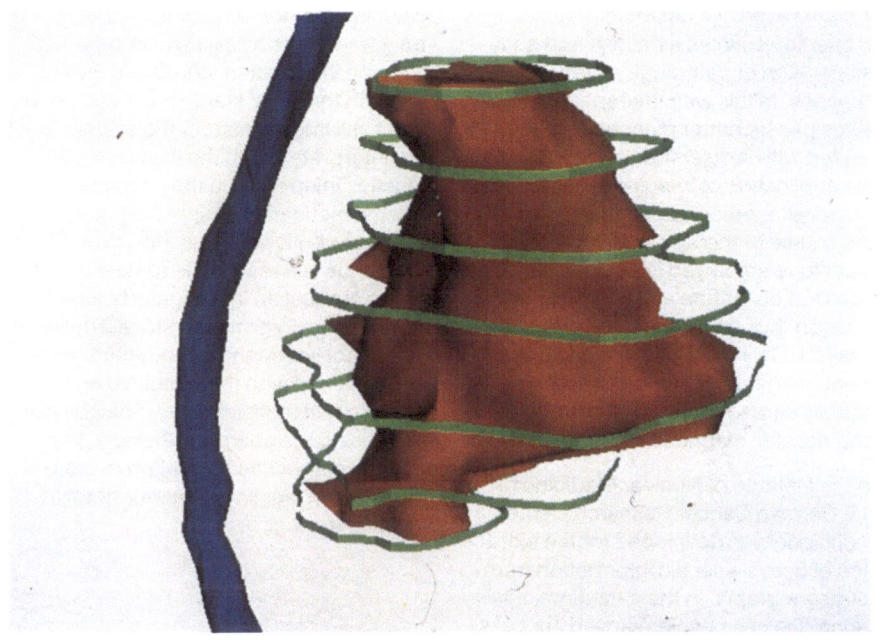

Fig. 113

Selected publications

Schlegel, W., Scharfenberg, H., Doll, J., Hartmann, G., Sturm, V., Lorenz, W. J.: Threedimensional Dose Planning Using Tomographic Data. In: Proceedings of The Eighth International Conference on the Use of Computers in Radiation Therapy, Toronto, July 9–12, 191–196, IEEE Computer Society Press, Silver Spring (1984).

Bauer, B., Schlegel, W., Boesecke, R., Doll, J., Hartmann, G., Lorenz, W. J.: Threedimensional Planning of Conformation Therapy. In: Computer Aided Radiology 85 (H. Lemke, ed.), Springer Verlag (1985).

Fig. 114

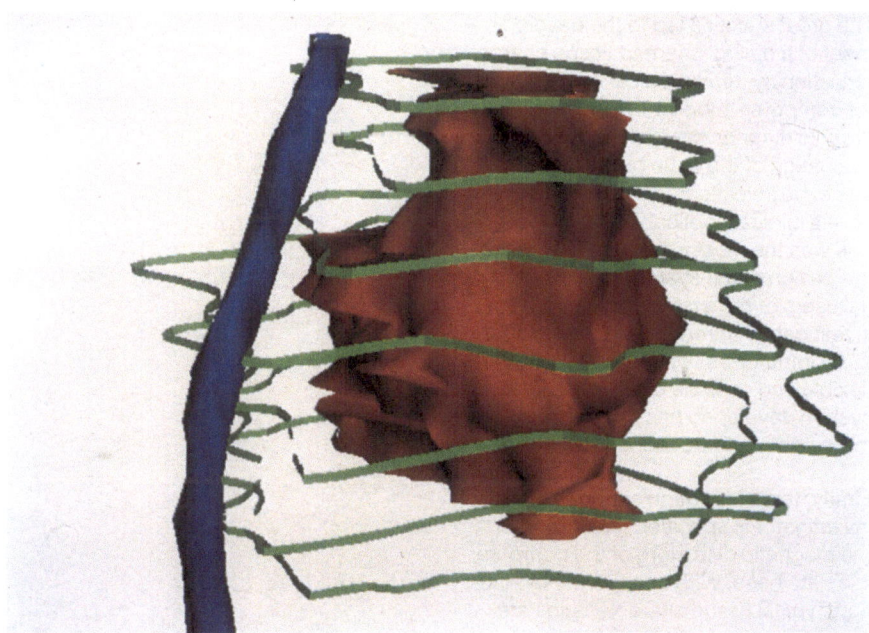

## 5.9 Computer-Assisted Echographic Tissue Characterization

by Dieter Schlaps

In recent years, the information obtained from imaging techniques has substantially increased in importance in the diagnostic appraisal of a patient. This was made possible only by the breath-taking development of micro-electronics. To a growing extent, the manifold increase in the computing capacity with simultaneous reduction in costs has allowed the integration of inexpensive and efficient microcomputers into the imaging systems for computer tomographic reconstruction and general improvement of images.

The classical X-ray technique is still the most important imaging investigation in view of its share of 92% in the total of all image diagnosis investigations. Besides this, the modern imaging techniques such as computer tomography, thermography, ultrasonography, scintigraphy, positron emission tomography and the recently developed nuclear magnetic resonance are now gaining increasing importance. In view of these technical innovations and improved forms of therapy, there are signs that a change is now taking place in medical imaging diagnostics. This is characterized by a greater interest in the quantitative characterization of biochemical and physiological tissue properties and thus goes beyond a morphological description of the tissue.

A comprehensive description of tissue properties enables a precise and early recognition of pathological tissue changes. In this way, therapeutic measures can be better planned and executed with regular therapy follow-up by the application of imaging techniques. However, a precondition for monitoring the course of therapy is that the imaging technique employed is noninvasive, i. e. does not constitute a risk for the patient and can thus be repeated as often as desired. Only a few of the techniques mentioned fulfill these requirements, namely ultrasonography, thermography and nuclear magnetic resonance.

In the Institute of Nuclear Medicine of the German Cancer Research Center, a technique was developed for the extraction of tissue-specific information from ultrasonograms. In the meantime, this technique has been employed successfully in several clinical studies with more than 500 patients and healthy subjects. The great success led to the development of a dialog-oriented tissue characterization system (medical workstation for computer-supported ultrasonographic diagnosis) which enables rapid evaluation of the state of the organ tissue to be investigated. As wide as possible a clinical applicability of the technique was the most important criterion in the design of the system. Since potential users of the system would wish to investigate different clinical questions, the computer-assisted system had to be flexible and capable of learning. The system developed has taken these requirements into account.

Firstly, the information sought for by the investigator is specified and stored in the magnetic disc store of the computer in a data base. With each new examination, typical tissue characteristics are calculated automatically from the ultrasonogram recorded and compared with the information stored in the data base. In the initial stage, the investigator must still largely instruct the system in the interpretation of the tissue characteristics inferred from the image texture. After investigation of approximately 20 patients per tissue class, however, the technique is already able to describe the tissue state of an investigated patient from its own information store. The investigator-independent, quantitative result obtained with this sensitive and specific test method is very valuable for appraising the course of therapy, the general diagnostic evaluation of a patient and for training ultrasonographic investigators.

## Conventional Ultrasonographic Diagnosis

In ultrasonographic diagnosis, the vehicle of physical information is sound radiation. By beaming in a longitudinal pressure wave, the sound is reflected, absorbed, refracted and scattered in the tissue structures. Of these physical effects, however, only the sound reflection can be observed directly. Sound absorption, scattering and refraction can only be detected together and indirectly as a general loss of echo intensity. The imaging systems scan the body region to be investigated line by line with a location-variable transducer and produce a two-dimensional section image from the reflected echo signals (Fig. 115 a–d). The application flexibility of the technique is almost unlimited, since the instruments are very handy and tomograms can be defined in all sectional directions. Three-dimensional information must be calculated by stacking several two-dimensional tomograms in the computer. The spatial resolution is dependent on the direction and depth in ultrasonography, but can generally be considered as very good, amounting to less than 1 mm. A major advantage of ultrasonographic diagnosis is the excellent time resolution, since up to 50 images per second can be produced. Conventional ultrasonographic diagnosis is a focal point of investigations for the visualization of the blood flow and object movements. The evaluation of unmoved organs and in particular of tissue alteration is in general very difficult and requires great experience on the part of the investigator. The conventional image interpretation is based above all on the anatomical evaluation of the body region investigated, on the evaluation of the mobility of organs and on the discovery of pathological tissue areas.

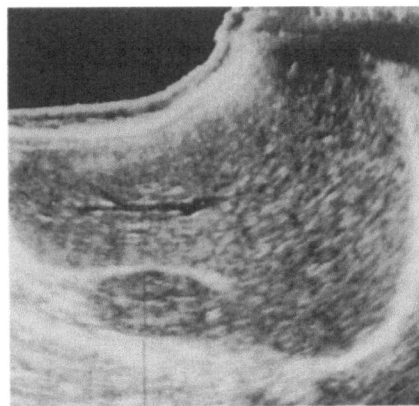
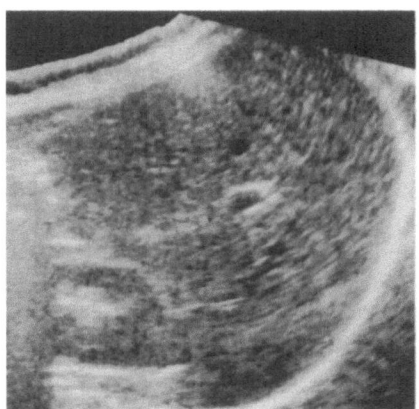
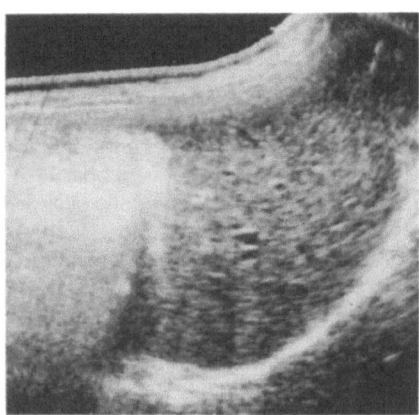
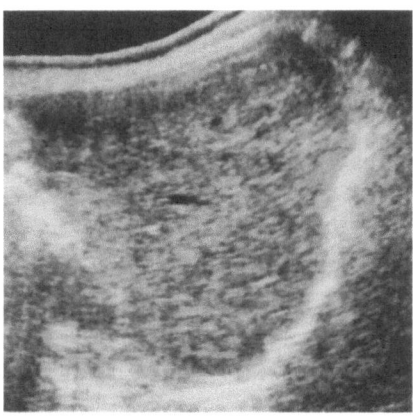

Fig. 115 a
Left section of the right lobe of the liver; here a normal liver (longitudinal section)

Fig. 115 b
Fatty degeneration of the liver with fibrosis

Fig. 115 c
Fatty liver

Fig. 115 d
Cirrhosis

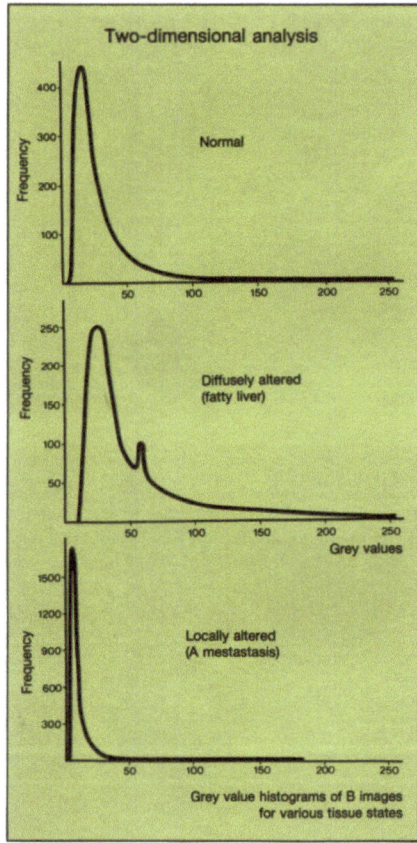

**Two-dimensional analysis**

Normal

Diffusely altered
(fatty liver)

Grey values

Locally altered
(A mestastasis)

Grey value histograms of B images
for various tissue states

Fig. 116

## Computer Echography

The objective of computer echography is a quantitative characterization of complex ultrasonographic information. As has been known since the psychophysical experiments by Bela Julesz, image texture information is only partially accessible to the human eye. For this reason, mathematical procedures have been developed which register and describe the spatial distribution of the ultrasonographic image texture with statistical models of different levels of complexity. Each model has a set of key parameters which characterize the image texture in the context of the model assumptions.

1. Parameters from conventional diagnosis. This group of parameters quantifies certain echographic phenomena which are also used in conventional ultrasonography for the diagnostic evaluation of the investigated organs. Such characteristics are, for example: sharpness of edge contours, enhancement and attenuation effects.

2. General characteristics of the echo distribution. These parameters describe the overall distribution of the echo (grey levels). Fig. 116 shows for example the grey value histograms of a normal liver, a fatty liver and a hepatic metastasis. The grey level distribution of the fatty liver is markedly displaced into the region of high intensities ("bright liver").

3. Texture parameters (spatial distribution of the echo). These parameters detect the spatial variation of the grey values in the image. As was shown in the psychophysical experiments of Bela Julesz, the human eye only has a limited capacity for differentiating image textures possessing different statistical correlations with their environment. With

the aid of the computer, these statistical properties of texture can be determined very precisely. As was shown in several publications, the computer is far superior to the human eye in distinguishing this class of image textures. The computer-assisted analysis of ultrasonograms utilizes this fact.

For the purpose of presentation of the properties of selected texture parameters, a test picture was generated in the institute's own computer VAX-11/780 (Fig. 117). The picture was subdivided into 16 segments to which an additive noise of various intensities was added. In each of these 16 segments of the phantom picture, the parameters "contrast" (Fig. 118), "mean grey value" (Fig. 119) and "variance of the grey values" (Fig. 120) are determined and coded in grey shades. Grey shade 0 (black) corresponds to the lowest of the 16 parameter values and grey shade 255 (white) to the highest parameter value.

It becomes evident from Figs. 117–120 that the different parameters support each other in a complementary manner in the description of the texture characteristics. For this reason, in a similar way groups of informative parameters, which enable the distinction of different tissue states, must be found for quantifying the ultrasonographic image information.

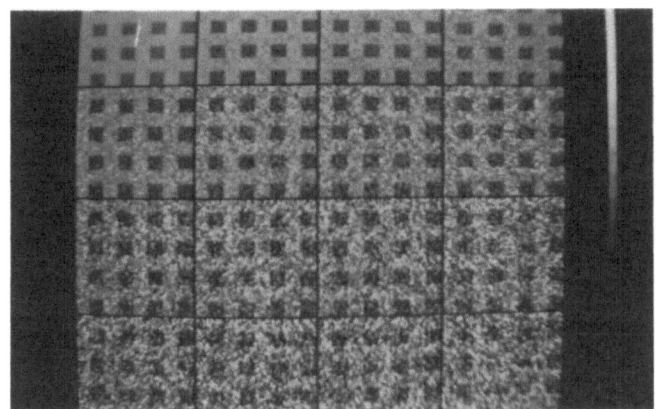 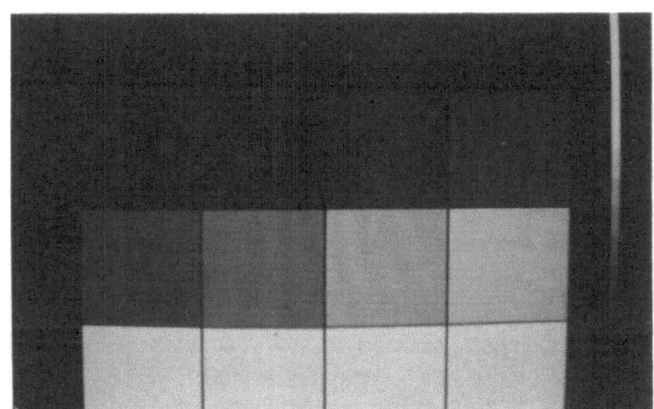

Fig. 117
Series of test pictures. Intensity of additive smoking
increasing from the left at the top to the right at the
bottom

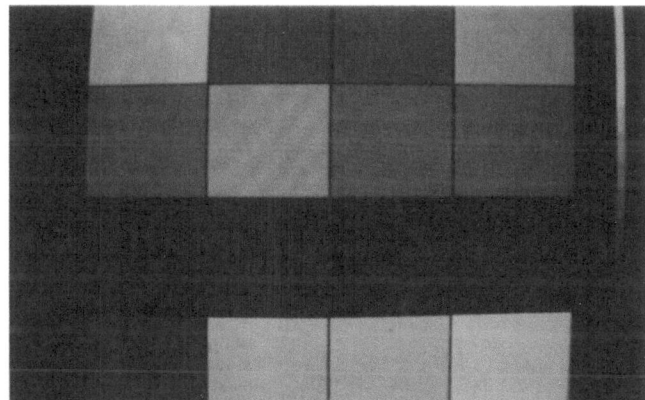

Fig. 118
Parameter "contrast" for each picture segment of
Fig. 116

Fig. 119
Parameter "mean grey value"

Fig. 120
Parameter "variants of the grey values"

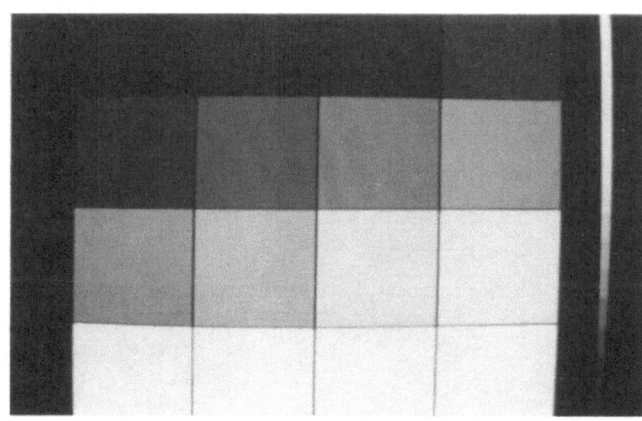

Tab. 10. Conventional analysis of ultrasonograms of the liver
(N = 40, overall diagnostic accuracy 83%)

| Histology | Results | | |
| --- | --- | --- | --- |
| | Normal | Diffuse Alteration | Tumor Tissue |
| Normal | 9 | 8 | 1 |
| Diffuse Alteration | 2 | 18 | 0 |
| Tumors | 2 | 2 | 6 |

Tab. 11. Computer assisted analysis of ultrasonograms of the liver
(N = 40, overall diagnostic accuracy 95%)

| Histology | Results | | |
| --- | --- | --- | --- |
| | Normal | Diffuse Alteration | Tumor Tissue |
| Normal | 10 | 0 | 0 |
| Diffuse Alteration | 1 | 19 | 0 |
| Tumors | 0 | 1 | 9 |

In a comparative study, in which conventional subjective ultrasonographic diagnosis was compared with computer-assisted echography, the following observations could be made: on the basis of recognized criteria of diagnosis such as image brightness, sound attenuation, peripheral vascular picture, liver size, ascites and spleen size as well as in space-occupying lesions in the liver, three different investigators arrived at a diagnostic evaluation of the localization, delimitability, size and echo pattern. The overall diagnostic accuracy (percentage of correct diagnoses) was 83%. On the other hand, the precision of the computer-assisted technique was 95% (see Tab. 10 and 11).

## Medical Workstation for Computer-Assisted Ultrasonographic Diagnosis

A decisive factor for a greater popularity of computerized echographic methods in medical diagnosis is, of course, the cost-benefit ratio of the technique employed.

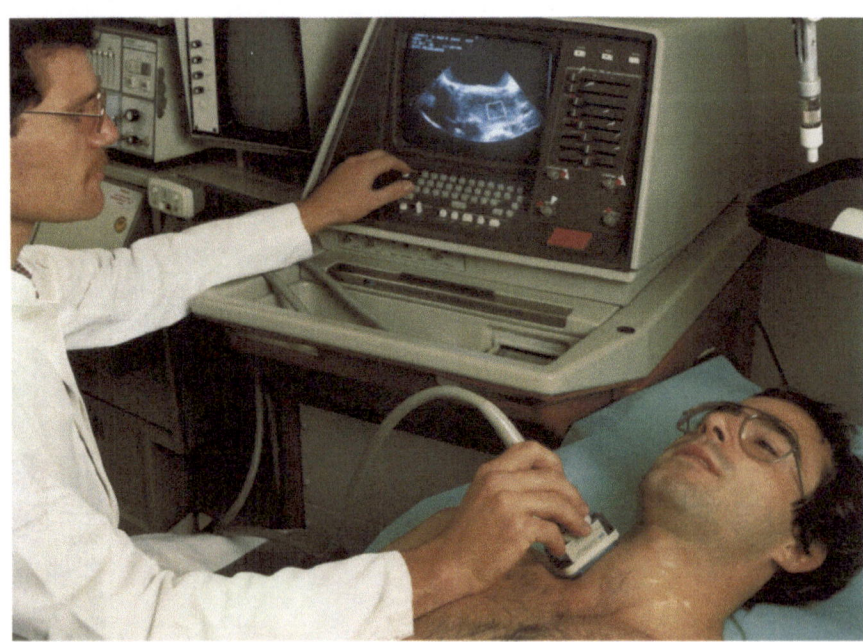

Fig. 121
Medical workplace for computer-supported ultrasonographic image analysis

In collaboration with the company Hewlett Packard in Andover, Mass., USA, a medical workstation was hence developed for computer-assisted ultrasonographic image analysis. The HP 1000 microcomputer used is connected to a HP 77070 A realtime electronic sector scanner and allows acquisition of the ultrasonographic picture and selection of tissue regions of interest (Fig. 121). After recording the ultrasonogram, the complete set of texture parameters is calculated. Afterwards, the most informative parameters are used for a diagnostic classification of the patient investigated, and a suggested diagnosis is worked out.

The suggested diagnosis constitutes a statistical appraisal, since it contains the probabilities with which the patient investigated can be classified into the different tissue classes. In the calculation of these probabilities, both the patient-specific image analysis results and the institute-specific information on the frequency of occurrence of various tissue diseases are taken into consideration.

At the end of the investigation, a diagnostic report is printed which is filed with the other clinical data and test results in the patient file and used for diagnostic evaluation. The medical workstation for computer-assisted ultrasonographic diagnosis can hence be interpreted as a quantitative, largely investigator-independent diagnostic test procedure of good specificity and sensitivity. Its diagnostic value is to be rated as very high.

To open up the system to other imaging techniques (computer tomography, nuclear magnetic resonance and positron emission tomography) and integration of a learning data base into the medical workplace system, a broad spectrum of new possibilities arises:

By the quantification of image information, the information collected at one center can be transferred to another center equipped with the same system. The research results of a scientific institution would thus benefit other institutions working in the same field.

General therapy follow-up can be carried out in an optimal way with such a system, since all relevant tissue differentiation data of the patient are also available on-line from previous investigations. Individual forms of therapy can be investigated for their success with appropriate tests of the statistical trend analysis.

It is not of help to progress in medicine if one succumbs to an uncritical fascination for the computer and the possibilities it opens up. The knowledge, overall impression and judgment of the investigating physician remains decisive even in this field of medical diagnosis. Nevertheless, it would be presumptious to reject the assistance in objective image diagnosis presented here. Even with critical consideration, a further improvement of diagnosis and therapy follow-up can be achieved by objective image analysis.

Dr. Dieter Schlaps
Biophysics and Medical
Radiation Physics,
Institute of Nuclear Medicine

In collaboration with

Dipl. Ing. Adolf Lorenz
Prof. Walter J. Lorenz
Dr. Ivan Zuna
Biophysics and Medical
Radiation Physics,
Institute of Nucleas Medicine

Prof. Gerhard van Kaick
Dr. Dorothea Lorenz
Dr. Ulrich Raeth
Special Oncological
Diagnostics and Therapy,
Institute of Nuclear Medicine

Prof. Bernhard Kommerell
Department of Gastroenterology,
Hospital for Internal Medicine, University of Heidelberg

Hewlett Packard, Medical Division, Andover, Massachusetts, USA

European Communities Converted Action on Ultrasonic Tissue Characterization

Selected publications

Julesz, B.: Experiments in the visual perception of texture, Scientific American 232, 34–43 (1975).

Julesz, B.: Textons, the elements of texture perception, and their interactions, Nature 290, 91–97 (1981).

Smith, S. W., Wagner, R. F., Sandrik, J. M., Lopez, H.: Low contrast detectability and contrast/detail analysis in medical ultrasound, IEEE Trans. Sonics Ultrasonics SU-30, 164–173 (1983).

Räth, U., Schlaps, D., Limberg, B., Zuna, I., Lorenz, A., van Kaick, G., Lorenz, W. J., Kommerell, B.: Diagnostic accuracy of computerized B-scan texture analysis and conventional ultrasonography in diffuse parenchymal and malignant liver disease, Journal of Clinical Ultrasound 13, 87–99, (1985).

## 5.10 Textural Analysis of Microscopic Images

by Dymitr Komitowski

The modern methods of image representation and image analysis have opened up novel, so far unknown possibilities of medical diagnosis. At the same time, they have initiated a transformation in the approach to diagnosis, the full repercussions of which will only become apparent in the future. Advances in the visual representation of disease processes and their description have become evident today on two levels:

- formally as an introduction of computer-controlled systems for the representation and characterization of forms of pathological manifestation and
- intellectually as a transition from the individual recognition and categorization of visual objects based on experience to their classification on the basis of mathematically defined features.

The qualitative jump from "what is the meaning of what I see" to the recognition of morphological patterns typical for pathological processes, using previously selected features is manifested most clearly in automatic image processing. The function of image processing is an objective and thus reproducible description of an object by means of quantitative features. Since the objective analysis of histological images is fundamental for histological diagnosis, the image processing techniques are gaining increasing significance in pathology. However, their application for the evaluation of histological images

gives rise to different problems. Some of these problems are related to the special optical features of the microscopical images, e. g., poor contrast, complexity or defocussed projections of objects outside the level of focus. Others concern the possibilities of the existing systems with regard to digital image processing. A general weakness of these systems is the amount of time required to evaluate the images. A compromise must thus be found in diagnostic practice between the accuracy of analysis and the time required.

Fig. 122
View of the entire image-processing system with the multiprocessor and the control panel on the right in the picture

The system of real-time analysis of histological images according to texture features developed in the Department of Histodiagnostics and Pathomorphological Documentation constitutes a step forward in the reduction of the time required. It enables the analysis of histological images in real time i. e. with the speed with which a videocamera presents the image to be investigated. Characteristic for this system is the possibility of effecting feature extraction in consequence of a learning process.

Our system consists of a light microscope which is equipped with a scanning table for an automatic movement of the slides and a motor-driven focus. The images produced by the microscope are transformed into electrical signals by a video camera. These are processed with the aid of computers. The transmission of the camera signals to the computer

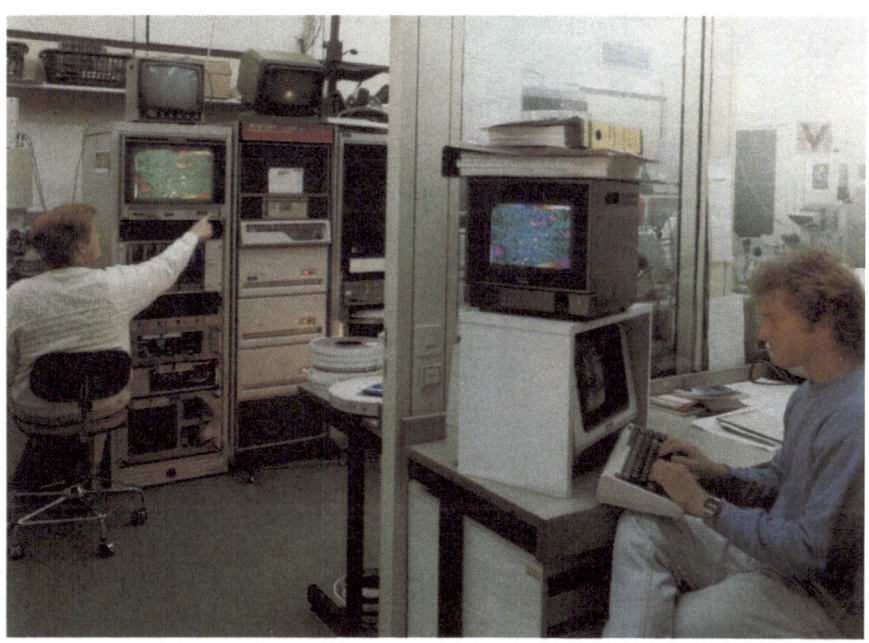

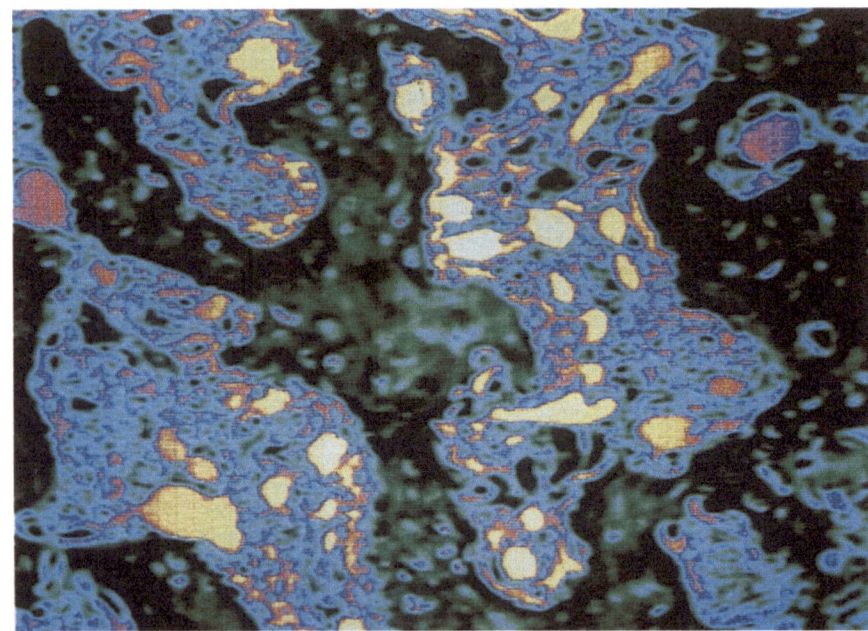

Fig. 123

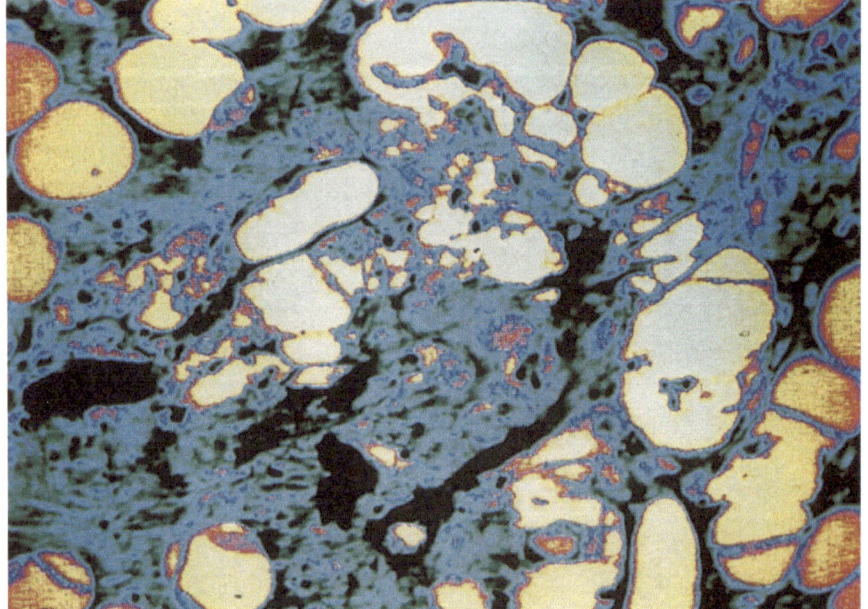

Fig. 124

takes place by video threshold value electronics which have the function of immediately extracting parameters from the current video signal characteristic for the image features. These serve as simple parameters for further description of the images. Since the extracted parameters only contain minimal spatial information, the possibilities of such a very fast, however inexact image analysis are restricted. For a preciser analysis, additional compact units for collecting and processing selected data (modules) are used.

One of them, the binary image module, is designated for storing and processing the information extracted from the video signal data in the form of binary images. These constitute a simplification of grey value images which differentiate two areas (tumor-positive and tumor-negative). These appeared separately from all other areas of the images. For processing binary images by computers, a longer time is necessary than that required for processing the video signal. The advantages are a better utilization of the spatial information of the images by using simple algorithms.

The third grey value image module enables rapid storage of the grey value data obtained by high resolution microscopy. For evaluation of this data, all the possibilities of digital image processing can be utilized. The full image information is available in the form of 256 grey levels with 1024 × 512 image points. For processing such a large amount of data (one image requires 500 kilobytes storage capacity), however, more time is necessary than for binary imaging.

The control of the microscope and the evaluation of the extracted parameters as well as the processing of binary and grey value images requires the use of an efficient computer. For these purposes, we have developed a multi-microcomputer configuration which constitutes the nucleus of the entire system.

The multi-microcomputer ("Heidelberg Polyp") consists of a theoretically unlimited number of microprocessors which permit a random access memory of four gigabytes (4,000,000,000 bytes). The individual processors are linked together by parallel computer buses so that both the parallel execution of programs as well as a reciprocal communication of the processors are possible in any direction and sequence desired. In this way, the necessary computer capacity can be provided by modular extension of the multi-microcomputer system. At present, the "polyp" system consists of six microprocessors with 12 megabyte storage capacity.

The great variability of the pathological problems to be solved by means of a quantitative analysis of histological images frequently requires an adaptation of sophisticated problem-specific programs. Because the multi-microcomputer system is only conceived for rapid execution of relatively simple programs, we have integrated in our system as a superordinate host computer a PTP 11/34 with 30 megabytes plate store and a magnetic type unit. The configuration of the entire system is shown in Fig. 122.

The outstanding feature of our system is its capacity to perform a selection of the extracted features by predetermined processing of the preparations and to adapt these optimally to the problems which have to be solved by means of

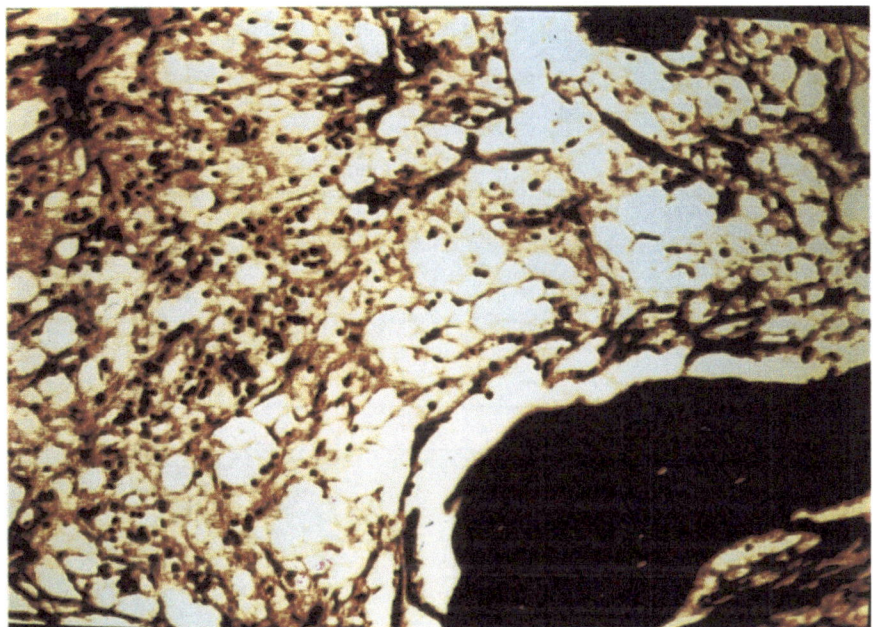

Fig. 125

quantitative analysis. This is carried out by comparing histological structures of test (learning) and investigation preparations. The features subsumed in a flexible matrix allow determination of the basic elements, repetition of which reproduces the entire histological structure and forms a texture characteristic for this structure. On the basis of the properties of the texture, various cell and tissue structures can be distinguished. With the incorporation of texture parameters, we have been able to recognize and register quantitatively the tumor regions which are still detectable microscopically as vital residues of a malignant tumor after pharmacotherapy. The consecutive analysis of serial sections provides the possibility of a three-dimensional reconstruction and thus a more precise description of the growth form of the tumor. This can be

analysed in detail in connection with other tissue elements, e. g., the blood vessels.

Our studies of human bone sarcomas represent an example of an evaluation of residual tumor regions based on texture parameters and, respectively, of the curative effect attained by chemotherapy. They were carried out on material from the Institute of Pathology, University of Münster and aim at an objective, completely automatic evaluation of the histological alterations occurring after chemotherapy. The effect of this therapy is regarded as a function of the size ratio between the vital and nonvital tumor regions. The image processing system has the function of reliably separating all the histological structures present in the preparations and of classifying them into three groups: vital

Tab. 12. Features

| Structures | Fibers | | Arrangement | | Cellularity | Nuclei | |
|---|---|---|---|---|---|---|---|
| | Density | Coarseness | Regular | Irregular | Density of Arrangement | Size | Optical Density |
| Osteosarcoma | ++++ | ++++ | – | +++ | +++ | ++++ | +++ |
| Necrotic | ± | – | – | | | – | – |
| Necrobiotic | ++ | – | – | | | – | – |
| Reparative | +++ | ++ | | | ++ | ++ | ++ |
| Cancelous Bone | – | – | – | | + | + | ++ |
| Bone Marrow | + | + | ++ | – | +++ | +++ | ++ |
| Cartilage | – | – | – | – | + | + | ++ |

Semiquantitative grading:

±) variable intensity;
+) low;
++) moderate;
+++) high;
++++) very high intensity.

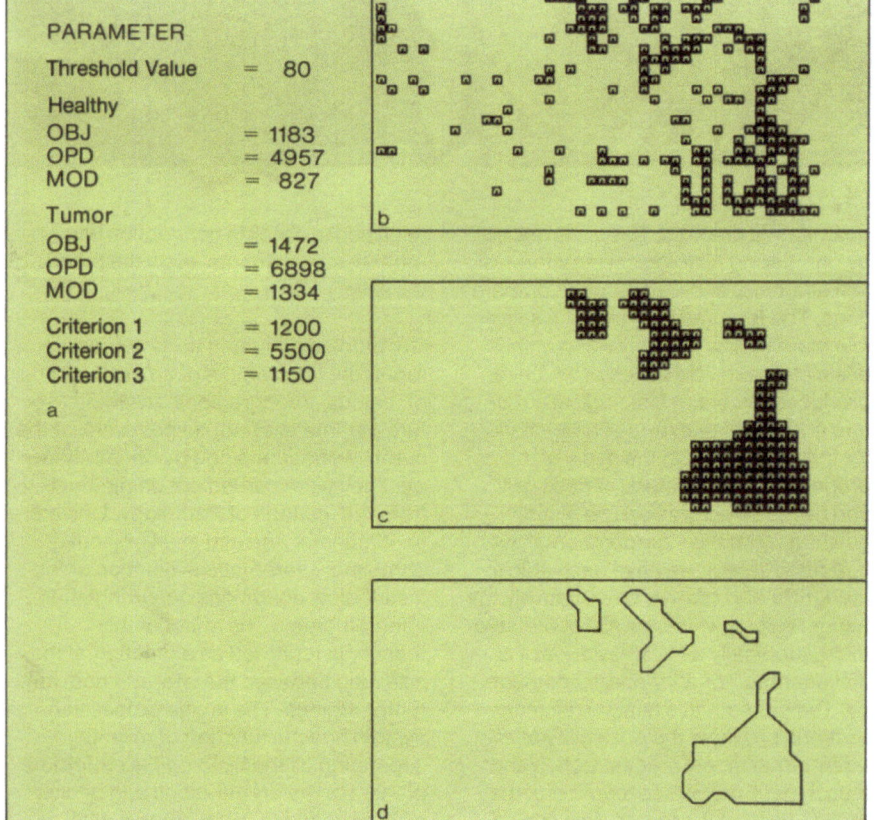

Fig. 126

tumor regions, nonvital regions and unchanged tissue comprising bone, cartilage and bone marrow. The microscopic investigations of the routinely performed histological preparations of osteosarcomas removed surgically after preoperative treatment show that all tissue structures, which can be detected in the removed bone, display identical basic textural elements. These are intensively stained cell nuclei, thin fibers and broad compact trabeculae. The different combination of these elements and differences in their appearance enable the elaboration of a broad spectrum of texture forms. Of special significance for the determination of these forms are differences in size, form and chromatin structure of the nuclei as well as the thickness, orientation and aggregation of the fibers. An analysis of the tissue structures observed shows that many texture forms are based on two basic patterns: fibers and trabeculae. These occur both in the vital and nonvital tumor regions and in the remaining bone tissues.

In the vital tumor regions, two histological forms of osteosarcomas are manifested: highly osteoneogenic forms with a trabecular texture (Fig. 123) and forms in which a fibrous texture dominates over bone texture (Fig. 124). The alterations of the tumor which have taken place in the subsequent therapy can be defined as necrotic and reparatory. The former are characterized by loss of the cell nuclei as a manifestation of the cell death caused by the treatment. The latter are (in general terms) of an inflammatory character and show a reticular fibrous texture (Fig. 125).

The texture of the unchanged bone and cartilage tissue, which is to be seen in any removed bone, can be designated as trabecular, whereas that of the bone marrow can be desginated as fibrous. The different histological tissue structures and their textural features are listed in Tab. 12. The table can serve as a decision matrix in order to select subjective parameters for the characterization of different texture patterns. These parameters are tested in the computer-controlled analysis of the test preparations in which no tumor tissue is to be demonstrated and in the investigation preparations which contain vital tumor regions. The analysis of the preparations shows that, in the discrimination of the characteristic vital tumor region textures, three features are significant: the number of individual objects within a structure (OBJ), their optical density (OPD) as well as the optical density of the objects of a certain size (MOD) (Fig. 126). The results of the image analysis in the application of the characteristics OBJ, OBD and MOD can be detected in a binary image which clearly delimits the vital tumor regions (Fig. 127). The map of the parts of the tumor remaining after the therapy served as a basis for the evaluation of the percentage of these parts in relation to the entire tumor. This is decisive in

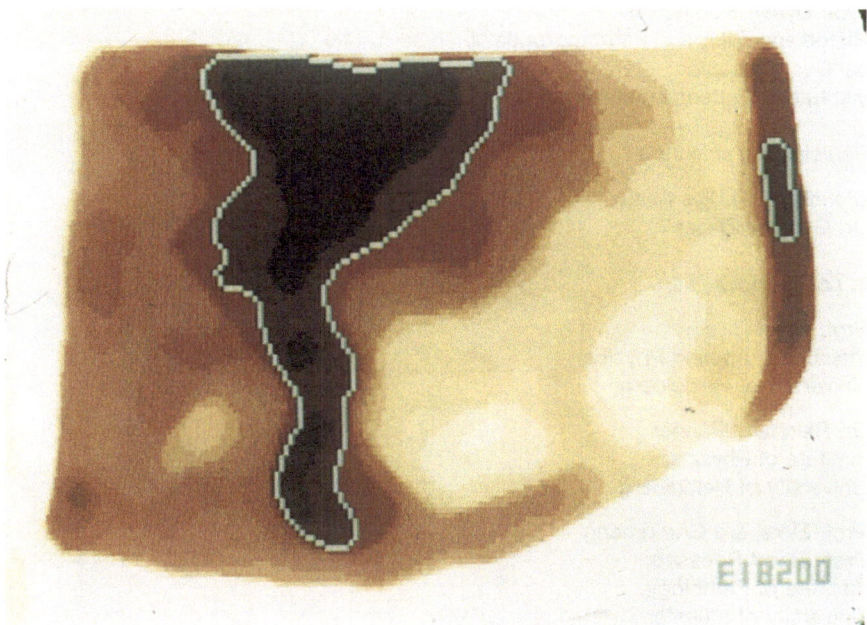

Fig. 127

the estimation of the therapeutic effect achieved. The completely automatic and objective analysis of a large number of serial preparations allows a reliable comparison of various methods of therapy. Our investigations show that the results attained are comparable with those of routine diagnosis during which serial sections are evaluated by usual microscopy.

The discrimination and description of the parts of the tumor surviving after therapeutic treatment is only a relatively simple example of an analysis of the histological images on the basis of textural parameters. The system developed in the Department of Histodiagnostics and Pathomorphological Documentation is also applied in other objects, e. g., detection of metastasis patterns, spreading of the tumors in connection with the

reaction of the connective tissue stroma or description of the chromatin structure of the nuclei according to textural characteristics. Its advantages are rapidity and great flexibility, which is based on the free programmability of the system and which insures optimal adaptation to the tasks of analysis.

Prof. Dymitr Komitowski
Histodiagnostics and Pathomorphologi-
cal Documentation,
Institute of Experimental Pathology

Participating scientists

Dipl. Phys. Tobias Müller
Dr. Gerhard Zinser

In colloboration with

Prof. Josef Bille
Institute of Applied Physics I,
University of Heidelberg

Dr. Reinhard Männer
Institute of Physics,
University of Heidelberg

Prof. Ekkehard Grundmann
Prof. Albert Roessner
Institute of Pathology,
University of Münster

Selected publications

Komitowski, D., Zinser, G.: Digital picture analysis for studying the development of experimentally induced osteosarcoma. J. Cancer Res. Clin. Oncol. 104, 229–236 (1982).

Komitowski, D., Zinser, G., Stute, D.: Digital picture analysis as an integral part of the information system for experimental oncopathology of the German Cancer Research Center. Meth. Inform. Med. 22, 69–74 (1983).

Zinser, G., Komitowski, D.: Segmentation of cell nuclei in tissue section analysis. J. Histochem. 31, 94–100 (1983).

Erhardt, A., Zinser, G., Komitowski, D., Bille, J.: Reconstructing 3-D light-microscopic images by digital image processing. Appl. Opt. 24, 10–15 (1985).

# Appendix

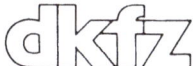

# Institutes

Fig. 128

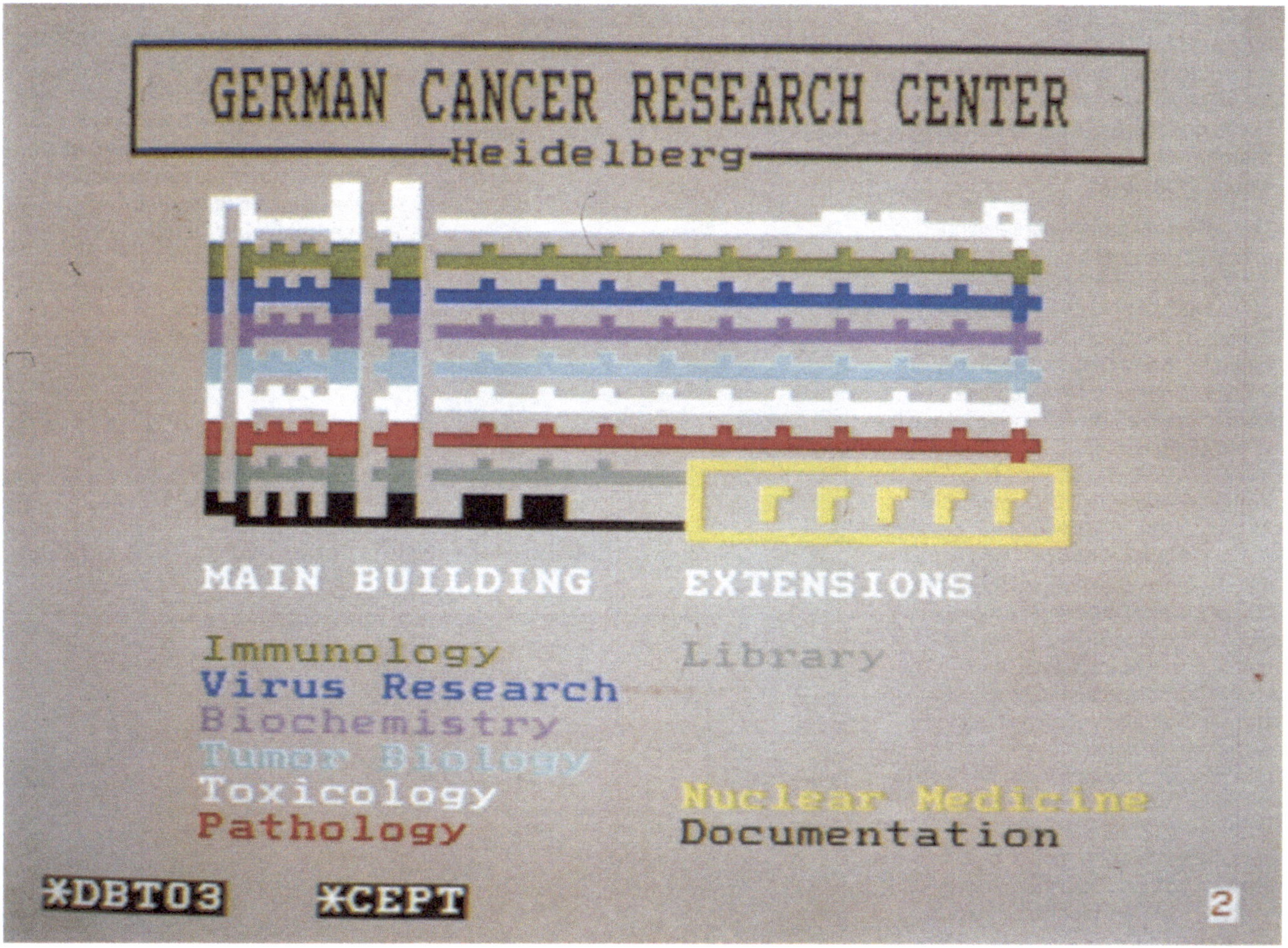

![GERMAN CANCER RESEARCH CENTER Heidelberg teletext graphic]

MAIN BUILDING    EXTENSIONS

Immunology       Library
Virus Research
Biochemistry
Tumor Biology
Toxicology       Nuclear Medicine
Pathology        Documentation

*DBT03   *CEPT

## Institute for Experimental Pathology

### Areas of Research

Cancer develops from cells which deviate from normal cells in their uncoordinated proliferation and defective differentiation. How do normal cells turn into cancer cells? How do cell proliferation and cell differentiation alter during carcinogenesis? How can the recognition of cancer cells and their precursors be improved? What properties of cancer cells determine their sensitivity to chemical or physical treatment procedures? These questions are central to the research work at the Institute of Experimental Pathology.

The individual projects are assigned to the research focal points: "Tumor Biology", "Mechanisms of Carcinogenesis" as well as "Cancer Diagnosis and Therapy". Above and beyond its own projects, the institute fulfills an important function for all research fields of the Deutsches Krebsforschungszentrum by virtue of the contribution by its department for "Histodiagnostics and Pathomorphological Documentation". As long as the diagnosis of tumors and tumor precursors can only be verified histologically, the morphological detection and classification of pathological tissue changes is not only the decisive basis of cancer therapy in humans, but is also an indispensable precondition for correct evaluation of many findings in experimental cancer research. The institute regards it as its special function to correlate defined morphological changes which are characteristic for carcinogenesis and cancer growth with results of other disciplines such as toxicology, virology, biochemistry or molecular biology.

Thus, besides conventional morphological and modern micromorphological techniques, such as electron microscopy and cytometry, cytochemical, biochemical and molecular biological methods are also used in the different departments and project groups of the institute. In addition, the institute runs a tumor bank which provides standardized investigation material to numerous research groups within and outside the Deutsches Krebsforschungszentrum. By means of a "Cancer Encyclopedia" which will be available as videotex, the institute makes a contribution to information and clarification of the public on the current state of cancer research.

The work in the four departments and the three project groups of the institute set up at the beginning of 1985 is concentrated in the following fields:

- Study of the sequence of cellular alterations in the development of various epithelial and mesenchymal tumor types, especially in the liver, skin, kidneys and bone;
- investigations on the mechanism of diaplacental carcinogenesis;
- studies of the interaction of viral and chemical carcinogenic factors in experimental skin carcinogenesis;
- investigations of the structure of enzymes which have a key role in the regulation of cell metabolism and the metabolism of foreign substances;
- investigations of regulatory disorders of carbohydrate metabolism during carcinogenesis in the liver and kidneys;

Fig. 129

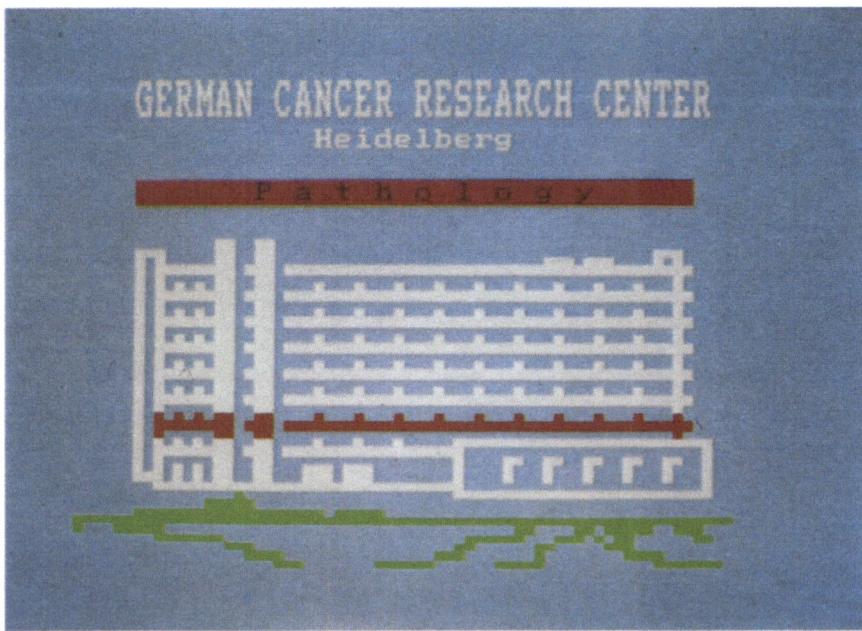

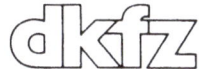

- investigations on the regulation of the differentiation in the skin and in teratocarcinoma cells;
- pathomorphological diagnosis and quantitative evaluation of experimental pathological findings with methods of image processing;
- testing of new parameters for the application of cytometry and image processing in "assisting diagnostics" of human tumors;
- further development of an information system of experimental oncopathology;
- development of cytometric techniques for quantitative and rapid analysis of chromosome alterations;
- study of the heterogeneity and therapy resistance of experimental and human tumors;
- investigations on the role of the liver in the body's own tumor defense.

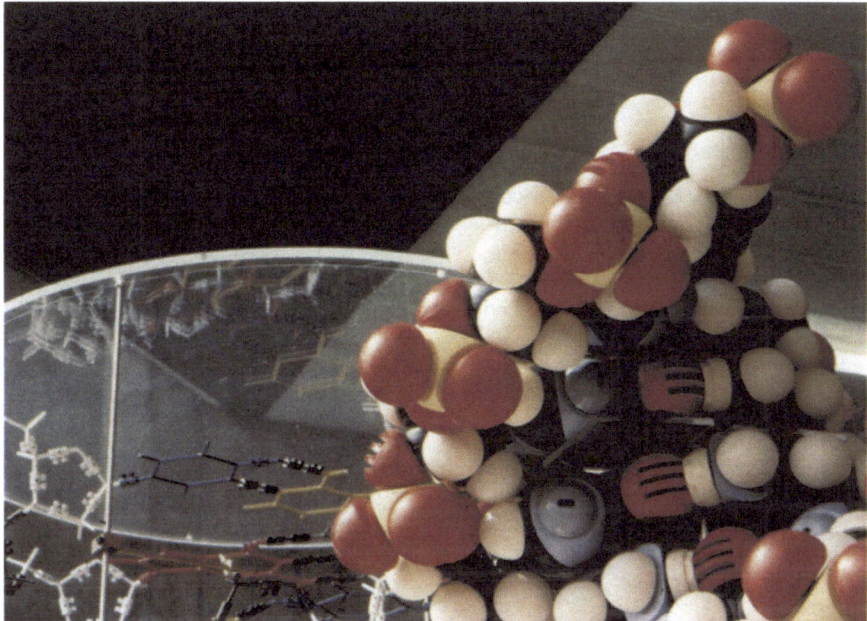

Fig. 130

Executive Director:

Prof. Peter Bannasch

Departments and their Heads:

Cell Pathology:
Prof. Peter Bannasch

Cell Biology:
Prof. Manfred Volm

Pathochemistry:
Prof. Volker Kinzel

Histodiagnostics and Pathomorphological Documentation:
Prof. Dymitr Komitowski

Project groups and their heads:

Cytometry and Chromosome Sorting, Tumor Bank:
Prof. Klaus Goerttler

Regulation of Differentiation:
Prof. Angel Alonso

Cancer Encyclopedia:
Prof. Klaus Goerttler
Dr. Rudolf Süss

## Institute of Toxicology and Chemotherapy

### Areas of Research

The function of the Institute of Toxicology and Chemotherapy is to detect carcinogenic chemical compounds in the human environment, to establish the degree of danger to man and the mechanism of action of carcinogenesis as well as the extent to which this can be influenced.

The institute contributes to the control of cancer disease by developing of new chemotherapeutical drugs and new animal experimental methods, investigating anticancer drugs as well as counselling in clinical treatment of tumor patients.

The institute participates in the research focal points of research "Carcinogenic Factors and Cancer Prevention" and "Therapy of Cancer Diseases".

The work of the institute is concentrated on

– the detection of carcinogenic substances in the human environment; substances which occur in food, air and water or which are used as drugs and of which the chemical structure suggests a suspicion of carcinogenic activity, are investigated as to whether they induce cancer in animals. This can have consequences for regulations.

– The investigation of chemical compounds for genotoxic action. It is a generally accepted theory that cancer diseases develop by changes in the cellular macromolecules important for inheritance. Chemical compounds which occur in the human environment or which serve as drugs are characterized in bacterial test systems and cell cultures of rat livers for their mutagenic (genetic substance-altering) properties. In this way, a preselection of substances is made which are later investigated for their carcinogenic action in mammals. Genotoxic metabolic products of carcinogenic substances are demonstrated with the test systems.

– Testing of the perinatal and prenatal effect of chemical compounds and viruses. For most tumors, which occur in children and adolescents (leukemias, tumors of the central nervous system, the kidneys and the connective tissue), the cause cannot be demonstrated epidemiologically. This can only be done by animal experiments. The similarity of infant tumors in humans and experimental animals shows that their causes are to be looked for in a lesion which is produced just before or immediately after birth by carcinogens (environmental poisons, viruses, drugs).

– Dose-effect relations in carcinogens; carcinogens or carcinogen combinations are administered in graduated doses to experimental animals. The chemical structure and the ingested dose of a carcinogen decide on the intensity and direction of its effect in the body. Experiments of this kind also allow inferences with regard to the effect of very tiny doses to which human beings are exposed.

Fig. 131

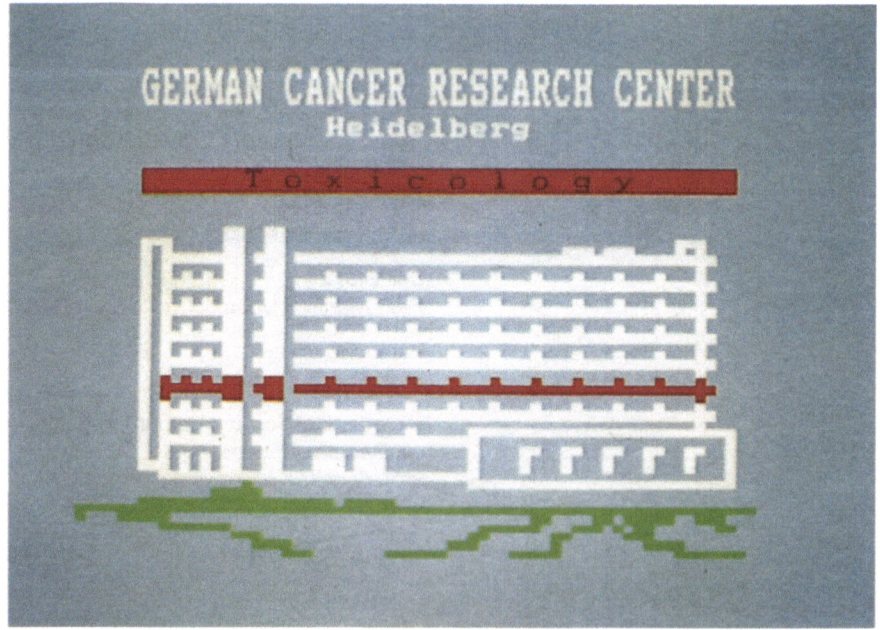

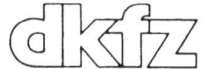

- Analysis of carcinogenic N-nitro compounds in the environment and body fluids of highly exposed people; N-nitroso compounds proved to be strong carcinogens in experiments in many animal species. They occur in foods, can be formed in the stomach from amines and nitrite and arise from volatile amines and nitrogen oxides in the air in certain industrial processes. The risk to individual persons exposed to N-nitroso compounds (above all at the place of work) can only be detected when the exposure in terms of duration and level (e. g. from contaminated food or air) can be related to the amounts of their metabolic and excretory products detectable in body fluids.

- The investigation of the mechanisms of action and the metabolism of N-nitroso compounds; uptake, transport and metabolism of carcinogens as well as the distribution of the metabolic and reaction products in the body and their excretion decide on the intensity of their carcinogenic action and the site of tumor development. Knowledge of these processes enables the elaboration of methods and substances to influence carcinogenesis.

- The influence of chemical carcinogenesis; substances which are suitable in terms of their chemical structure to inhibit the metabolism of carcinogenic compounds, to intercept metabolic products or to prevent their reaction with the macromolecules of the cell, are tested for their effectiveness in comparable animal experiments and biochemical experiments. The objective of this research is to prevent the carcinogenic action of chemical compounds (anti-carcinogenesis).

- Elaboration of animal experimental models for the toxicological and therapeutic investigation of anti-cancer drugs; the drugs used in the treatment of cancer patients can cause side effects which are frequently only recognized very late. Thus, depending on the administered dose, many chemotherapeutical drugs have an injurious effect on the bone marrow, heart, lungs or bladder. In the long term, other chemotherapeutical drugs are themselves carcinogenic. The side effects restrict the applicability of the substances. Animal tumors with properties similar to those of human tumors allow a short-term evaluation of the efficacy and side effects of known and new chemotherapeutical drugs and their combinations.

- Attempts to reduce the toxicity of anticancer drugs; besides the desired tumor-inhibitory effects, cancer chemotherapeutics also have adverse effects which limit their applicability. These effects are caused either by the substances themselves or their metabolic products in the body. All reactions which inhibit the vital biochemical and cellular processes of the body to a greater extent than tumor growth are undesirable. These reactions can be reduced or prevented completely by an administration of substances which either support the vital body functions or which intercept the metabolic products which are toxic for the entire body and cause their excretion. By means of animal experiments, therapeutic methods based on these insights have been developed which reduce the undesired effects of the anti-cancer drugs methotrexate and bleomycin. In this way, long-term tumor regression could be attained in patients with carcinomas in the head and neck region without the toxic side effects which are otherwise usual.

- Development of new cancer chemotherapeutical drugs; this highly expensive and personnel-intensive field can only be worked on at certain points, e. g. with the class of the chloronitrosourea compounds. In addition, screening is also carried out for substances or classes of substance which might open up new principles in cancer chemotherapy.

Executive Director:

Prof. Dietrich Schmähl

Departments and their Heads:

Carcinogenesis and Chemotherapy:
Prof. Dietrich Schmähl

Perinatal Toxicology:
Prof. Stanislav Ivankovic

Experimental Chemotherapy:
Prof. Hans Osswald

Metabolism of N-Nitroso Compounds:
Priv.-Doz. Dr. Manfred Wießler

Environmental Carcinogens:
Prof. Rudolf Preußmann

## Institute of Cell and Tumor Biology

### Areas of Research

Malignant growth is manifested by cell proliferation which kills the host by invasive and metastatic spreading. Investigations on the growth and division of cells, the regulation of cell functions and the nature of mutual influences on cells are of course the given fields of work in an institute concerned with cellular research in the context of cancer research. In 1980, three departments ("Molecular Biology of the Cell I and II" and "Membrane Biology and Biochemistry") were integrated into the institute, which led to the renaming of the Institute of Cell Research as "Institute of Cell and Tumor Biology". The fields of research at the institute, which are classified almost exclusively under the focal point research "Tumor Biology", were thus extended. The projects at the institute are concerned with the following problems:

– organization of the mitotic apparatus of the cell, description of the course of cell division on the ultrastructural and molecular level;
– investigations on the regulation of growth at the level of genome replication and via the regulation of cell function at the level of expression of genetic information;
– investigations on cell-cell interactions with various models such as invasion of tumor aggregates into receptor tissue;
– investigations on problems of metastasis in tumor lines with differing malignancy as well as investigations on the problem of cells "settling" on certain substrates;
– control of gene function in animal cells, transmission of genetic information from the genetic material in biological molecules;
– membrane behavior of the cell, behavior and formation of the cell surface in normal cells and during tumorigenesis;
– behavior of the cytoskeleton in normal and transformed cells;
– use of antibodies against cytoskeletal proteins for differential tumor diagnosis.

Executive Director:

Prof. Werner Franke

Departments and their Heads:

Membrane Biology and Biochemistry:
Prof. Werner Franke

Growth and Division of the Cell:
Prof. Neidhard Paweletz

Molecular Biology of the Cell I:
Prof. Günther Schütz

Molecular Biology of the Cell II:
Prof. Walter Keller

Biochemistry of the Cell:
Prof. Dieter Werner

Project Group:
Molecular Biology of Mitosis:
Prof. Herwig Ponstingl

Fig. 132

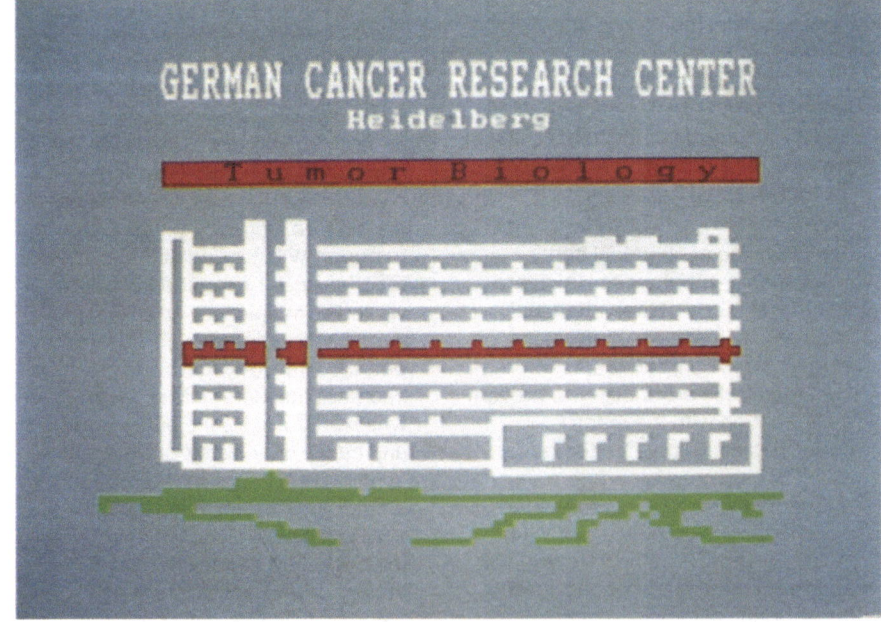

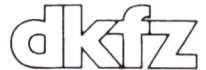

## Institute of Biochemistry

### Areas of Research

The institute is concerned with the exploration of the biological and biochemical basis of carcinogenesis, especially biochemical factors. Its research activities deal with the research focal points "Tumor biology", "Mechanism of Carcinogenesis", "Carcinogenic Factors" as well as "Diagnosis and Therapeutic Research". The work of the institute is mainly concentrated in the following fields:

– Exploration of the physiological basis of normal cells. Isolation, characterization and clarification of the mechanism of action of the tissue's own substances regulating cell division, especially in mouse skin in vivo and in vitro (chalons) as a model for regulation of growth and differentiation processes; biochemical mechanism of the action of humoral factors controlling proliferation, especially in connection with wound healing. Analysis of the influence of the factors on epidermal differentiation and keratinization.
– Exploration of the basis of neoplastic transformation of normal cells. Metabolism and mechanism of action of tumor initiators (polycyclic aromatic hydrocarbons, nitrosamines) and tumor promoters (diterpene esters, drugs, environmental chemicals, endogenous factors) on the model systems mouse skin and rat liver; interaction of the active form of solitary carcinogens with cellular macromolecules in simple biological model systems, especially biochemistry of the carcinogen-induced DNA repair and promoter-induced development of tumor cells. Investigation of

chromosome alterations and disorders of differentiation in spontaneous and promoter-induced malignant transformation of epithelial cells in culture.
– The occurrence and distribution of cocarcinogens, especially tumor promoters, in the environment and their chemical and biological characterization.

Executive Director:

Prof. Erich Hecker

Departments and their Heads:

Mechanism of Tumorigenesis:
Prof. Erich Hecker

Molecular Toxicology:
Prof. Werner Kunz

Biochemistry of Tissue-specific Regulation:
Prof. Friedrich Marks

Differentiation and Carcinogenesis in vitro:
Prof. Norbert Fusenig

Interaction of Carcinogens with Macromolecules in Biological Systems:
Dr. Dr. Heinz-Walter Thielmann

Fig. 133

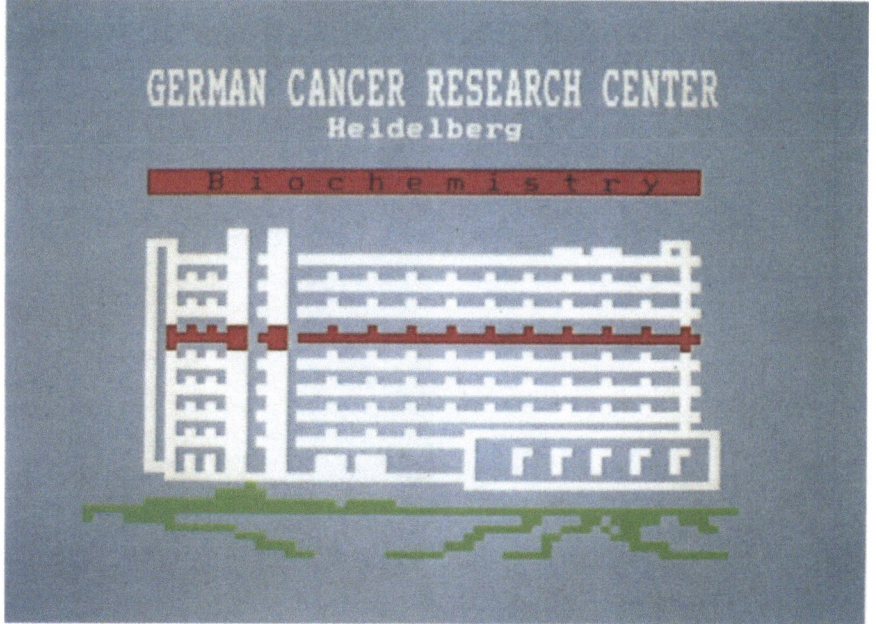

## Institute of Virus Research

### Areas of Research

The institute is engaged in the investigation of biological and molecular biological mechanisms of carcinogenesis induced by SV 40 and papilloma viruses, human pathogenic herpes viruses, retroviruses as well as cell transformation experiments with these viruses in cell culture, the search for the site of integration of the virus in the tumor cell, for virus-induced proteins and antigens in tumor cells, physical and biological gene mapping, biology of interferons and interferon inducers, electron microscopy, tumor induction in laboratory animals. A special focal point is the search for viruses as causative agents of tumors and leukemia in man; a further focal point is the investigation of antiviral and antitumoral substances.

Executive Director:

Prof. Klaus Munk

Departments and their Heads:

Human Tumour Viruses:
Prof. Klaus Munk

Molecular Biology of
DNA Tumour Viruses:
Prof. Gerhard Sauer

Tumour Virus Genetics:
Prof. Hans Christian Kaerner

Genome Modifications and Carcinogenesis:
Prof. Lutz Gissmann

Tumour Virus Immunology
Prof. Holger Kirchner

Fig. 134

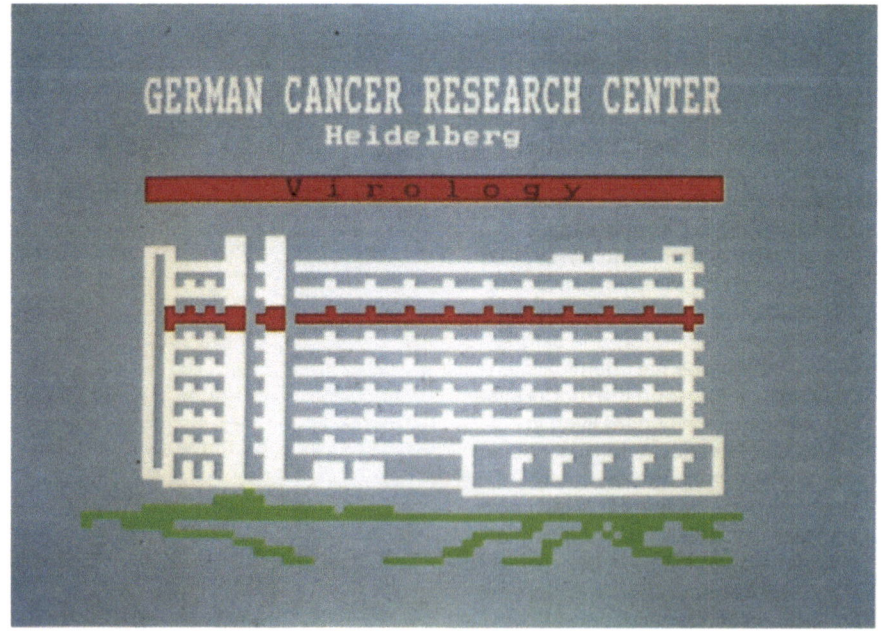

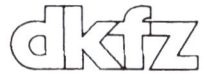

## Institute of Immunology and Genetics

### Areas of Research

The work of the institute is concentrated on new immunological methods of tumor diagnosis as well as on immunological concepts for tumor therapy and on the investigation of the biological mechanisms of cellular interactions and metastatic processes.

- A focal point of research is the production of monoclonal antibodies with specificity for tumor-associated antigens.
- Several projects are concerned with the regulation of the immune system: this includes the investigation of immunoregulatory products of tumor cells, identification and biochemical characterization of lymphokines and investigations on the immunogenicity of mutagenized tumor cell lines. In connection with the regulation of the immune system, antigen receptors and lymphokine receptors are also being investigated inter alia.
  A further focal point is the expression of membrane antigens on cells. In this connection, not only tumor-specific antigens, but also viral antigens and in particular histocompatibility antigens are being investigated. Inter alia, the role of these antigens in the immunological struggle between the host and the tumor is being investigated.
- Another focal point of the work of the institute are the mechanisms of tumor invasion and development of metastases.
- The development of new therapeutic concepts on an immunological basis is an important goal of research to which there are different approaches in all departments of the institute. These investigations take into account that in many cases tumor cells are recognized by the immune system so that they can be potentially eliminated, and that, on the other hand, so far unknown regulatory mechanisms can prevent protective immune responses against tumor cells.

Executive Director from 1984–1986:

Prof. Wulf Dröge

Departments and their Heads:

Immuno-Chemistry:
Prof. Wulf Dröge

Immuno-Genetics:
Prof. Peter Krammer

Somatic Genetics:
Prof. Günter Hämmerling

Cellular Immunology:
Prof. Volker Schirrmacher

Fig. 135

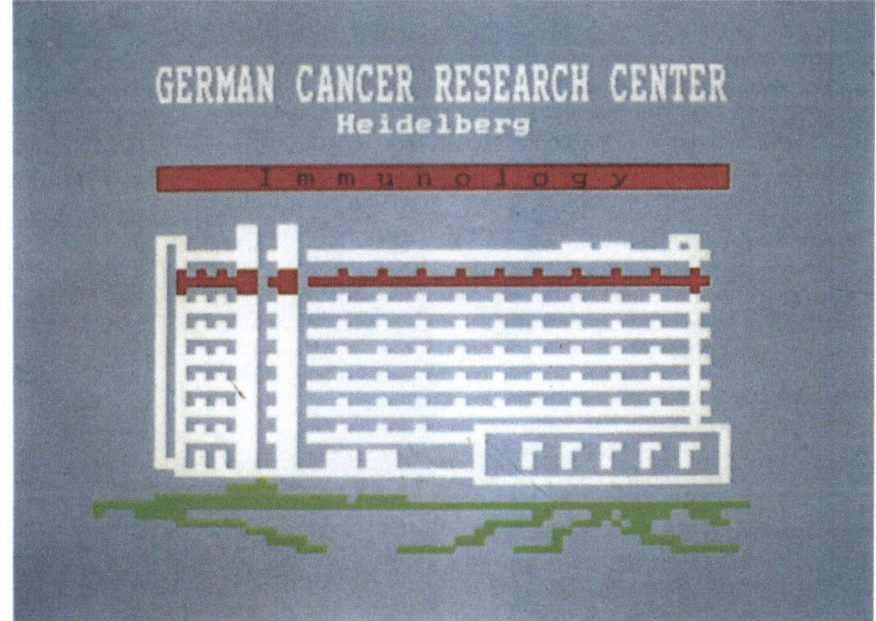

# Institute of Nuclear Medicine

## Areas of Research

Radiology is one of the most important scientific disciplines for diagnosis, therapeutic planning, treatment and follow-up of cancer. Besides the familiar radiological diagnosis and therapy techniques, the special designation "radiology" today also includes the new methods using nonionizing radiation such as ultrasound or electromagnetic waves for the purposes mentioned.

The task of the institute is to do radiological and nuclear medical research in the field of oncology. New radiological methods are therefore being developed for tumor diagnosis and therapy and are being evaluated in clinical studies. Exploration of carcinogenesis by ionizing radiation in humans is one of the fields of interest.

After the transfer of the department "Nuclear Medical Diagnosis" (Head: Prof. Peter Georgi) to the Radiological Center at the University of Heidelberg in 1984, the following research activities have priority:

- radiotherapeutic research
- magnetic resonance tomography and spectroscopy (MRT and MRS)
- positron emission tomography (PET)
- immunoscintigraphy

"Radiotherapy Research" is a cooperative research project which is being carried out together with clinical partners at the Mannheim-Heidelberg Tumor Center, especially at the Radiological and the Neurosurgical Hospitals of the University of Heidelberg. A constituent project of this research field will be concerned with the combined application of

radiotherapy and local hyperthermia in the treatment of brain tumors.

The research objectives of modern oncological diagnosis not only include the diagnosis and localization of a tumor, but also the investigation of its metabolism and microcirculation before and during therapy.

The work of the institute will in the future be supported by two new departments: Department of Tumor Biochemistry and Department of Applied Immunology.

Executive Director:

Prof. Walter J. Lorenz, Ph.D.

Departments and their Heads:

Special Oncological Diagnostics and Therapy:
Prof. Gerhard van Kaick, M.D.

Biophysics and Medical Radiation Physics:
Prof. Walter J. Lorenz, Ph.D.

Radiochemistry and Radiopharmacology:
Dr. Wolfgang Maier-Borst, Ph.D.

Biochemistry of Tumors:
(N.N.)

Applied Immunology:
(N.N.)

Fig. 136

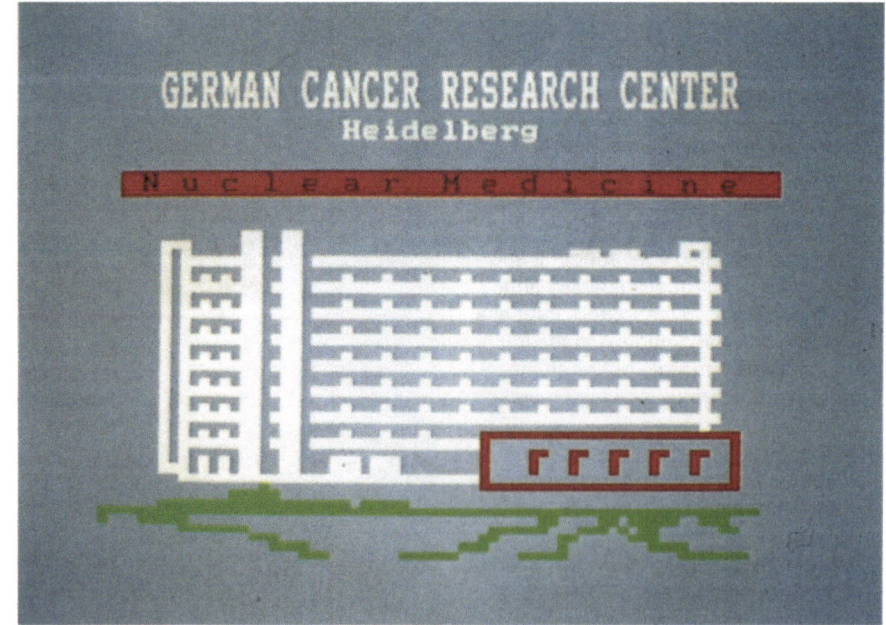

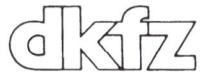

## Institute of Documentation, Information and Statistics

### Areas of Research

The broad spectrum of work at the Institute of Documentation, Information and Statistics is covered by four departments.

The Department of Cancer Documentation and Epidemiology is responsible, inter alia, for maintaining the epidemiological bone tumor registry for the Federal Republic of Germany. Bone tumors were chosen as a model for registration because, on the one hand, they are a rare tumor form which can be dealt with in organizational terms by a single central collection point in the Federal Republic and, on the other hand, because their cause remains largely unclarified. In addition, this department is carrying out retrospective and prospective epidemiological studies (as far as these are at all any longer possible in view of the present legal situation) and clinical cancer documentation projects (e. g. for the Tumor Center Heidelberg/Mannheim) are being advised. In the context of the working group of the Deutsches Krebsforschungszentrum, the department coordinates the standardized clinical documentation of all cancer patients in the Federal Republic of Germany (the "basic documentation" for tumor patients and the organ-specific tumor documentation based thereon).

Together with the French Cancer Research Center in Paris the working group Literature Documentation in this department is jointly responsible for the literature information system CANCER-NET (formerly SABIR C). This covers the entire international cancer literature and has been jointly developed by the two institutes.

The mathematical formulation of theoretical models, which describe the essential aspects of cancer growth and spreading, is the field of work of the Department of Mathematical Models. The mathematical and biological model concepts developed are illustrated and largely explored by computer simulation as numerical experiments. The staff of the department cooperate closely with scientists oriented toward biological theory on the one hand and "applied" mathematicians on the other hand in order to obtain a basis for the development and treatment of mathematical models. The results obtained correspond to confirmed experimental data and serve to elaborate theories and to support new hypotheses.

The Department of Biostatistics has the function of advising experimental scientists of the center and clinical researchers of the Heidelberg/Mannheim Tumor Center with regard to optimal use of the available facilities in order to obtain a maximum of information with as low an effort as possible. The basis of this many-sided work is intensive scientific research in the field of mathematical-statistical methods in order to be able to carry out problem-specific data analyses on this basis.

The functions of central data processing were transferred to a central facility of the Deutsches Krebsforschungszentrum in 1985.

Fig. 137

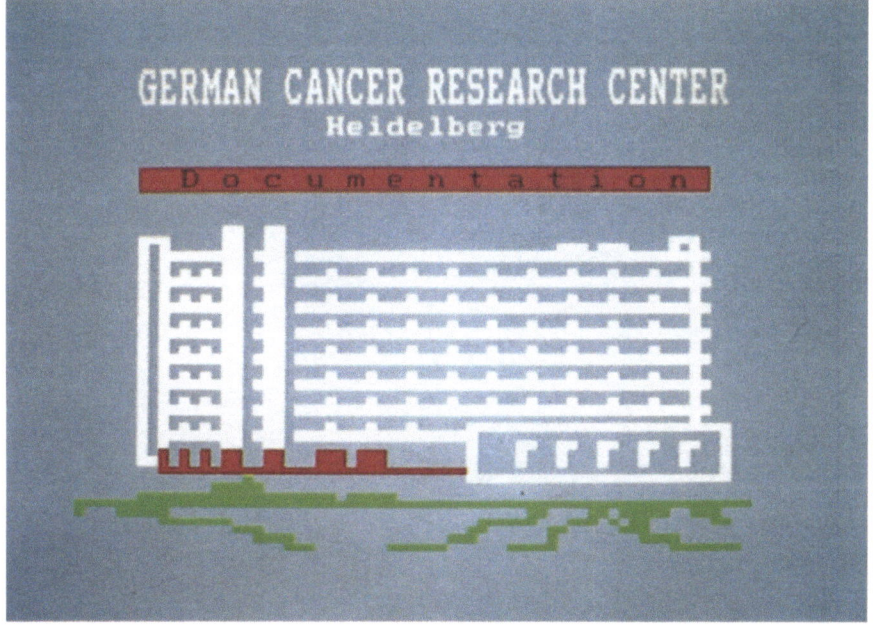

The Department of Medical and Biological Information is working on problems of bioenergetics, image processing, analysis of biological sequences, information processing in the health service, and is concerned with producing software systems which belong to the "fourth generation".

With its departments of Cancer Documentation and Epidemiology as well as Biostatistics, the institute participates in the focal research area "carcinogenic factors and cancer prevention". Above and beyond this, all departments are engaged in further research activity in the public interest. The "Clearing-House for On-Going Research in Cancer Epidemiology", developed jointly with the International Agency for Research on Cancer (Lyon), the reference center for German-speaking countries in the international project for standardization of medical terminology of the Council for International Organizations of Medical Sciences (CIOMS), the coordination of multiclinical field studies for the validation of the TNM system (tumor, node, metastasis) of the Union Internationale Contre le Cancer (UICC) and the development of a thesaurus for oncology in cooperation with the Centre National de la Recherche Scientifique in Villejuif (Paris) are to be mentioned in particular.

Executive Director:
Prof. Jürgen Wahrendorf
(1. 5. 86)

Departments and their Heads:

Cancer Documentation and Epidemiology:
Prof. Jürgen Wahrendorf
(1. 5. 86)

Mathematical Models:
Prof. Petre Tautu

Biostatistics:
Prof. Ernst Weber

Medical and Biological Informatics:
Priv. Doz. Dr. Claus O. Köhler

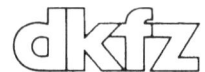

# Central Facilities

## Central Library

The work of the Central Library encompasses the collection, cataloguing and provision of the scientific literature relevant for the Deutsches Krebsforschungszentrum.

Besides this, the Central Library looks after the eight research libraries maintained in the various departments and allocates the German-language journals for evaluation in the in-house data base CANCERNET.

The literature collection by the library is focused on the entire literature on cancer. In addition, literature which is oriented toward the research activities in the Center, above all that from the disciplines biochemistry, genetics, immunology, molecular biology, radiation medicine, environmental research, virology and cell research, is collected.

At present, 830 journals are subscribed to. Total stocks comprise about 43,000 volumes. In the eight institute libraries, 180 journals and 9,000 books are available in addition.

The holdings of the Central Library and the institute libraries are listed in an alphabetical and in a key word catalog in the form of card indexes; in addition, searches for authors and for key words can be carried out via a data monitor connected to the Center's own computer.

Since 1979, lists of new acquisitions have been published every two months and lists of journals as required. These lists are distributed within the Center and to interested outside institutes and scientists.

The reading room has seats for 52 readers. The books and bound journals are arranged in subject groups in open access. The most recent journal issues are arranged alphabetically in a display of periodicals. Books can be taken out for one week within the building; journals cannot be borrowed, but three copying machines (one of them a coin-operated copier) are available (about 1.7 million copies in 1984); in addition, a microfiche monitor with copy-back facility is available.

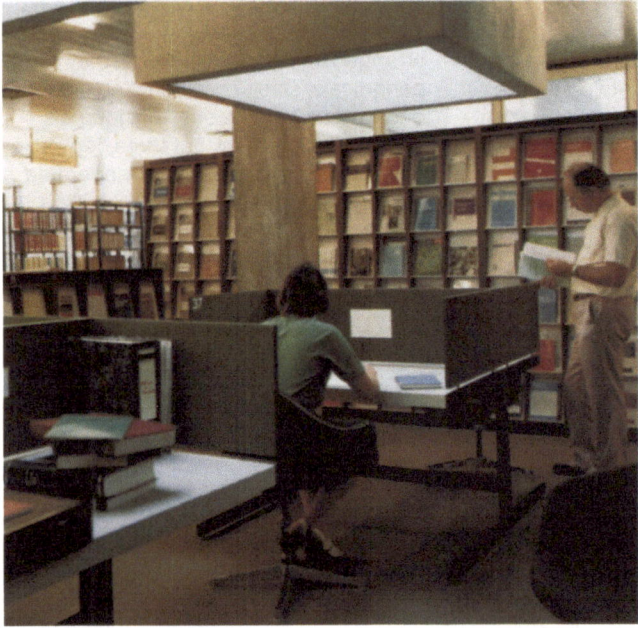

Fig. 138 a
Central library

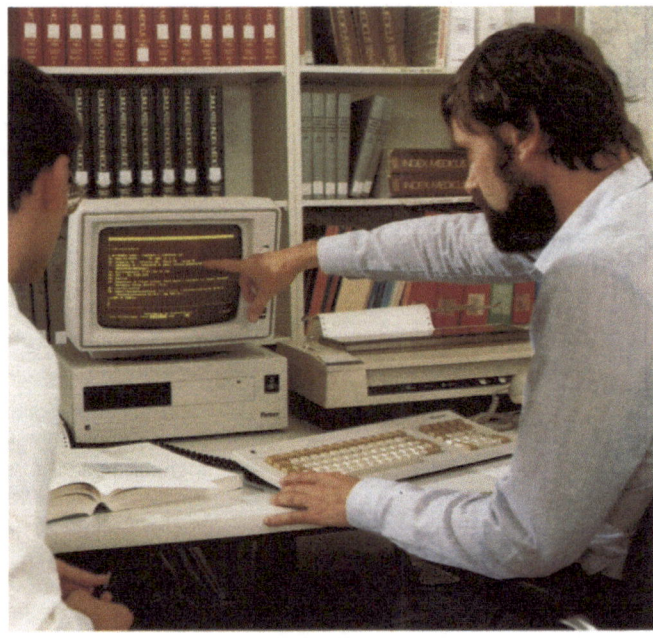

Fig. 138 b
Users and information procurement in the online
literature research

The job of the information center, which is an annex of the Central Library, is to provide the researchers at the Deutsches Krebsforschungszentrum with the bibliographic information they need. It thus supports them in bibliographic searches and supplements their own information obtained from colleagues. Bibliographic information is mainly offered by searching on-line data bases. About 60 of these data files (also including factual data banks which allow direct information without recourse to the literature) are being used at present. Almost the entire spectrum of oncologically relevant and multidisciplinary data bases are thus available. The bibliographic files among these represent a total of almost 100 million items. The on-line connections comprise the data base supplier DIMDI (German Institute for Medical Documentation and Information) in Cologne, the Information Service for Energy, Physics and Mathematics in Karlsruhe, Dialog Information Services in Palo Alto, California, as well as the in-house data base CANCERNET.

Apart from the staff of the Deutsches Krebsforschungszentrum, the library and the information center are also available to scientists and students of the University of Heidelberg as well as to other external researchers dealing with cancer-related problems.

Opening times of the library:
Monday to Friday: 9 a.m. to 10 p.m. and
Saturday:          9 a.m. to 12 a.m.

Service times of the information center:
Monday to Friday: 9 a.m. to 12 a.m. and
                  2 p.m. to 5 p.m.

Head of the library:
Christa Pinkernell

Deputy Head of the library:
Rolf-Peter Kraft

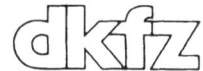

Selection of the data bases available in the information center

| Data base | Specialty |
| --- | --- |
| BIOSIS (Biosciences Information Service) | entire biological sciences |
| CA Search (Chemical Abstracts Search) | chemistry, biochemistry |
| Cancerlit (Cancer Literature) | oncology |
| CANCERNET | oncology |
| Cancerproj (Cancer Research Projects) | oncology, research projects currently in progress |
| Clinprot (Clinical Cancer Protocols) | clinical studies, cancer chemotherapy, factual data bank |
| Embase (Excerpta Medica Data Base) | biological medicine, pharmacy |
| FSTA (Food Science and Technology Abstracts | nutrition and food sciences |
| INIS (International Nuclear Information System) | nuclear medicine |
| MEDLARS (Medical Literature Analysis and Retrieval System) | biological medicine |
| Scisearch (Science Citation Index Search) | total exact sciences, multidisciplinary |
| Toxline (Toxicology Information On-line) | toxicology, invironmental research |

## Central Animal Laboratory

Advance in biochemical research is the cornerstone to improvement in human (and animal) health and welfare. Biomedical research still requires experimental animals. Animal experiments have made major contributions to our knowledge on biological processes, especially on the understanding of cancer. However, it is still urgently necessary to carry out fundamental and applied research in order to develop methods for improved diagnosis, treatment and prevention.

The German Cancer Research Center recognizes both a scientific and the ethical responsibility in animals keeping. Everyone who works with animals must share the responsibility for their general well-being. The central animal laboratory is responsible for ensuring that all animals used in research are housed and used in compliance with the Animal Protection Law. The animal laboratory is a professionally managed unit comprising experienced veterinarians, diagnostic laboratory technicians and trained animal keepers. The manager of the laboratory is directly responsible to the Management Board with regard to the observation of all legal and other regulations. Besides general animal management, the animal laboratory has an advisory function in the application of techniques designed to preserve the health and physical well-being of the animals it looks after. It is supported in this by two important bodies, the animal protection commission founded in the Center in 1985 and the Department of Biostatistics.

The primary role of the animal protection commission is to weigh the employment of experimental animals against the be-

nefit which may result from new knowledge. Recent experience in other centers has shown that the critical awareness of the scientists concerned is made more acute by the work of such a commission. Whereas the statutory regulations constitute a basis for controlling animal experiments, the commission established in the Cancer Research Center will be responsible for their detailed interpretation.

Biostatistics plays a major role in the planning of scientifically based experiments. The proviso that a minimum of animals must be used is just as important as the employment of an adequate number of animals, so that the results of each experiment are reliable. This greatly reduces the necessity of trial repetition. Statistical methods of analysis also help to evaluate and thus control those variables inherent in all animal experiments.

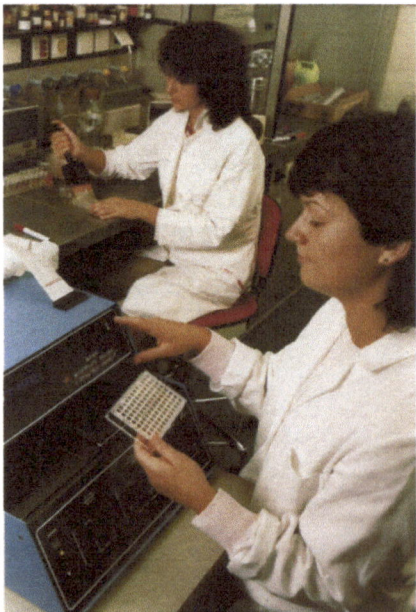

Many variables influence animals and their reaction to the effects of the environment to the same extent as they affect our daily life. Protection from diseases, regular and balanced diet, control of climate and maintenance of important biological rhythms are just as important as careful handling and clean cages. The Animal Laboratory has an intensive program for health surveillance based upon a regular surveillance of microbiological status. This means that not only clinically sick animals are examined but that the presence of sub-clinically infections is also closely monitored.

In the past two years, a rebuilding programme for the main animal laboratories has been planned. The objectives are to reduce still further the incidence of spontaneous disease and to improve the climatic control of the holding rooms. These measures, it is hoped, will reduce the variability in experimental results and thus lead to a reduction in the number of animals required.

Head:
Dr. Peter Eaton

Deputy Head:
Dr. Werner Nicklas

Fig. 139
The animals in the animal laboratory are regularly checked for their state of health. Here laboratory assistants evaluate a test (ELISA),with which freedom from infections is demonstrated

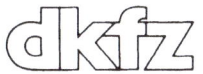

# Central Spectroscopy

The Central Spectroscopy Department (ZAGS) serves all departments of the Cancer Research Center and assists in research activities that require spectroscopic analytical methods.

The work carried out involves the recording of infrared, ultraviolet, mass and nuclear magnetic resonance spectra. Such spectra are required for the identification, characterization, structure elucidation and purity determination of natural products and other compounds employed in cancer research.

The main emphasis is on collaboration with departments of the Deutsches Krebsforschungszentrum whose research activities comprise fields of chemical analysis and the chemistry of natural substances (carcinogens, cocarcinogens and their metabolic products) as well as the synthesis of organic compounds.

Besides the measurement and evaluation of the spectra, a further function of the ZAGS is the documentation and archiving of the measured spectra by means of electronic data processing. For complete characterization of a compound, the chemical structure must be stored in a form which can be processed digitally. With regard to the interpretation of the spectra and the identification of substances, the spectral data must be supplemented with relevant reference spectra. These are derived in part from our own measurements as well as from the literature or commercially available data banks. Thus, important preconditions for the computer-assisted analysis of spectra are created.

The spectroscopic information system SPEKTREN has been developed which requires practically no special expertise of the user. These programs enable recall and output of spectra on the monitor or plotters, printout of the substance name, molecular weight, the empirical formula as well as the two-dimensional representation of the stored chemical structure. Furthermore, SPEKTREN allows an automated analysis by means of spectral comparison. Correlations between spectroscopic features and chemical structure can be derived with mathematical techniques. These correlations can be used for interpretating the spectra and for structure elucidation of unknown substances.

In addition to the routine application of analytical methods, the ZAGS is dedicated to exploring the possiblities of applying the latest spectroscopic techques to research problems in biology and biochemistry.

With the introduction of a novel ionization method (liquid SIMS) in mass spectroscopy, significant advances in trace analysis and the analysis of polar compounds could be made, allowing the investigation of substances that previously could not be analyzed.

Fig. 140
The sample of a chemical substance in solution is introduced into the magnet of a nuclear magnetic resonance instrument in order to be able to measure the nuclear magnetic resonance spectrum of the substance. This spectrum provides information on the structure of the compound

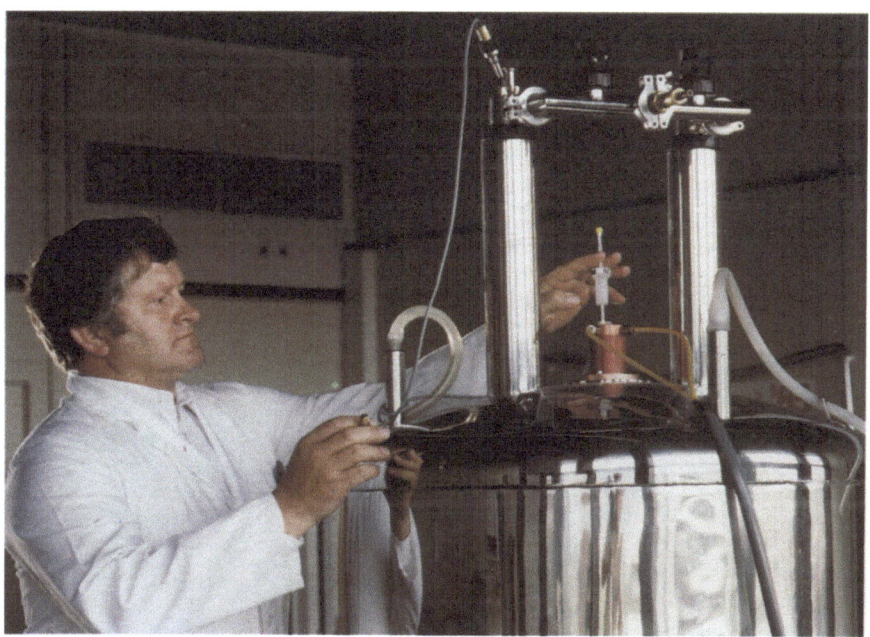

In the area of nuclear magnetic resonance spectroscopy, the efficient observation of nuclei such as 19-F, 31-P, 15-N in addition to $^1H$ and $^{13}C$ has become possible due to the acquisition of a high-field NMR instrument (AM 500) in 1983/1984. This spectrometer features the highest commercially available field strength and outstanding detection sensitivity as well as full flexibility in applying new pulse sequences for two-dimensional NMR. This allows the complete characterization of small quantities of complex organic compounds. Many interesting biochemical problems can now be investigated including the identification and quantification of particular metabolites in cell suspensions and tissue samples.

Head:
N. N.

Deputy Head:
Dr. Hans Josef Opferkuch

## Central Service of Radiation Protection and Dosimetry

In the exploration of carcinogenesis and cancer control carried out on a broad basis, use of radioactive substances or of ionizing radiation as tools is indispensible. Health protection at the Deutsches Krebsforschungszentrum therefore requires that all work with potential risk from ionizing radiation must be regulated and monitored by appropriate organizational and instrumental measures and precautions.

Fig. 141
The equipment of finger rings with thermoluminescence dosimeters with which the dose exposure of the hands of staff is detected

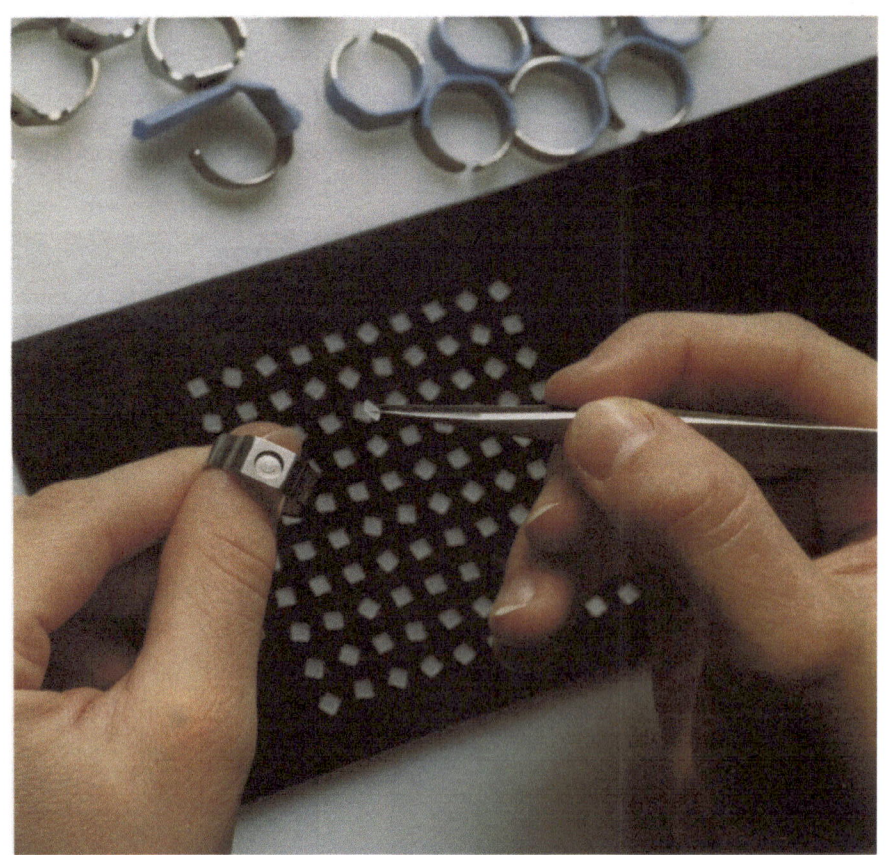

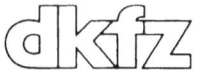

At the Deutsches Krebsforschungszentrum, these functions are conferred on the "Central Service of Radiation Protection and Dosimetry". It is responsible for the following items:

1. Protection of the workers in the laboratories;
   - radiation protection surveillance by dosemeters for whole-body and part-body exposure
   - incorporation and contamination measurements
   - documentation
2. Counselling of the staff at the Deutsches Krebsforschungszentrum in all questions arising in work with ionizing radiation.
3. Checking, maintenance and calibration of radiation protection instruments.
4. Drawing up a balance of the radioactivity employed
   - that obtained from external manufacturers (Tab. 13)
   - that produced internally (Tab. 14)
   - radioactive waste management
   - documentation
5. Monitoring the environment
   - thermoluminescence dosimetry in the environment

- measurement of the long-living beta activity in rain water
- monitoring of emission of radioactive gases and aerosols
- analysis of the activity of the waste water in the central collection facility.

Table 15 contains an overview of the personal doses measured in 1984 in the staff, broken down according to the individual institutes.

Besides the specific radiation protection monitoring functions, some more fundamental questions and problems within the field of radiation protection are also treated. These are radiation protection dosimetry in the presence of neutron fields, which entail a far greater risk to health than gamma rays, and the aspects of radiation protection in therapeutic application of ionizing radiation with patients. The motivation for this is that besides the desired radiation of the tumor, the patient himself must be protected from an undesired irradiation.

Tab. 13 The main radionuclides obtained from external manufacturers

| | |
|---|---|
| Tritium | Chromium 51 |
| Carbon 14 | Iodine 125 |
| Phosphorus 32 | Gallium 67 |
| Sulphur 35 | Molybdenum 99 |
| Yttrium 90 | Indium 111 |
| | Iodine 123 |
| | Iodine 131 |
| | Xenon 133 |
| | Thallium 201 |

Tab. 14 The main radionuclides produced in the Deutsches Krebsforschungszentrum

| Reactor TRIGA II | Compact cyclotron |
|---|---|
| Bromine 80 m | Carbon 11 |
| Copper 64 | Nitrogen 13 |
| Iodine 128 | Fluorine 18 |
| Krypton 85 m | Bromine 77 |
| Manganese 56 | Rubidium 81 |

Tab. 15 Distribution of the personal doses measured at the Deutsches Krebsforschungszentrum in controlled areas in 1984 (permissible doses: 15 or 50 mSV, respectively)

| Institute | Exp. Pathol. | Toxic. and Chemotherap. | Cell- and Tumor-Biology | Biochem. | Virus Res. | Immunol. and Genetics | Nuclear Med. | Other |
|---|---|---|---|---|---|---|---|---|
| (Milli-Seevert) | | | | | | | | |
| 0–<1.5 | 88 | 44 | 107 | 63 | 148 | 125 | 133 | 61 |
| 1.5–<5 | – | – | – | – | – | 22 | 19 | 2 |
| 5–<10 | – | – | – | – | – | – | 4 | – |
| 10–<15 | – | – | – | – | – | – | – | – |
| 15–<20 | – | – | – | – | – | – | 1 | – |

These studies are carried out in close collaboration with the Department of Biophysics and Medical Radiophysics, Institute of Nuclear Medicine.

Head:
Dipl. Phys. Otto Kraus

Deputy Head:
Dipl. Phys. Dr. Günther Hartmann

## Reactor

The research reactor TRIGA Heidelberg II was put into operation seven years ago in the new buildings of the DKFZ. One year before, the predecessor TRIGA Heidelberg I had been closed down and put out of service. It had been in operation since 1966.

The TRIGA Heidelberg II was largely a novel design. Only the fuel elements from the TRIGA Heidelberg I were transferred and reused.

The TRIGA Heidelberg II is a very reliable irradiation facility easy to operate. It shows very little susceptibility to disturbances and is run and maintained by a small team of three staff members supported by the institute's own precision mechanical workshop.

The reactor is used primarily for neutron activation analysis. Apart from neutron activation, there is no suitable method to determine small traces of various elements in a tissue sample, i. e. as compared to atomic absorption, several elements can be detected at a time by neutron activation and subsequent gamma spectroscopy.

The in-core irradiation positions are used mainly for production of radionuclides for investigations in nuclear medical diagnosis, for material research, and for other labelling procedures.

Since the start of operation in February 1978, an energy of 2,307,000 kilowatts was released in the TRIGA Heidelberg II up to December 31st 1984. In this period, 3,079 experiments were carried out with a total of 14,206 individual irradiation samples.

The reactor was in operation for radiation experiments of 180 days per year on an average. On about 80 days per year, tests were carried out mostly in the presence of representatives of the TÜV (State Technical Supervisory Department). In addition, about 20 days per year are required for repair and maintenance work. The daily radiation time rose continuously from 4.7 hours a day in 1978 to 9.5 hours a day in 1984. Likewise, there has been a general trend towards more radiation tests and longer irradiation times per experiment in recent years.

After the FR 2 reactor in the Nuclear Research Center in Karlsruhe was closed down, the irradiations carried out by external users rose continuously, so that the use of the TRIGA Heidelberg II is still increasing.

Responsible Head of the Facility:
Prof. Walter Lorenz, Ph.D.

Operational Manager:
Dr. Wolfgang Maier-Borst, Ph.D.

Deputy Operational Manager:
Otto Krauß, M.Sc.

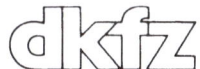

# Cyclotron

The compact cyclotron accelerates light atomic nuclei (protons, deuterons, $^3$He and $^4$He ions) to energies which are sufficient to start nuclear reactions on low-Z isotopes with high yields.

## Applications

Today, the work of the cyclotron facility is largely concerned with the production of radionuclides (mainly short-lived) for quantitative nuclear medical cancer diagnosis and for the development of new radiochemical and radiopharmaceutical methods. Beams of fast neutrons and charged particles are likewise available for experiments in other fields of research (biology, chemistry, radiation physics).

The compact cyclotron affiliated to the Institute of Nuclear Medicine was developed from 1968 to 1971 by the company AEG Telefunken in the context of a cooperative project supported by the Federal Ministry for Research and Technology. Purchase of the cyclotron and the basic equipment of the beam handling system were funded by the Volkswagenwerk Foundation.

The facility is also used by guest scientists of the Center, the University of Heidelberg and other scientific institutes home and abroad on the basis of joint projects or in informal cooperation. This in principle is possible for any research group.

The staff consists of a leading physicist, a chief operator and three technicians. For maintenance of the equipment, for repairs, constructions and new developments, a precision-mechanical workshop and the electronic laboratory of the institute provide assistance.

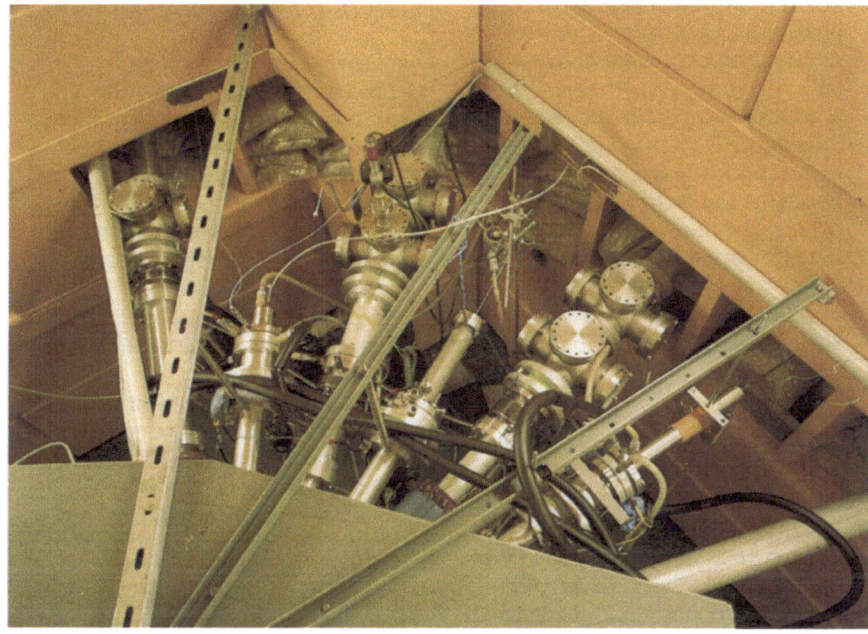

Work in recent years has concentrated on:

– Radioisotope production, especially production of $^{11}$C, $^{13}$N and $^{18}$F. These correspond chemically to the elements carbon, nitrogen and hydrogen occurring in organic matter. They thus allow labelling organic compounds (e. g. sugars, amino acids, fatty acids etc.) without alteration of the biochemical properties, and allow physiological processes in the living body to be rendered visible without disturbance by means of nuclear medical procedures. Their special property of emitting positrons (positively charged electrons) in radioactive decay is utilized by positron emission tomography (PET) for the quantitative measurement of certain metabolic steps. The Institute has carried out intensive preliminary work

Fig. 142
A system of ray tubes conducts the accelerated atomic nuclei from the compact cyclotron to several "targets". These are specialized for various functions, e.g., for the production of radionuclides for nuclear medical diagnostics or for the production of rapid neutrons and charged particles for radiobiological experiments. The photo shows the ray tubes radiating from the circuit-break magnet and three targets in the space in between for production of oxygen 15 (on the left), carbon 11 (middle) and fluorine 18 (on the right)

in this field for about five years and will be able to put a whole-body positron emission tomograph into operation at the beginning of 1986. In correlation with other techniques, it is intended to help to characterize and evaluate the behavior of tumors and normal tissue under the action of therapeutic measures.

- For other nuclear medical and analytical investigations, further (in some cases long-lived) isotopes ($^{75}Br$, $^{77}Br$, $^{81}Rb$, $^{121}I$ etc.) are also produced for users in-house or outside the Center. In the context of the cooperation contract between the Deutsches Krebsforschungszentrum and the Heidelberg University Hospital, $^{81}Rb-^{81m}Kr$ generators as well as $^{13}N$ glutamate is supplied to the Radiological Hospital of the University.

- The preclinical phase of the cooperative project "Therapy with Fast Neutrons" was brought to an end. In this, three external groups (from the Institute of Biophysics, University of the Saarland in Homburg/Saar, and from the Gesellschaft für Strahlen- und Umweltforschung (GSF), Department of Radiation Physics in Frankfurt/Main, as well as the Institute of Radiation Protection, Neuherberg) had been collaborating. The clinical application (today in close collaboration with the Heidelberg University Radiological Hospital) was transferred to the fast neutron generator KARIN, which is superior to the rigid low-energy cyclotron neutron beam with regard to radiation quality and mobility. The latter continues to be reserved for dosimetric reference measurements.

Head of the Facility:
Prof. Walter Lorenz, Ph.D.

Operational Manager:
Gerd Wolber, Ph.D.

## Central Data Processing

Almost all departments of the Deutsches Krebsforschungszentrum use programs and computing capacity of central computers which are accessible directly via terminals at the place of work. The spectrum of applications comprises the following focal points:
- Recording of laboratory data, e. g., by digitalization
- Keeping of data banks, e. g., for DNA sequences, for spectra, animals and literature.
- Statistical analysis, e. g., of laboratory and animal trials.
- Image processing, e. g., for cell and organ sections.
- Simulations and calculations, e. g. for cell growth models and interactions between molecules.
- Presentation of the results by text processing, graphs, diagrams.

The Department of Central Data Processing (ZDV) supports the users in their data processing applications by the adaptation of instrument interfaces for recording of laboratory data with microcomputers, by transport of data to the appropriate evaluation computer or terminal, by the operation of centrally available computers and the provision of programs for user groups. The tasks include in addition the training and counselling in the use of data processing, programming and result presentation. Users, who wish to employ personal computers in order to carry out individual data processing independently, are supported by the ZDV in the selection, configuration and operation of their computer on site. The Central Data Processing operates two computers of the type IBM 4381 with the operation systems VM/CMS and TSS in two operator shifts. Eight microcomputers, some per-

Fig. 143
Control panel of the two central computers

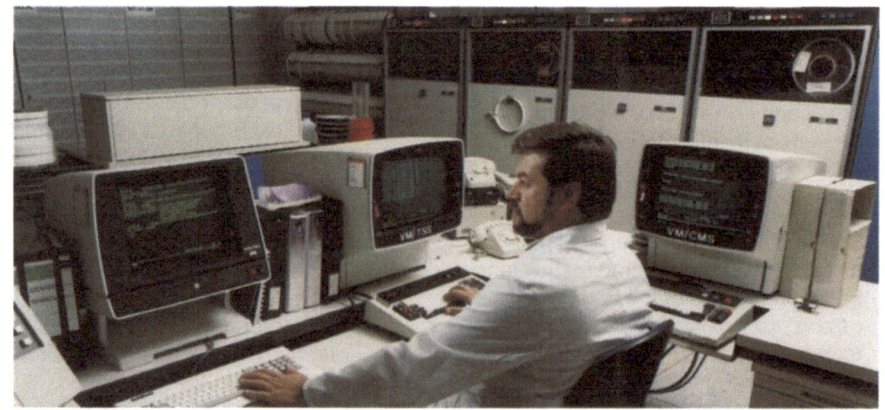

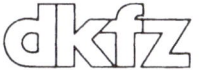

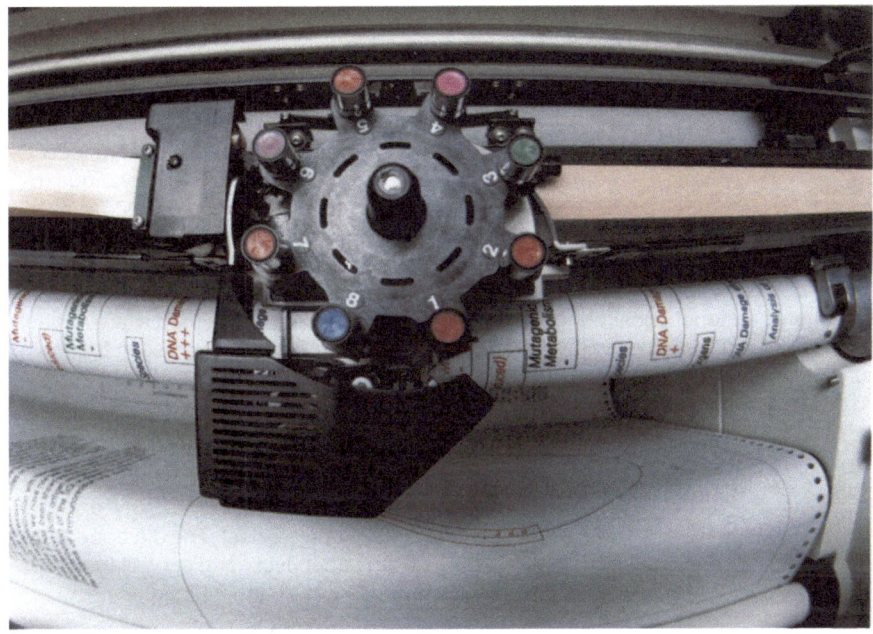

Fig. 144
Scientific results are documented graphically with
this electronic drawing instrument

sonal computers and about 130 terminals in the Deutsches Krebsforschungszentrum are connected. External, directly connected users are institutes
and clinics of the University of Heidelberg. Via the data networks of the Bun-
despost (Datex-L, Datex-P), access to
the computers of the Deutsches Krebsforschungszentrum is also available to
other authorized users. Recently, a
worldwide data and information exchange, especially with other research
facilities and universities, is possible for
all users by connecting computer to the
EARN computer network. Direct computer links are available to the University
Computer Center, to the Center for
Molecular Biology and to the European
Laboratory for Molecular Biology in
Heidelberg.

The program languages available on the
computers of the ZDV are Basic, Pascal,
APL, PL/1, Fortran and Spitbol. The following generally recognized software
packets are implemented for statistics:
SAS, SPSS; for data banks: SQL; for
graphics: Tellagraph; for word processing: Script. The program packages developed by the Deutsches Krebsforschungszentrum also have a large spectrum of use, e. g., for statistics: Adam;
for data banks: INDA; for image processing: PIC; for DNA sequence analysis: BSA; for data transmission:
ODIF/ODIX.

The Central Data Processing gives support to all scientific research activities
and service facilities in the Deutsches
Krebsforschungszentrum with regard to
the use of the computer as a tool of
modern research and has hence been
organized as a central facility since the
beginning of 1985.

Head:
Dr. Kurt Böhm (acting)

## Safety

Works doctors and safety engineers are appointed in accordance with the Industrial Safety Law. In order to ensure medical care of the staff, the Deutsches Krebsforschungszentrum cooperates with the "Industrial Medical Center" in Eppelheim.

Counselling on safety technology and checks are carried out by the "Safety Division" which is under the direct supervision of the scientific director. The work of the safety division extends from planning new buildings and building alterations to inspecting places of work and counselling staff handling carcinogenic substances and is involved in the disposal of dangerous wastes.

In addition, the installation of effective protective measures dealing with dangerous working materials and pathogenic material, monitoring the air at places of work is important. Air measurements are carried out routinely and on request. Monitoring biological safety includes the maintenance of a serum bank.

For the information of staff, advanced training sessions are held on various topics of industrial safety. Problems in work organization, experimental studies, and animal experiments are dealt with individually and in group discussions. Audiovisual media (e.g. video) are used to improve the dissemination of information.

There is close contact and exchange of experience with external facilities (e. g., major research institutions, the European Molecular Biology Laboratory (EMBL), universities). The dialogue with health supervisory and surveillance authorities is also maintained.

Head:
Dipl. Ing. Edgar Heuss
(Safety Engineer)

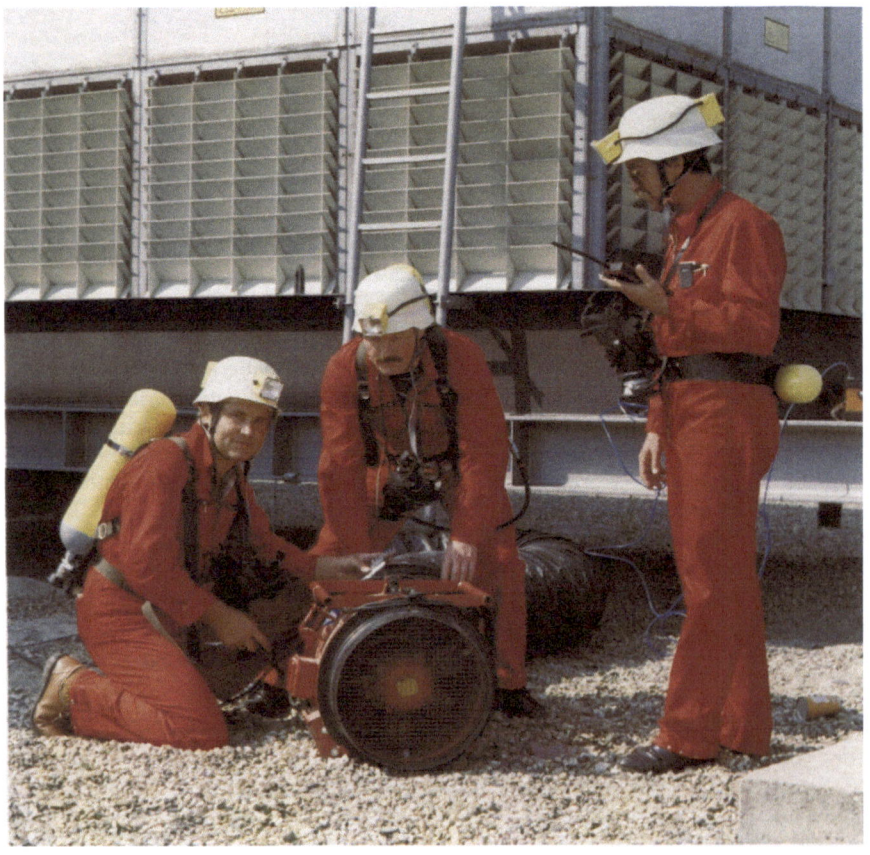

Fig. 145
Work's fire brigade in an operational exercise with breathing protection and aspiration instrument

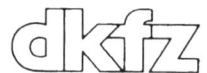

# Evaluation of Results

According to its statutes it is the function of the Deutsches Krebsforschungszentrum to carry through cancer research. The center plans and designs its scientific program in the light of this obligation. Public funds are used almost exclusively to carry through the research program, necessitating an efficient and as successful an application as possible. Evaluation of results is hence a recognized element in the research process and is one of the tasks of the responsible organs acting on the part of the Cancer Research Center. Expertises based on site visits by external visiting committees are a major prerequisite for decisions on the promotion of research activities and disciplines as well as the establishment of scientific focal points.

According to the statutes, above all the Scientific Committee of the Board of Trustees carries out this function. In the report period, the Board of Trustees has subjected to a detailed expert evaluation the Institutes of Toxicology and Chemotherapy, Experimental Pathology, Cellular and Tumor Biology as well as Virus Research with additional expert opinions. The time sequence of the site visits is such that each of the eight institutes is evaluated once about every five years. Supplementary to the external evaluations by the Scientific Committee, the Scientific Council and the Management Board carried out an internal evaluation of the research programs and individual activities of the scientists of all divisions as a well-founded basis for the design of future programs in view of reductions in available resources.

Evaluations on the basis of presentations have been the basis for changes in contents and structure in the Deutsches Krebsforschungszentrum. New project groups have been formed, divisions have been reduced in size or enlarged, new divisions with new contents, taking into account the current scientific developments, have been installed. Other divisions have been dissolved, the staff being allocated newly defined functions. An overview of the reorientation in the individual fields is given in the introduction to this book by Prof. Harald zur Hausen. To a limited extent, budget funds have been used since 1982 to form an internal pool of materials in order to support selected research activities more intensively in an internal application procedure.

The high number of research projects (over 150), which have been applied for in the organizations promoting research and which have been financed by these organizations, as well as the continuous publication of the research results in recognized scientific journals are further elements of a scientific evaluation of the results.

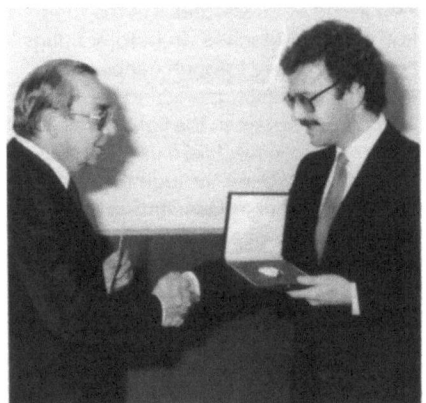

Fig. 146
Award of the Domagk-Prize for 1984

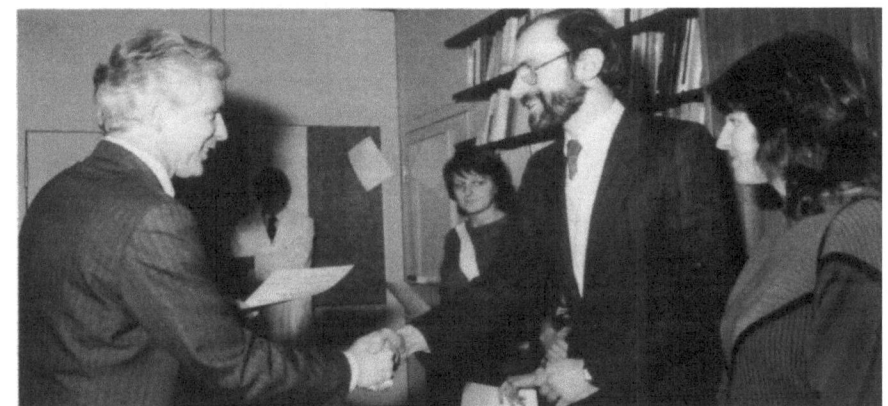

Fig. 147
Award of the Walther and Christine Richtzenhain
Prize for 1983

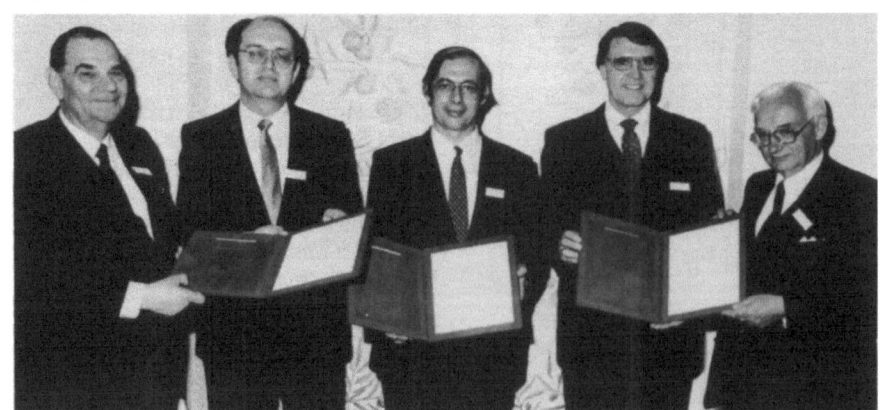

Fig. 148
Award of the Ernst Jung Prize for 1984

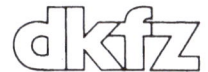

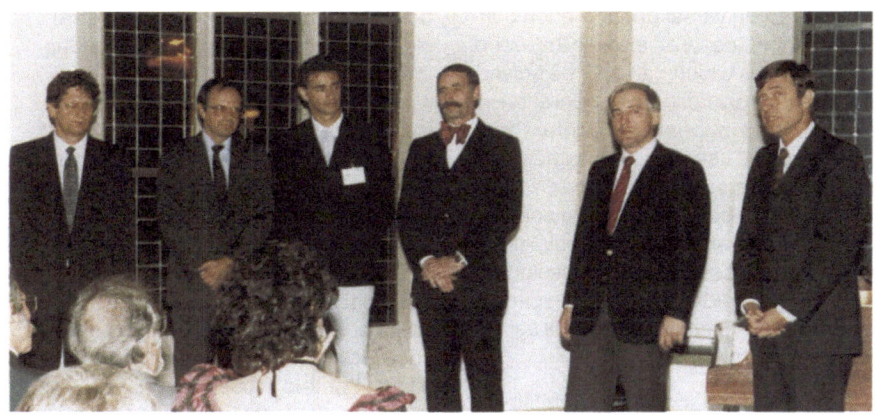

Fig. 149
Award of the Farm Italia Carlo Erba Prize for 1985 for the result of a combined project between the Chest Hospital in Heidelberg-Rohrbach and the German Cancer Research Center. Prof. Gerhard Nagel, Göttingen, (on the right) during his laudation

## Distinctions, Appointments

Once again, numerous prizes have been conferred on scientists of the Deutsches Krebsforschungszentrum for their scientific achievements:

1983 Meyenburg prize (Prof. Dr. Lutz Gissmann); 1983 Redel prize (Michael Dieter Kramer), 1983 Walter and Christine Richtzenhain prize (Dr. Beatrice Neuer, Dr. Dorothea Ziegelmüller, Dr. Lynn Graf, Dr. Dieter Schlaps); 1984 Domagk prize (Prof. Dr. Lutz Gissmann); 1984 Ernst-Jung prize (Prof. Werner Franke jointly with Prof. Klaus Weber, Max Planck Institute of Biophysical Chemistry, Göttingen); 1984 Annual Award of the Foundation of Research in Dermatology (Dr. Hermlita Winter, Dr. Mitsuru Kinjo, Dr. Jürgen Schweizer, Dr. Gerhard Fürstenberger); 1985 Lila-Gruber Cancer Research Award (Prof. Harald zur Hausen); 1985 Farmitalia Carlo Erba prize (two groups: Prof. Manfred Volm, Priv. Doz. Dr. Klaus Wayß, Dr. Jürgen M. Mattern, Dr. Jaroslav Sonka, Deutsches Krebsforschungszentrum, with Prof. Peter Drings, Prof. Ingolf Vogt-Moykopf, Thorax Clinic Heidelberg-Rohrbach, Prof. Richard Herrmann, Leading Physician in the Westend Hospital, Berlin, with Prof. Werner Kunz and Prof. Hans Osswald, Deutsches Krebsforschungszentrum).

Prof. Otto Westphal was awarded the 1983 Karl Heinrich Bauer medal for special services in cancer research. Prof. Harald zur Hausen received an honorary doctorate of the University of Chicago, USA.

Prof. Volker Schirrmacher was invited to accept a professorship for experimental cancer research at the University of Essen. Prof. Walter Keller was invited to accept a post as divisional head at the National Institutes of Health, Bethesda, Maryland. Neither appointment was accepted.

## Publications

The results of the scientific work of the Deutsches Krebsforschungszentrum are published regularly in scientific journals. Since its foundation in 1964, around 4066 publications have appeared in scientific journals (666 in 1983/1984 alone), about 408 diplomas, doctoral and lectureship theses (58 in 1983/1984) and 1009 other publications, including books or handbook contributions in 1983/1984. Members of the staff at the Center presented their results at meetings in more than 5027 oral or poster contributions.

The publications of the staff members of the Center are continuously registered and published annually in a bibliographic list "Publications from the Deutsches Krebsforschungszentrum". The list is available to interested persons on request.

The staff office "Press and Public Relations" of the Deutsches Krebsforschungszentrum is concerned to ensure that the general public are continuously informed of the results of our work.

# National and International Collaboration

Cancer as a universal phenomenon confronts cancer research all over the world with problems which can only be solved by close interdisciplinary cooperation in a national and international context and by the specific use of the available financial and personnel resources. The extremely complex problems of cancer research necessitate a multidisciplinary approach to research encompassing practically all fields of biological sciences and exact sciences as well as some social sciences.

In the implementation of its scientific program, the Deutsches Krebsforschungszentrum, therefore, collaborates on a national and international level with a large number of scientists and research institutions.

With its program integrated into that of the Federal German Government "Research and Technology in the Service of Health", the Deutsches Krebsforschungszentrum also participates in programs of research promoting organizations as well as combined research projects of the Federal Ministry of Research and Technology, the Federal Ministry of Youth, Family and Health Affairs, and the Federal Ministry of the Interior, the Federal Office for Environmental Affairs and the World Health Organization (WHO). There is a close collaboration with other large-scale research institutions, federal research institutes and a large number of university institutes and hospitals, especially of the University of Heidelberg.

The appointment of scientists from the Center and active collaboration in executive and working committees of the large international societies and organizations working towards the goal of cancer control is a decisive aspect of international cooperation and coordination. Thus scientists of the Center are elected members of the Council of the International Union against Cancer (UICC, Geneva) and of the Committee for International Cooperation (CICA) of the UICC, of the International Cancer Research Center (IARC, Lyon), of the Advisory Board of the European Cancer Society (EACR), of the National Academy of Sciences, USA, and subcommittees of the Council of the International Organizations for Medical Sciences (CIOMS, Geneva). The cancer research centers in the world have formed the organization of European Cancer Institutes and coordinate questions of joint interest at regular intervals.

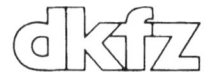

The scientists of the Center are members in numerous international and national federations of their specialist disciplines. To a continuously increasing extent, they are responsible or partly responsible for organizing large international and national congresses, symposia and workshops (cf. section on Events). In the national context, there is collaboration in commissions and subcommittees of the German Research Association (Environmental Research, Dyestuffs Commission, Foreign Substance Commission, Hinterzarten Circle, Experimental Animal Research, Primate Research, Toxicity Evaluation of Carcinogenic Effects. etc.), in working groups and the Commission of the German Cancer Society, e. g. in the section Experimental Cancer Research and in the Commission for the Investigation of Anticancer Drugs with Doubtful Effect, in commissions of the Trade Cooperative Associations, in advisory boards of the Federal Minister for Youth, Family and Health Affairs, of the Federal Minister for Research and Technology and the Federal Minister of the Interior. Scientists of the Deutsches Krebsforschungszentrum are elected experts of the German Research Association and write expert reports for a large series of research promotion programs of national and foreign institutions. Projects of the Deutsches Krebsforschungszentrum are integrated into three special research programs of the Deutsche Forschungsgemeinschaft (cancer and resistance, stochastic mathematical models and medical virology-tumorigenesis and tumor development).

The close integration of the scientists of the Deutsches Krebsforschungszentrum into international scientific exchange is manifested inter alia in their work as editors or co-editors of scientific journals of their specialties. 81 scientific journals are supported by the regular collaboration of research workers of the Deutsches Krebsforschungszentrum on the editorial board, including for example the International Journal of Cancer, Journal of Molecular Biology, Experimental Cell Research – European Journal of Immunology, Immunobiology, Journal of Cancer Research and Clinical Oncology, Cell and Biochemistry.

In the report period, scientists of the Center were appointed into the executive committees or presidia of the German Society of Medical Physics, the section for Experimental Cancer Research of the German Cancer Society, the International Federation of Cell Biology and the European Cell Biology Organization, the German Society for Immunology and the Metastasis Research Society, to name only a few.

The Deutsches Krebsforschungszentrum also holds the chair in the Commission for Cancer Research of the Arbeitsgemeinschaft der Großforschungseinrichtungen.

## Bilateral Agreements

The year 1986 was the ten year anniversary of the contractual agreement between the government of Israel, represented by the National Council for Research and Development and the Federal German Government, represented by the Deutsches Krebsforschungszentrum, to carry out joint research projects in the field of cancer research. These were all projects which had so far been carried out on the German side in the Institutes of Virus Research, Immunology and Genetics, Biochemistry, Cell and Tumor Biology, Nuclear Medicine and Experimental Pathology. On the Israeli side, they had been carried out by scientists of Ben Gurion University, Beer-Sheba, Tel Aviv University, the Hebrew University of Jerusalem, the Weizman Institute of Science, Rehovoth, Technicon Haifa and the Hadassah University Medical School, Jerusalem. Each research promotion period comprises three years. A detailed appraisal of the projects by the German-Israeli Scientific Program Committee takes place in workshops. New projects initiated in 1985. The Deutsches Krebsforschungszentrum considers this cooperation as an especially effective instrument for supplementing the research program through multidisciplinary cooperation with competent partners abroad.

In addition, the Deutsches Krebsforschungszentrum has established a contractually agreed Clearing-House of On-Going Research in Cancer Epidemiology in the context of the International Cancer Research Data Bank Program of the US National Cancer Institute. The main function of the Cancer Research Center in the context of this international project is the processing of information received on projects in progress in the field of cancer epidemiology.

In 1985, the tenth edition of the Directory of On-Going Research in Cancer Epidemiology, which is published jointly, appeared.

In the last two years, the offers of foreign institutions of cancer research to develop and implement or to extend joint research programs together with the Deutsches Krebsforschungszentrum have appreciably increased. In this connection, there are contacts with the People's Republic of China, with India, Hungary, the USA, Saudi-Arabia, the Tanzania Tumor Center and Italy. Joint symposia were held with these partners and the focal points of joint scientific interests were defined. In some cases, there has already been cooperation over many years, e. g., with Japan and France.

## International Scientific Exchange

In 1983 and 1984, a total of 219 guest scientists were working at the Deutsches Krebsforschungszentrum (1981/1982: 252).

The intensity of international and national cooperation in the Deutsches Krebsforschungszentrum thus continued to remain at a high level.

These visits of guest scientists over a limited time provide them on the one hand with an insight into certain disciplines, and on the other hand, enables them to learn techniques in which the scientists of the Deutsches Krebsforschungszentrum are pre-eminent; more over, they serve to recruit scientists with specific know-how which is complementary to the scientific work at the Deutsches Krebsforschungszentrum. A further objective of international cooperation is the development and implementation of joint projects and programs in the fields of cancer research.

In 1983, 122 guest scientists from 24 countries (in 1982: 97 guest scientists from 25 countries) including 30 female guest scientists were working at the Deutsches Krebsforschungszentrum. The foreign guests included one Humboldt prize-winner, four recipients of postgraduate grants and 15 other scholarship holders who chose the center as their place of research.

In 1984 there were 94 foreign guests from 23 countries, 67 of whom were working in the Center for at least three months. The guests included 13 postgraduate scholarship holders, including four of them with scholarships from the Humboldt Foundation.

The number of long-term guest stays has appreciably risen, whereas the number of brief guest stays has decreased. Among the foreign guests, there were 20 women.

The guest house, opened in 1977 with a total of 15 apartments, was fully booked continuously in both years with a total of 222 guests (1981/1982: 198 guests).

The second guest house opened in 1981 with eight completely equipped flats (seven three-room flats, one two-room flat) was occupied by a total of 28 guest scientists and their families in the two report years. It was thus used to capacity.

In the seminar room of the guest house, 16 events for a total of 250 participants took place in 1983. In 1984, there were 25 events (workshops, postgraduate training seminars, talks for journalists) for a total of 867 participants.

The scholarship holders were supported by the Humboldt Foundation, the World Health Organization (WHO), the German Academic Exchange Service (DAAD), the German Research Association (DFG), the Minerva Foundation, the Max Planck Society, the NTNFC (Norges Teknisk Naturvitenskapelige Forskningrad/Oslo), industrial and other sources. As a rule, scholarship holders choose the laboratory, in which they would wish to work on the basis of whether they would find qualified support for their research project. Since the Deutsches Krebsforschungszentrum comprises practically all disciplines of the exact sciences which may contribute to exploration of cancer, it is very attractive for scholarship holders and guests from home and abroad.

The exchange of the most recent scientific information at the Deutsches Krebs-

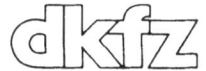

forschungszentrum is also especially supported by the program of colloquia in which scientists from Germany and all over the world regularly present papers. In 1983/1984, papers were presented by 317 scientists from 24 countries. This program of colloquia is part of a joint lecture program of the Heidelberg Scientific Institution which informs on all scientific lectures in all scientific institutions in the form of monthly computer printouts which can be obtained from all Heidelberg research facilities.

## Heidelberg/Mannheim Tumor Center

Heidelberg was the location of the first international cancer congress and seat of the first university cancer research institute in Europe founded in 1906 by - Professor Vincenz Czerny. Heidelberg thus has a long tradition in the battle against cancer. This tradition was continued by the establishment of the oncological working group in Heidelberg in 1966 and by the foundation of the Tumor Center in 1979.

The liaison between the hospitals in Heidelberg and Mannheim and the Cancer Research Center as Tumor Center has proved its effectiveness. The main objective was the best possible care of tumor patients in the hospitals and in the region. As close a link as possible with hospitals of the surrounding area is aimed at. In addition, new impulses for diagnosis and therapy of malignant diseases should result from the research programs carried out between hospitals, theoretical institutes and the Deutsches Krebsforschungszentrum.

Partners for clinically relevant research and direct application of new knowledge in the care of patients are the Deutsches Krebsforschungszentrum and the University of Heidelberg with its hospitals in Heidelberg and the medical faculty at the Mannheim Municipal Hospital as well as with the hospital in Rohrbach (Heidelberg-Rohrbach Thorax Clinic) of the Landesversicherungsanstalt Baden as financing body.

In terms of the basic demands which must be met by a tumor center, the prerequisites of the Heidelberg/Mannheim Tumor Center are optimal:

- The center combines basic and clinical research and enables training and postgraduate education in diagnostic and therapeutic methods on an interdisciplinary basis in the diagnosis and treatment of malignant diseases.
- Optimal facilities for basic research are available through the institutes of the University and the Deutsches Krebsforschungszentrum.
- Hospitals and research facilities with a high level ensure the scientific-clinical and technical liaison with centers at home and abroad.
- Research projects of prevention and early diagnosis are a constituent part of the program.
- A local cancer registry provides the statistical basis for data processing and evaluation of the results both in clinical care and in research.
- A large number of scientific events ensures reciprocal contact between the partners of the center and doctors in the region.
- The center has a central administrative office which enables coordination of the activities between the various partners.
- The structure of the center allows optimal use of financial resources both for research and for highly specialized patient care.
- The attractiveness of the clinical facilities of the center allows a large number of tumor patients to benefit from the practical application of theoretical-clinical research work. This knowledge can be further developed by a consultation program with the region.

The objectives of the Tumor Center are conceived and promoted by the executive committee (Chairman: Professor Christian Herfarth) as central coordination and management unit.

The central objectives of the Tumor Center are formulated. According to the classical rules of the Comprehensive Cancer Center in the USA, they comprise the typical features:

– Establishment of guidelines for diagnosis and therapy of the individual tumors, i.e. also for malignant systemic diseases, for special problems of metastases and chemotherapy. The guidelines are published as a manual for the Tumor Center and the region. In the meantime, almost all tumor types are described in accordance with certain criteria. In 1983/ 1984, recommendations on breast cancer and non-Hodgkin lymphomas were published. Overall, seven recommendations have been published in the last five years. They can be obtained in the administrative office.

– Elaboration and functional application of a documentation system which includes both basic documentation and the special tumor documentation. The general registration of all tumor patients in the Tumor Center and the central storage of the data was made possible by the link-up of four node computers (Rohrbach, Mannheim, Old and New University Hospital in Heidelberg) with a central computer of the Tumor Center. In all participating hospitals of the Tumor Center, terminals and printers are available for data storage and recall of data, e.g. in the form of an automatized medical report.

– Development of models for follow-up and special oncological outpatient departments. The prerequisites for

this were ensured. The operated patients are completely registered; a controlled appointment and reminder system was built up. Close collaboration with outside institutions was established both with the surrounding hospitals and with the medical practitioners doctors and special tumor outpatient clinics.

– Cooperative therapy studies and programs for a series of tumors are a further objective. In view of the necessity of forming large-scale controlled therapy groups, research projects are also to be promoted which are linked not only in interdisciplinary terms in the context of the center, but also outside it with other tumor centers and organizations, e.g., with the European Organization for Research on Treatment of Cancer (EORTC), with the Swiss Working Group for Clinical Cancer Research (SAKK) and with the oncological working groups of the German Cancer Society.

– Work in the Tumor Center must include the results and plans of basic research. A focal point in this respect is research on tumor biology and tumor immunology, problems of tumor sensitivity testing, enteropoiesis (cell-forming system of the esophagus and gastrointestinal tract) and hematopoiesis (formation of the red blood cells). The major interdisciplinary research programs between theoretical institutes of basic research and the hospitals should also be concentrated in these fields in the future.

– Supraregional and international collaboration is promoted not only with other tumor centers in the context of the Working Group of German Tumor Centers (ADT), but also with the large-scale institutions of clinical cancer re-

search (National Cancer Institute, USA, Swiss Working Group for Clinical Cancer Research, European Organization for Research on Treatment of Cancer and working groups of the various specialist disciplines in the German Cancer Society).

– Postgraduate training in the field of clinical oncology in regional and supraregional seminars and colloquia are regarded as a major task. Thus, a series of meetings take place every year. Special events to be emphasized from those which took place in 1983 and 1984 are:
Progress or Stagnation in the Diagnosis and Therapy of Gastric Carcinoma? (5. 2. 1983)
Prostate Carcinoma and Malignant Testicular Tumor (15. 10. 1983)
Local Tumor Recurrence – A Challenge to Cooperative Therapeutic Planning (4. 2. 1984)
Metastases of Gastrointestinal Carcinomas – Diagnosis and Therapy (10. 11. 84)
Oncology for the Family Doctor (1. 12. 1984)
In collaboration with the surgical working group oncology and the internal medical working group for oncology, an international symposium was held:
Therapeutic Strategies in Primary and Metastatic Liver Cancer (17.–19. 9. 1984)

– Cooperation with the region by the establishment of "oncological" telephones in an effort to build up regional therapy studies is being further intensified. A constant advisory service on special oncological problems is thus provided for hospitals in the region.

– A future task will be to define clear responsibilities and the addresses for inquiries for the individual tumors and

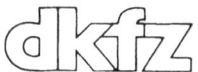

malignant systemic diseases in order to ensure standards and focal points for the region.

A major focal point of the Heidelberg/ Mannheim Tumor Center is to be seen in the cooperation with the Deutsches Krebsforschungszentrum. Coordinated and cooperative research programs on prevention, diagnosis and therapy, and above all programs of basic research on clinical questions will be promoted in this way. New knowledge, i.e. results of basic research, will thus be rapidly applied in practice. Just as the close cooperation with the Deutsches Krebsforschungszentrum gives rise to new knowledge, we aim at the same time at being active throughout the region by close contacts with the hospitals of the region and the medical practitioners.

Characteristic for the development of the Heidelberg/Mannheim Tumor Center is, therefore, also the fact that in the past years research projects have been concentrated on cooperative special programs. After a large number of small projects had been at the forefront at the beginning, following a five-year pilot phase, the Tumor Center has now placed accents on specific focal areas based on a particular scientific profile and documented by special areas of concentration in patient care. Naturally, a large number of individual oncological projects and clinical studies are being carried out and promoted at the hospitals and oncological units of the Tumor Center. However, the cooperation between the Deutsches Krebsforschungszentrum and the hospitals is concentrated in the field of the large-scale projects which were selected on the basis of their evaluation by a committee of international experts. Four cooperative clinical-theoretical large-scale projects were created:

A. Investigations about the individualized evaluation of progress and prognosis as well as therapy of the colorectal carcinoma
(coordinator: Prof. Peter Schlag, Surgical Hospital, University of Heidelberg)

with the following subprojects:

1. Analysis of the invasive and metastatic spreading of human colorectal carcinomas
(Project heads: Prof. Volker Schirrmacher, Institute of Immunology and Genetics, Deutsches Krebsforschungszentrum, and Prof. Peter Schlag, Surgical Hospital, University of Heidelberg).
2. Quantitative detection of the individual cell cycle phases of colorectal carcinomas on the basis of impulse-cytophotometric investigations
(Project heads: Dr. Georg Feichter, Institute of Comparative and Experimental Pathology, University of Heidelberg, Prof. Klaus Goerttler, Institute of Experimental Pathology of the Deutsches Krebsforschungszentrum, Prof. Peter Schlag, Surgical Hospital, University of Heidelberg).
3. Determination of the proliferative capacity of a tumor
(Project heads: Priv.-Doz. Dr. Michael Betzler, Surgical Hospital, Prof. Burghard Bohn, Institute of Biochemistry II, University of Heidelberg, Priv.-Doz. Dr. Hans-Peter Geisen, Surgical Hospital, University of Heidelberg, Prof. Holger Kirchner, Institute of Virus Research, Deutsches Krebsforschungszentrum).
4. Isolation of single cells by means of carrier-free cytophoresis and flow-cytometric determination of binding parameters for surface markers
(Project heads: Prof. Burghard Bohn, Institute of Biochemistry II, Prof. Reinhard Brossmer, Institute of Biochemistry II, University of Heidelberg).
5. Determination of immunological parameters in patients with colorectal carcinomas
(Project heads: Priv.-Doz. Dr. Michael Betzler, Surgical Hospital, Priv.-Doz. Dr. Hans-Peter Geisen, Surgical Hospital, University of Heidelberg, Prof. Holger Kirchner, Department of Tumour Virus Immunology in the Institute of Virus Research, Deutsches Krebsforschungszentrum).

6. Qualitative and quantitative characterization of colorectal carcinomas by means of xenogenic antisera, monoclonal antibodies and lectins with the goal of individualized prognosis and progress observation
(Project heads: Dr. Peter Möller, Institute of Pathology, University of Heidelberg, Prof. Herwart Otto, Institute of Pathology, University of Heidelberg, Dr. Armin Quentmeier, Surgical Hospital, Priv.-Doz. Dr. Heinrich Schmidt-Gayk, Surgical Hospital, University of Heidelberg).
7. Monoclonal antibodies against tumor-associated antigens of colorectal carcinoma
(Project heads: Dr. Gerhard Moldenhauer, Department of Somatic Genetics, Institute of Immunology and Genetics, Deutsches Krebsforschungszentrum, Prof. Günter Hämmerling, Department of Somatic Genetics, Institute of Immunology and Genetics of the Deutsches Krebsforschungszentrum, Prof. Peter Schlag, Surgical Hospital, University of Heidelberg).

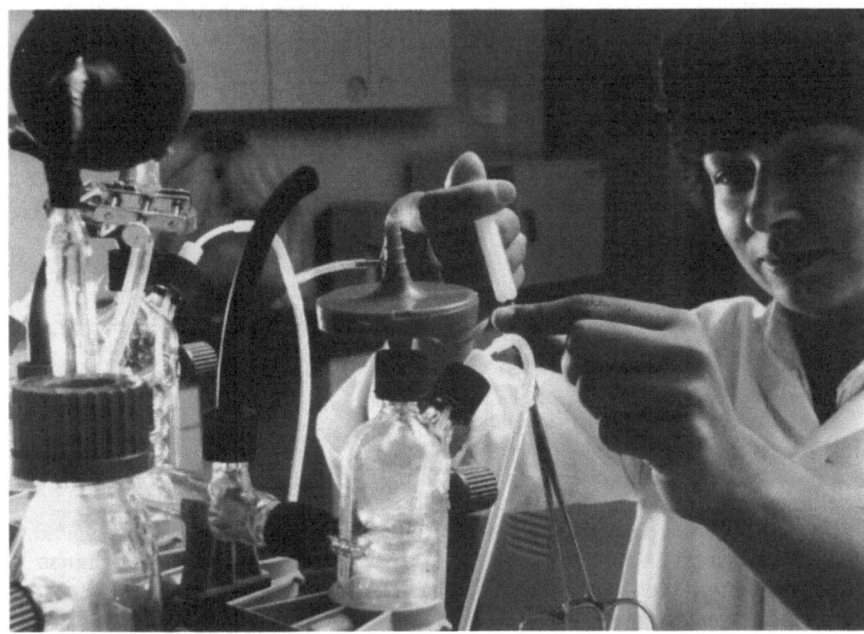

Fig. 150
Determination of the number of antibody-forming white blood cells in the context of a research project of the Heidelberg-Mannheim Tumor Center, here in the Chest Hospital in Heidelberg-Rohrbach

8. In vitro investigations of tumor colony formation in colorectal carcinomas and the influence of cytostatics
(Project heads: Prof. Peter Schlag, Surgical Hospital, Dr. Dagmar Flentje, Surgical Hospital, University of Heidelberg).

9. Individualization and modification of chemotherapy with 5-fluorouracil in colorectal carcinomas
(Project heads: Prof. Richard Herrmann, Medical Division, University of Heidelberg, Dr. Rüdiger Port, Institute of Biochemistry at the Deutsches Krebsforschungszentrum).

10. Perfusion studies and pharmacokinetic investigations on hepatic metastases of colorectal carcinomas
(Project heads: Prof. Peter Georgi, Radiological Hospital, University of Heidelberg, Dr. Wolfram Knapp, North Rhine-Westfalia Heart Center, Bad Oeynhausen, Dr. Bernd Kober, Institute of Nuclear Medicine, Deutsches Krebsforschungszentrum, Project Group Radiotherapy, Radiological Hospital, University of Heidelberg).

11. Model investigations on locoregional chemotherapy
(Project heads: Dr. Martin Berger, Institute of Toxicology and Chemotherapy, Deutsches Krebsforschungszentrum, Prof. Dietrich Schmähl, Institute of Toxicology and Chemotherapy, Deutsches Krebsforschungszentrum, Dr. Rolf Bartkowski, Surgical Hospital, University of Heidelberg, Prof. Christian Herfarth, Surgical Hospital, University of Heidelberg, Prof. Peter Schlag, Surgical Hospital, University of Heidelberg).

B. Bronchial carcinoma: diagnosis, pathophysiology and therapy (coordinator: Prof. Peter Drings, Rohrbach Hospital, Thorax Clinic of the Landesversicherungsanstalt Baden).

The following subprojects are to be mentioned:

1. Value of bronchoalveolar lavage (BAL) in the diagnosis of pulmonary tumors
(Project head: Dr. Heinrich David Becker, Rohrbach Hospital).

2. Interactions of tumors with cultivated endothelial cells of human pulmonary capillaries and human monoclonal antibodies (cold agglutinins) as markers for pulmonary tumors as compared to normal cells
(Project head: Prof. Werner Ebert, Rohrbach Hospital).

3. Mechanisms of action, character and origin of circulating and local factors

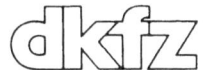

with inhibitory effect on cellular defense processes in patients with lung cancer
(Project head: Priv.-Doz. Dr. Hans-Georg Manke, Rohrbach Hospital).

4. Influence on the immune system of malignant tumors of the lower respiratory tract
(Project head: Priv.-Doz. Dr. Dr. Klaus Kayser, Institute of Pathology, University of Heidelberg).

5. Ferritins and isoferritins in malignant diseases. Studies on patients with lung cancer, breast cancer, neuroblastoma and leukemia for evaluation of the serum ferritin levels found to be clinically raised, the biological interactions of the cell with ferritin and the biochemical and molecular characteristics of this molecule
(Project head: Dr. Marianne Huntsberry-Dörner, Medical Hospital, University of Heidelberg).

Fig. 151
Investigation of the interaction between pulmonary endothelial cells and tumor cells in the Chest Hospital in Heidelberg-Rohrbach

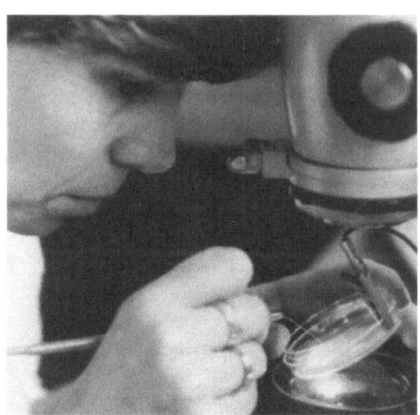

C. Malignant lymphoma and leukemia – new approaches in diagnosis and therapy of leukemia and malignant lymphomas: biological and immunological basis
(coordinator: Dr. Bernd Dörken, Medical Policlinic, University of Heidelberg).

The following subprojects are carried out within this large-scale project:

1. Autologous bone marrow transplantation
(Project head: Dr. Martin Körbling, Medical Policlinic, University of Heidelberg).

2. Production of monoclonal antibodies against tumor-specific superficial antigens and B-cell differentiation antigens in lymphatic leukemia and malignant lymphomas
(Project head: Dr. Bernd Dörken, Medical Policlinic, University of Heidelberg).

3. Production of individual-specific monoclonal antibodies against idiotype determinants of membrane immunoglobulins in lymphatic leukemia and malignant lymphomas
(Project head: Dr. Gerhard Moldenhauer, Institute of Immunology and Genetics, Deutsches Krebsforschungszentrum).

4. The enzymes of purine metabolism in the differentiation of normal lymphocyte precursors and in malignant lymphatic cells
(Project head: Priv.-Doz. Dr. Anthony Ho, Medical Policlinic, University of Heidelberg).

5. Classification of human leukemias by biochemical and immunological characterization of surface structures on leukemic and normal lymphatic cells capable of differentiation
(Project head: Dr. Reinhard Schwartz, Institute of Immunology and Genetics, Deutsches Krebsforschungszentrum).

6. Lymphokin receptors on human T leukemias and T-cell lymphomas
(Project heads: Priv.-Doz. Dr. Peter Krammer, Institute of Immunology and Genetics, Deutsches Krebsforschungszentrum, Dr. Klaus-Michael Debatin, Pediatric Hospital, University of Heidelberg).

7. Investigation of the biology of prophylactic treatment of the central nervous system in leukemias in the animal model
(Project head: Dr. Rolf Ludwig, Pediatric Hospital, University of Heidelberg).

D. Brain tumors
(Coordinator: Prof. Volker Sturm, Surgical Hospital, University of Heidelberg).

Subprojects:

1. Stereotactic brain tumor therapy
(Project heads: Prof. Volker Sturm, Department of Neurosurgery, Surgical Hospital, University of Heidelberg, Prof. D. Walter J. E. Lorenz, Department of Nuclear Medicine, Deutsches Krebsforschungszentrum).
2. Elaboration of an individual prognosis of human brain tumors by correlation of histological, immunocytochemical and impulse-cytometric data
(Project head: Dr. Karl Schwechheimer, Institute of Neuropathology, Institute of Comparative and Experimental Pathology).

These projects have repercussions in the research fields tumors of the respiratory tract, gastrointestinal tract and of the hematopoietic system. Further large-scale projects are foreseen. The members of the Tumor Center are convinced that the formation of these cooperative focal point research projects results in intensive use of the arsenal of methods, theoretical and clinical knowledge, so that personal research initiatives and specific clinical care of carcinoma patients are especially promoted.

Besides the large-scale projects, the following four individual projects are promoted in the Heidelberg/Mannheim Tumor Center:

1. Investigations on serial sections of the breast to improve and rationalize histopathological workup
(Project head: Dr. Axel Müller, Gy-necological Hospital and Institute of Pathology, University of Heidelberg).

2. Detection of blood group antigens and autologous antibodies against tumor-associated antigens in bladder tumors and renal cell carcinomas
(Project head: Prof. Kurt Dreikorn, Surgical Hospital, Priv.-Doz. Dr. Ernst Rauterberg, Institute of Immunology and Serology, Dr. Axel Schäfer, Institute of Immunology and Serology, all University of Heidelberg).

3. Cytoskeleton differentiation markers for improvement of diagnosis of skin tumors
(Project head: Prof. Werner Franke, Institute of Cell and Tumor Biology, Deutsches Krebsforschungszentrum, Prof. Ernst G. Jung, Dermatological Hospital, Mannheim Clinic, University of Heidelberg).

4. Investigations on the immunoregulation of paraprotein-forming human lymphocytes in vitro by means of anti-idiotypic antibodies
(Project head: Dr. Jürgen Brust, Institute of Immunology and Serology, University of Heidelberg).

The Heidelberg/Mannheim Tumor Center with its close link between hospitals and the Deutsches Krebsforschungszentrum is an optimally integrated center for research and therapy. A sign of positive development is, among other things, the fact that the agreement between the partners of the Tumor Center was revised to take into account the current situation and signed again in December 1984. The spirit of this contract, namely to attain progress in patient care by cooperation between a large number of clinical and theoretical units, has remained the same.

## Coordinating Committee for Cancer Research of the Arbeitsgemeinschaft der Großforschungseinrichtungen

The Working Group of the Arbeitsgemeinschaft der Großforschungseinrichtungen (AGF) of the Federal Republic of Germany comprises 13 institutions with a total of around 16,000 staff members. It regards its function inter alia as a rational coordination of research work closely related in terms of topic, in which several large-scale research facilities are participating. The Coordinating Committee for Cancer Research was constituted in 1983. About 1,500 staff in institutions of the AGF are devoted to cancer research. Cancer research is concentrated at the Deutsches Krebsforschungszentrum (DKFZ) in Heidelberg, but important contributions are also being made by various other large-scale research institutions. This is reflected by the membership composition of the Committee. One member of the Coordinating Committee comes from the Society of Biotechnical Research (GBF) in Braunschweig-Stöckheim, one member each from the Nuclear Research Facility in Jülich (KFA) and the Nuclear Research Facility in Karlsruhe (KFK); the Gesellschaft für Strahlen- und Umweltforschung (GSF) in München-Neuherberg is represented by two members, and the Deutsches Krebsforschungszentrum with three members:

Prof. Peter Bannasch, DKFZ (Chairman)
Prof. Ludwig E. Feinendegen, KFA
Prof. Wolfgang Gössner, GSF
Prof. Ulrich Hagen, GSF
Prof. Harald zur Hausen, DKFZ
Prof. Peter Herrlich, KFK
Prof. Peter Mühlradt, GBF
Prof. Dietrich Schmähl, DKFZ

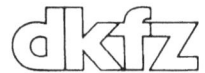

Dr. Horst Metzler of the Deutsches Krebsforschungszentrum looks after the organization of the committee.

In the first year of its existence, the committee first of all carried out a survey of the work performed in the field of cancer research in the AGF and has defined the focal points of future work: "Cancer research in the AGF. Present state of cancer research and list of research activities" (available on request).

In a publication sent to the Federal Ministry for Research and Technology, this report was supplemented by specifications of fields of work in which the committee sees research areas especially worthy of promotion. These include "molecular and classical tumor cytogenetics", "early cellular alterations in carcinogenesis", "metastatic spread and invasive growth", "monoclonal antibodies in tumor diagnosis and therapy" and "experimental radiotherapy and chemotherapy". The committee expressly pointed out that the necessary establishment or extension of this research facility is not possible without provision of additional funds.

For the promotion of international collaboration in cancer research, the Coordinating Committee represented German interests in the preparation of the second Indian-German Symposium which took place in Bombay in February 1985 under the auspices of the Indian Council of Medical Research. Fourteen German scientists from the institutes of the AGF, the Max Planck Society and the Universities of Essen, Hamburg, Kiel and Mainz participated in the symposium. In accordance with the wishes of the Indian hosts, a broad spectrum of current problems was treated at the symposium, which focused on the question of causes, etiology and possibilites of controlling the types of cancer which are especially frequent in the Indian population. This applies, for example to oral cavity cancer, which has clearly been shown to be caused by the chewing of tobacco usual in India, to cervical cancer and liver cancer as well as malignant diseases of the blood and lymphatic tissue. In the opinion of all participants, the symposium was very successful. After the symposium, members of the German delegation visited the Indian cancer research centers in Bombay, Madras, Calcutta and New Delhi besides some other research facilities, e.g., the Center of Cellular Molecular Biology and the National Institute of Nutrition in Hyderabad. The German scientists were not only able to explore the possibilities of cooperation with Indian partners on the spot. The extensive experience gathered at the symposium in Bombay and during the information visits to various institutes formed an excellent basis of the final conference with the Indian Council of Medical Research in New Delhi, at which concrete plans for Indian-German projects in cancer research were discussed. A concentration of cooperation on a few fields of work, in which the exchange of research concepts and methods appears especially desirable, was agreed:

– Genesis of cancer induced by environmental chemicals and food additives
– cause and etiology of cancer types which predominate in India, e.g., cervical cancer, hepatic cancer, breast cancer and cancer of the blood
– fundamental mechanism of growth and differentiation of which the exploration is important for the understanding of all kinds of cancer.

The possibilities of implementing the projects presented so far are being checked at present on the Indian side by the Indian Council of Medical Research, and on the German side by the AGF Coordinating Committee for Cancer Research.

Above and beyond the described activities, the Coordinating Committee is planning scientific events which are concerned with current problems of cancer research and at the same time will present a report on the contribution of the AGF to the solution of these problems. The first symposium of this kind will take place in 1986 in Heidelberg under the title "Cancer risks: strategies for elimination". The AGF Coordinating Committee is deliberately taking up a topic for which there is great public interest.

Cooperations of the Deutsches Krebsforschungszentrum with Hospitals and Institutes at Home and Abroad in the Field of Clinical and Experimental Oncological Research (February 1986)

## Institute of Experimental Pathology

Sequential analysis of neoplastic transformation of epithelial and mesenchymal cells.
Cooperations:
Department of Pathology, Nagoya City University Medical School, Japan.
Institute of Pathology, University of Wuhan, People's Republic of China.

Cellular and molecular mechanisms of hepatocarcinogenesis.
Cooperations:
Laboratory for Experimental Oncology, Indiana University, USA.
Department of Pathology, Nagoya City University, Japan.
Institute of Physiology, University of Toulouse, France.
Institute of Pathology, University of Munich.
Department of Radiology, University of Chicago, USA.

Induction and resistance of tumors.
Cooperations:
Gynecological Hospital of the University, Freiburg.
Rohrbach Hospital Thorax Clinic, Heidelberg.
Cologne University Medical School/University of Texas, San Antonio, USA.

Cellular mechanisms of cytostatic resistance.
Cooperations:
Gynecological Hospital of the University, Heidelberg.
Rohrbach Hospital Thorax Clinic, Heidelberg.

Pathomorphological diagnosis of experimentally induced cancers.
Cooperations:
National Cancer Institute, Bethesda, USA.
Department of Pathology, USC School of Medicine, Los Angeles, USA.
Department of Psychology, University of Missouri – St. Louis, USA.
Institute of Pathology, University of Münster.

Information system of experimental oncopathology and register of experimental tumors.
Cooperations:
Registry of Experimental Cancers, National Cancer Institute, USA.

Protein kinase and substrates at the surface of human cells.
Cooperations:
Institute of Virology, Gießen.
Institute of Neurobiology, University of Heidelberg.
Institute of Biological Chemistry, Padua, Italy.

Bioregulation of the catalytic subunit cAMP-dependent protein kinase.
Cooperations:
Institute of Physiology, University of Heidelberg.
Institute of Pharmacology, University of Heidelberg.

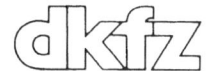

Weizmann Institute, Rehovot, Israel.
University of California, Davis, USA.
University of Melbourne, Australia.

Control of foreign substance-metabolizing key enzymes by protein kinases and effect of carcinogens on the protein-phosphorylating regulation apparatus of the cell.
Cooperations:
Institute of Toxicology, University of Mainz.
Imperial Cancer Research Fund, Medical Oncology Unit, Edinburgh, Great Britain.
Max-Planck Institute of Biophysical Chemistry, Göttingen.

Project: Cytometry with affiliated tumor bank.
Cooperations:
Institute of Anthropology and Human Genetics, University of Heidelberg.
Memorial Sloan Kettering Cancer Center, New York, USA.
Pediatric Hospital of the University, Heidelberg.
Gynecological Hospital of the University, Heidelberg.
Rohrbach Hospital Thorax Clinic, Heidelberg.
University Medical School, Heidelberg.


Institute of Toxicology and Chemotherapy

Experimental chemotherapy.
Cooperations:
3rd Medical Hospital Munich, Großhadern.
Institute of Pharmaceutics, University of Regensburg.
European Organization for Research on Treatment of Cancer.
Study Group of the Federal Ministry of Research and Technology: Drug development and testing for cancer chemotherapy.

Investigations of chemical carcinogens for biological effects in various short-term test systems.
Cooperations:
Federal Institute of Meat Research, Kulmbach.
Universities of Berlin, Freiburg and Hamburg.
Society for Radiation and Environmental Research, Neuherberg.
Federal Institute of Nutrition, Karlsruhe.
Frederick Cancer Research Center, Frederick, Massachusetts, USA.

Comparison of the pathogenetic mechanisms and possibilities of therapy in perinatal or adult phases of tumors of the digestive tract.
Cooperations:
Surgical Hospital, University of Heidelberg.

Chemotherapeutic characterization of new cytostatics; development of new approaches to therapy.

Cooperations:
Max-Planck Institute of Biophysical Chemistry, Göttingen.
Göttingen University Medical School.
Human Genetics, University of Kaiserslautern.
Freiburg University Medical School.
National Cancer Institute Laboratory, Brussels, Belgium.
European Organization for Research on Treatment of Cancer, Screening and Pharmacology Group.
Members of the Study Group of the Federal Ministry for Research and Technology: Drug development and testing for cancer chemotherapy.
University of Kaiserslautern.
Medical Policlinic of Heidelberg University.
Institute of Immunology and Serology, University of Heidelberg.

Occupational exposure to nitrosamines.
Cooperations:
Senate commission for testing of substances damaging to health of the German Research Association.
Factory inspectorates.
Various industrial medical institutes of German universities.

Biological monitoring of nitrosamines.
Cooperations:
Industrial medical institutes.

Analysis of nonvolatile N-nitroso compounds.
Cooperations:
International Agency for Cancer Research, Lyon, France.

Quantification of endogenous nitrosation and of precursors of N-nitroso compounds.
Cooperations:
Surgical Hospital, University of Heidelberg.
Food Chemistry, University of Kaiserslautern.
International Agency for Research on Cancer, Lyon, France.

Carcinogenic and cytostatically acting alkyl-aryl triazenes: metabolism and activation.
Cooperations:
Oncological Institute, Prague, CSSR.
Paterson Laboratories, Christie Hospital and Holt Radium Institute, Manchester, Great Britain.

International Agency for Research on Cancer, Lyon, and Petrov Institute, Leningrad, USSR.
Cancer Chemotherapy Group, Department of Pharmacy, University of Aston, Birmingham, Great Britain.
Department of Biochemical Pharmacology, Institute of Cancer Research, Sutton, Surrey, Great Britain.

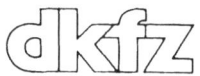

Medical Research Council Toxicology Laboratory, Carshalton, Great Britain.
Institute of Pharmacology, University of Trieste, Italy.

Development of new nitrosourea cytostatics.
Cooperations:
Department of Internal Medicine, University of Freiburg.
Screening and Pharmacology Group of the European Organization for Research on Treatment of Cancer.
Institute of Biochemistry II, University of Heidelberg.
Members of the Study Group: Drug development and testing of the Federal Minister of Research and Technology.

Modification of N-nitrosamine carcinogenesis by anticarcinogens.
Cooperations:
Institute of Toxicology, University of Düsseldorf.

Investigations on the biochemical basis of the combination of antineoplastic chemotherapeutics with nucleosides.
Cooperations:
Ludolf Krehl Hospital, University of Heidelberg.

Improvement of chemotherapy of carcinomas of the head and neck region.
Cooperations:
Tata Memorial Cancer Centre, Bombay, India.


Institute of Cell and Tumor Biology

Cellular control mechanisms in cell division.
Cooperations:
Department of Biological Science, Stanford University, Hopkins Marine Station, Pacific Grove/California, USA.
Department of Biological Science, Florida State University, Tallahassee, Florida, USA.
European Molecular Biology Laboratory, Heidelberg.
Centre of Cell and Chromosome Research, University of Calcutta, India.

Model experiments on the problem of invasion and metastatic spreading.
Cooperations:
Rohrbach Hospital Thorax Clinic, Heidelberg.

Cytoskeleton and karyoskeleton of normal and transformed cells for tumor diagnostics (basis of tumor diagnostics with antibodies against cell type-specific proteins).
Cooperations:
Max Planck Institute of Biophysical Chemistry, Göttingen.
Institute of Pathology, University of Graz, Austria.
Institute of Pathology, University of Geneva, Switzerland.

Institute of Biology, University of Geneva, Switzerland.
Weizmann Institute, Rehovot, Israel (cooperation with Israel in Cancer Research).
Institute of Neurobiology, University of Heidelberg.
Department of Biology, University of Chicago, Chicago, USA.
Rohrbach Hospital Thorax Clinic, Heidelberg.
Imperial Cancer Research Fund, London, Great Britain.

Membranes and redox components of the mammary gland and the mammary tumors.
Cooperations:
Department of Biochemistry, University of Maryland, College Park, Maryland, USA.
Department of Biochemistry and Nutrition, Virginia State University, Blacksburg, Virginia, USA.
Institute of Pathological Anatomy, University of Vienna, Austria.

Structure and function of chromatin: mechanisms of gene activity and regulatory interventions.
Cooperations:
Hershey Medical Center, Hershey, Pennsylvania, USA.
National Institutes of Health, Bethesda, Maryland, USA.
Molecular Genetics, University of Heidelberg.
University of Tennessee, Oak Ridge, Tennessee, USA.

Characterization of transcription units and transcription products in lamp-brush chromosomes.
Cooperations:
University of Chicago, USA.
University of St. Andrews, Scotland.

Relatedness, formation and functions of plasma membrane-associated electron transport systems in animal cells.
Cooperations:
Department of Biological Sciences, Purdue University, West Lafayette, Indiana, USA.
Department of Biochemistry, University of Maryland, College Park, Maryland, USA.

Interactions of proteins from intermediate filaments with other cell constituents.
Cooperations:
European Molecular Biology Laboratory, Heidelberg.
Weizmann Institute of Science, Rehovot, Israel.

Correlation of DNA sequence and chromatin structure of primary transcription units.
Cooperations:
Institute of Biochemistry, University of Würzburg.
Institute of Physiological Chemistry, University of Marburg.
Institute of Molecular Biology, University of Zürich, Switzerland.
Laboratory of Molecular Biology, University of Cambridge, England.
Institute of Biochemistry, University of Würzburg.

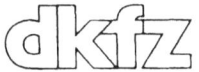

Systems of intracellular $Ca^{2+}$ regulation, use of monoclonal antibodies.
Cooperations:
Endocrinology, University of Heidelberg.
Institute of Physiology I, University of Heidelberg.
Stanford University, Pacific Grove, California, USA.
Florida State University, Tallahassee, USA.
Pacific Biomedical Research Center, University of Hawaii, Honolulu, USA.

Control of gene function by steroid hormones.
Cooperations:
Institute of Physiological Chemistry, University of Marburg.

Cloning of mRNA for preproneurophysin I and II.
Cooperations:
Institute of Physiological Chemistry, University of Heidelberg.
Institute of Physiological Chemistry, University of Marburg.

Structure and expression of the chick lysozyme gene.
Cooperations:
Institute of Physical Chemistry, University of Marburg.

Expression of the genes for tryptophan oxygenase and tyrosine aminotransferase after transfer into homologous and heterologous cells.
Cooperations:
University of Munich.

Correlation of the structure and function of the Dictyostelium genes.
Cooperations:
Max Planck Institute of Biochemistry, Munich-Martinsried.
Molecular Biology Center, Heidelberg.
Max Planck Institute of Molecular Genetics, Berlin.

Structures and function of the dechromatinized cell nucleus.
Cooperations:
Special Research Field 136 (Cancer Research) of the German Research Association, University of Heidelberg.
Institute of Cell Biology, University of Essen.
Department of Microbiology, University of Tel Aviv, Israel (cooperation with Israel in Cancer Research).

Genome alterations of mutated tumor cells.
Cooperations:
Institute of Human Genetics, Homburg/Saar.
Institute of Applied Physics, University of Heidelberg.
Institute of Anthropology and Human Genetics, University of Heidelberg.
Instituto de Investigaciones Bioquimicas "CAMPOMAR", Buenos Aires, Argentina.

Mechanism of mitosis.
Cooperations:
Department of Biochemistry, University of Wyoming, Laramie, USA.
Institute of Immunology and Serology, University of Heidelberg.
Department of Dermatology, University of Heidelberg.
Munich University Medical School.
Gießen University Medical School.

Localization of the binding sites of cytostatics on tubulin, test of a photo-reactive derivative for the feasibility of therapeutic use.
Cooperations:
Department of Pharmacology, University of Indiana, Indianapolis, USA.
University of Texas, San Antonio, USA.
Weizmann Institute of Science, Rehovot, Israel (cooperation with Israel in Cancer Research).

## Institute of Biochemistry

Metabolism and mechanism of action of initiators of carcinogenesis, polyfunctional aromatic hydrocarbon type.
Cooperations:
Institute of Toxicology, University of Mainz, Special Research Field 302, "Control factors of tumorigenesis".
Institute of Microbiology, Darmstadt Technical University.
Baylor College of Medicine, Department of Pharmacology, Texas Medical Center, Houston, Texas, USA.

Metabolism and mechanism of biochemical action of initiation promoters of carcinogenesis: polyfunctional diterpene type.
Cooperations:
Fraunhofer Institute, Hannover.
Institute S. Stefan, Ljubljana, Yugoslavia.
National Cancer Center, Research Institute, Tokyo, Japan.

Tumor promoters of the diterpene ester type as cancer risk factors.
Cooperations:
Institute of Pharmaceutical Biology, University of Munich.
Institute of Honey Research, Bremen.
Institute of Bee Research, Celle.
Istituto di Entomologia Agraria dell'Università di Napoli, Portici, Italy.
Kunming Institute of Botany, Academia Sinica, Kunming, People's Republic of China.
Phytochemical Laboratory, Kunming Institute of Botany, Academia Sinica, Kunming, People's Republic of China.
Cancer Research Institute, Tata Memorial Centre, Bombay, India.
Graduate School, Prince of Songkla University, Thailand.

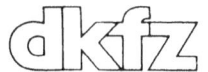

Antineoplastic action of polyfunctional diterpenes.
Cooperations:
National Cancer Institute, Screening Laboratory, Institute Jules Bardet, Brussels, Belgium.
Department of Dermatology, Kiryat Hadassah, Jerusalem, Israel.
Kunming Institute of Botany, Academia Sinica, Kunming, People's Republic of China.
Director, Phytochemical Laboratory, Kunming Institute of Botany, Academia Sinica, Kunming, People's Republic of China.

Molecular and cellular progress parameters of chemical hepatocarcinogenesis.
Analysis of mechanisms and quantitative principles of initiation and promotion as a basis of risk appraisal.
Cooperations:
Institute of Molecular Pharmacology, University of Mainz.
Imperial Cancer Research Fund, Medical Oncology Unit, Edinburgh, Great Britain.
Institute of Toxicology, University of Tübingen.
Max Planck Institute of Biophysical Chemistry, Göttingen.
Institute of Toxicology, University of Tübingen.

Expression of marker enzymes and oncogenes in preneoplastic and neoplastic liver cells.
Cooperations:
MacArdle Laboratory for Cancer Research, Madison, Wisconsin, USA.

Biochemical basis of antineoplastic combination chemotherapy.
Cooperations:
Heidelberg University Medical Hospital.
Heidelberg University Surgical Hospital.

Biochemistry of epidermal hyperplasia.
Cooperations:
New York State University, Syracuse, New York, USA.
Centre International de la Recherche Dermatologique, Valbonne (France).
Institute of Biological Chemistry, University of Heidelberg.
Dermatological Hospital, University of Heidelberg.
Heidelberg University Medical Hospital, Department of Clinical Pharmacology, Heidelberg.
Dermatological Hospital, University of Munich.

Mechanism of action of tumor promoters.
Cooperations:
Western Regional Research Center, Berkeley, California, USA.
Oak Ridge National Laboratory, USA.
University of Düsseldorf.
International Agency for Research on Cancer, Lyon.
Weizmann Institute, Rehovot, Israel (cooperation with Israel in cancer research).

Endogenous tumor promoters.
Cooperations:
Max-Planck Institute, Bad Nauheim.
Weizmann Institute of Science, Rehovot, Israel.

Carcinogenesis of keratinocytes in vitro.
Cooperations:
Hebrew University, Jerusalem, Israel (cooperation with Israel in cancer research).
Institut Suisse de Recherches Expérimentales du Cancer (ISREC), Lausanne, Switzerland.

Disturbances of differentiation during carcinogenesis.
Cooperations:
Max-Planck Institute of Biochemistry, Munich.
Dermatology Division, University of Munich.
Department of Dentistry, University of Iowa, USA.
Cosmital Research Laboratory, Fribourg, Switzerland.
Department of Anatomy and Oral Biology, University of Michigan, Ann Arbor, USA.
Department of Microbiology, University of California, Irvine, USA.

Chromosome alterations and gene activation during carcinogenesis.
Cooperations:
Dermatological Hospital, University of Heidelberg.

Institute of Anthropology and Human Genetics, University of Heidelberg.

Biochemical analysis of DNA repair defects in Xeroderma pigmentosum.
Cooperations:
Dermatological Hospital, Mannheim Municipal Hospitals.
Oak Ridge National Laboratory, Oak Ridge, USA.

Induction of biological functions ("SOS functions") by carcinogens.
Cooperations:
Technion Haifa, Israel.

## Institute of Virus Research

Mechanisms of oncogenesis by herpes simplex virus and cytomegalovirus.
Latency and persistence of these viruses in vitro and in vivo.
Cooperations:
University of Michigan, Ann Arbor, USA.
Institute of Virology, University of Erlangen.
Federal Research Institution for Virus Diseases of Animals, Tübingen.
Institute of Virology, University of Frankfurt.
University Policlinic, Heidelberg.
Surgical Hospital, University of Heidelberg.

1. Structure and function of virus- and tumor-specific components;
2. Characterization of human syncytial retrovirus (HSFV).

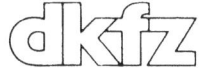

Cooperations:
Institute of Medical Virology, University of Heidelberg.
European Molecular Biology Laboratory, Heidelberg.
Federal Health Office, Berlin.
Nuclear Research Center, Karlsruhe.

Molecular biology of the papilloma viruses.
Cooperations:
Virchow Hospital, Berlin.
Gynecological Hospital, University of Heidelberg.
Biomedical Center, Uppsala, Sweden.
Institute of Clinical Virology, Erlangen.

DNA rearrangements during proliferation of herpes simplex virus. Origin and structure of defective HSV genotypes, amplification of DNA sequences in the HSV genome.
Cooperations:
University of Michigan, Ann Arbor, USA.

1. Restriction of virus multiplication by variant virus particles in HSV;
2. Expression of integrated hepatitis B virus DNA.
Cooperations:
University of Michigan, USA.

Herpes virus DNA replication.
Cooperations:
Sidney Farber Cancer Institute, Harvard Medical School, Boston, USA.
Institute of Virology, Glasgow, Great Britain.

Neuropathogenicity of HSV in the mouse model of HSV infection.
Cooperations:
University of Michigan, USA.

Role of papilloma viruses in human tumors.
Cooperations:
Gynecological Hospitals of the Universities: Ulm, Freiburg, Heidelberg, Düsseldorf.
Dermatological Hospitals of the Universities: Freiburg, Aachen.

Genome structure and gene expression of human papilloma viruses.
Cooperations:
Max-Planck Institute for Breeding Research, Cologne.

B-lymphotropic papovavirus.
Cooperations:
Center for Molecular Biology, Heidelberg.

DNA amplification and tumorigenesis.
Cooperations:
Institute of Virology, University of Freiburg.
Université libre, Brussels.

Investigations on virus-host cell interactions of the Epstein-Barr virus.
Cooperations:
University of Heidelberg.
International Agency for Research on Cancer (IARC), Lyon, France.

Reference Center for papilloma viruses pathogenic in humans.
Cooperations:
Diakonissenkrankenhaus, Freiburg.
University Hospital, Ulm.
Dermatological Hospital, University of Freiburg.
Danish Cancer Registry, Copenhagen, Denmark.
International Agency for Research on Cancer, Lyon, France.

Primary resistance to virus infections.
Cooperations:
University of Erlangen.
Institut Curie, Orsay, France.
Dermatological Hospital Mannheim, University of Heidelberg.

Interferon inducers and immunostimulants.
Cooperations:
University of Marburg.
University of Wisconsin, USA.

Interferon gamma.
Cooperations:
Institute of Microbiology, University of Turin, Italy.
Department of Molecular Pharmacology, Hanover University Medical School.
Bayer Research Center, Wuppertal.

Antiviral mechanisms of interferons.
Cooperations:
Jerusalem (cooperation with Israel in cancer research).
National Cancer Institute, Bethesda, USA.

Structure of viral and cellular chromatin.
Cooperations:
European Molecular Biology Laboratory, Heidelberg.

## Institute of Immunology and Genetics

Immunobiology of metastatic spreading.
Cooperations:
Immunochemistry Research, Evanston University, Evanston, USA.
Department of Experimental Internal Medicine, University of Cologne.

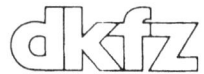

Molecular genetic investigations on metastatic spreading of tumors.
Cooperations:
European Molecular Biology Laboratory, Heidelberg.

Biological, biochemical, molecular biological and genetic analysis of lymphokins, their receptors and target cells in mice and man.
Cooperations:
Department of Experimental Hematology, Society for Radiation and Environmental Research, Munich.
University of Marburg.
Pediatric Hospital, University of Heidelberg.
Department of Microbiology, University of Texas, Dallas, USA.
University of Michigan, Ann Arbor, USA.

Tumor growth and histocompatibility antigens.
Cooperations:
(Cooperation with Israel in cancer research).
European Molecular Biology Laboratory, Heidelberg.

Structure of immune response antigens.
Cooperations:
Yale University, USA.
European Molecular Biology Laboratory, Heidelberg.

Receptors on T lymphocytes.
Cooperations:
University of Münster.
Weizmann Institute, Rehovot, Israel.

Monoclonal antibodies against tumor-associated antigens.
Cooperations:
Medical Policlinic, University of Heidelberg.
Institute of Pathology, University of Heidelberg.
Surgical Hospital, University of Heidelberg.
Radiological Hospital, University of Heidelberg.
Sloan-Kettering Institute for Cancer Research, New York, USA.

Function of main histocompatibility antigens.
Cooperations:
European Molecular Biology Laboratory, Heidelberg.
Sloan-Kettering Institute for Cancer Research, New York, USA.
Stanford University Medical School, USA.
Johns Hopkins University, Baltimore, USA.
National Institute of Health, Bethesda, USA.

Identification of antigens of the main histocompatibility complex.
Cooperations:
National Institute of Health, Bethesda, USA.

## Institute of Nuclear Medicine

Nuclear magnetic resonance tomography in cancer research (medical part).
Cooperations:
Radiological Hospital, University of Heidelberg.
Department of Radiodiagnostics, Surgical Hospital, University of Heidelberg.
Department of General Surgery, Surgical Hospital, University of Heidelberg.
Department of Urology, Surgical Hospital, University of Heidelberg.
Department of Neurosurgery, Surgical Hospital, University of Heidelberg.
Department of Endocrinology, Medical Policlinic, University of Heidelberg.
Rohrbach Hospital Thorax Clinic, Heidelberg.

Echographic diagnostics and computer echoography in oncology.
Cooperations:
Department of Endocrinology, Medical Policlinic, University of Heidelberg.
University Gynecological Hospital, Heidelberg.
Institute of Pathology, University of Heidelberg.
Medical Hospital, Department of Internal Medicine IV (Gastroenterology), University of Heidelberg.
Rohrbach Hospital Thorax Clinic, Heidelberg.
Surgical Hospital, University of Heidelberg.

Computer tomography in oncological diagnostics, planning of therapy and follow-up.
Cooperations:
Rohrbach Hospital Thorax Clinic, Heidelberg.
Department of Neurosurgery, Surgical Hospital, University of Heidelberg.
Radiological Hospital, University of Heidelberg.

Nuclear medical diagnostics and therapy, including positron tomography in oncology.
Cooperations:
Department of Nephrology, Rehabilitation Center, Heidelberg.
Department of Urology, Surgical Hospital, University of Heidelberg.

Stereotactic therapy of brain tumors.
Cooperations:
Department of Neurosurgery, Surgical Hospital and Radiological Hospital, University of Heidelberg.
Further Cooperations:
Study Group Brain Metabolism, Institute of Pathochemistry and General Neurochemistry, University of Heidelberg.
Department of Neuropathology, University of Heidelberg.
Haukeland Sjukehuset, Neurosurgery Department, Bergen, Norway.
Brain Tumor Research Center, University of California, San Francisco, USA.
Department of Neurological Surgery, University of Michigan, Ann Arbor, Michigan, USA.

Investigations on optimization of therapy of cancer diseases with various kinds of radiation – Collaborative project of the Departments 810, 820 and the Radiological Hospital, University of Heidelberg.

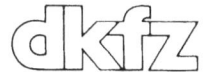

German Thorotrast study.
Cooperations:
Institute of Biophysics, University of the Saarland, Homburg.
Institute for Radiation Hygiene of the Federal Health Office, Munich-Neuherberg.
Institute of Pathology, Municipal Hospital, Ludwigshafen.


Physics in radiodiagnostics and magnetic resonance (MR).
Cooperations:
Radiological Hospital, University of Heidelberg.
Department of Neurosurgery and Department of Urology, Surgical Hospital, University of Heidelberg.
Rohrbach Hospital Thorax Clinic, Heidelberg.
Department of Gastroenterology, Medical Hospital, University of Heidelberg.
Department of Endocrinology, Medical Policlinic, University of Heidelberg.
Department of Oncological Surgery, Surgical Hospital, University of Heidelberg.
Radiology Center, Municipal Hospitals, Mannheim.
Institute of Cancer Research, Royal Marsden Hospital, Sutton, Great Britain.
European Communities Concerted Action on Ultrasonic Tissue Characterization.


Physics in nuclear medicine and positron emission tomography.
Cooperations:
Rohrbach Hospital Thorax Clinic, Heidelberg.
Institute of Applied Physics, University of Heidelberg.


Physics in radiotherapy.
Cooperations:
European Organization for Research on Treatment of Cancer (European Clinical Neutron Dosimetry Group).
Universities of Essen, Hamburg, Munich and Münster.
Institute of Radiobiology, Society for Radiation and Environmental Research, Neuherberg.


Development and application of computer-supported techniques in oncological radiology.
Cooperations:
Radiological Hospital, University of Heidelberg.
Department of Neurosurgery, Surgical Hospital, University of Heidelberg.
Institute of Technical Information Science, Technical University of Berlin.
Department of Physics, Daniel de Hoed Cancer Clinic, Rotterdam, Netherlands.


Investigations on radiation-induced carcinogenesis.
Cooperations:
Institute of Radiation Hygiene, Federal Health Office, Munich.
Nuclear Medical Division, Steglitz Hospital, Berlin.
Institute of Pathology, Municipal Hospitals, Ludwigshafen.

Development of techniques for the visualization and labeling of organic biomolecules.·
Cooperations:
Society for Nuclear Research, Karlsruhe.
Nuclear Research Facility, Jülich.
Chemical Institute, University of Heidelberg.
Medical Hospital, University of Heidelberg.

Development of radiolabeled drugs for nuclear medical diagnosis and therapy.
Cooperations:
Surgical Hospital, University of Heidelberg.

Radiolabeled drugs for positron scintigraphy of tumors.
Cooperations:
Rohrbach Hospital Thorax Clinic, Heidelberg.

Labeling of organic compounds with $^{11}$C or $^{18}$F.
Cooperations:
Institute of Chemistry, University of Heidelberg.
Institute of Chemistry, University of Göttingen.
Max Planck Institute of Medical Research, Heidelberg (Organic Chemistry).

In vivo investigation of membrane receptors.
Cooperations:
Medical Hospitals, University of Heidelberg.
Baylor College, Houston, USA.

Characterization of tumors with monoclonal antibodies: differentiation, progression, prognosis and in vivo localization.
Cooperations:
Dermatological Hospital, University of Münster.
1st Medical Hospital, University of Mainz.
Radiological Hospital, University of Heidelberg.
Department of Immunology, 1st Medical Hospital, University of Hamburg.
Ludwig Institute of Cancer Research, Lausanne, Switzerland.
Surgical Hospital, University of Heidelberg.
Dermatological Hospital, University of Heidelberg.

Cellular immune defense mechanisms in metastasizing spontaneous tumors.
Cooperations:
Surgical Hospital, University of Heidelberg.
Institute of Genetics and Toxicology, University of Karlsruhe.
Institute for Agricultural Research, Cambridge, Great Britain.
Weizmann Institute of Science, Rehovot, Israel (cooperation with Israel in cancer research).
Karolinska Institute, Stockholm, Sweden.
Institute of Immunopathology, University of Verona, Italy.

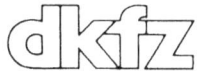

## Institute of Documentation, Informatics and Statistics

Epidemiological bone tumor registry; Working Group on Bone Tumors.
Cooperations:
The Working Group on Bone Tumors comprises as permanent members 12 bone tumor reference centers from the Federal Republic of Germany and eight bone tumor reference centers from abroad (German Democratic Republic, Switzerland, Austria, Hungary, CSSR and Poland).

Descriptive epidemiological studies.
Cooperations:
State Statistical Offices of the Federal States.

CIOMS nomenclature project.
Cooperations:
About 450 scientists from the German speaking world (Federal Republic of Germany, German Democratic Republic, Austria, Switzerland).

Clearing-House for On-Going Research in Cancer Epidemiology.
Cooperations:
National Cancer Institute, Bethesda, USA.
International Agency for Research on Cancer, Lyon, France.

Clinical cancer documentation, e.g., Working Group of the German Tumor Centers (ADT, TNM field studies).
Cooperations:
ADT and Federal Tumor Centers, numerous partner hospitals in the context of TNM studies.

Analytical epidemiological studies.
Cooperations:
Vienna Bone Tumor Registry.
International Agency for Research on Cancer, Lyon, France.
Institute of Medical Documentation and Statistics, University of Mainz.
Professional Trade Association of the Metal-Processing Industry.
Institute of Pathology, University of Göttingen.
Federal Health Office, Berlin.

International cancer literature information system/CANCERNET.
Cooperations:
Centre National de la Recherche Scientifique, Villejuif, France.

Analysis, improvement and reconstruction of organizational structures in cancer diagnosis, therapy and follow-up.
Cooperations:
Heidelberg/Mannheim Tumor Center.
Tumor Registry of the State of Salzburg, Austria.
Department of Transplantation Immunology, Institute of Immunology and Serology, University of Heidelberg.

Development and application of mathematical, information science and quantum theoretical methods for the analysis of biopolymers.
Cooperations:
Los Alamos National Laboratory, Los Alamos, USA.
European Molecular Biology Laboratory, Heidelberg.
Molecular Biology Center, Heidelberg.
Max Planck Institute of Medical Research, Heidelberg.
Institutes of the University of Heidelberg.

Development of dialog-capable systems with methods of information theory and pattern recognition to support analytical and diagnostic techniques in cancer research.
Cooperations:
Institute of Applied Physics I, University of Heidelberg.
University Computing Center, University of Uppsala, Sweden.
AI Laboratory, Massachusetts Institute of Technology, Cambridge, USA.
Hadassah Medical School, Hebrew University, Jerusalem, Israel.

Statistical methods for planning animal experiments taking into account the course of the tumor process.
Cooperations:
Biostatistics Unit, International Agency for Research on Cancer, Lyon, France.
National Cancer Institute, Bethesda, Maryland, USA.
Medical Hospital (Gastroenterology), University of Heidelberg.

Statistical models in carcinogenesis and cocarcinogenesis.
Cooperations:
International Agency for Research on Cancer, Lyon, France.

Statistical methods for clinical studies.
Cooperations:
Heidelberg/Mannheim Tumor Center.
Working Group on Breast Cancer (10 hospitals).
Working Group on Gastrointestinal Tumors (15 hospitals):

Mathematical-statistical analysis of experiments in cell biology.
Cooperations:
Max Planck Institute of Immunobiology, Freiburg.
Federal Research Institute for Virus Diseases of Animals, Tübingen.

Production and further development of statistical software (nonstandard software).
Cooperations:
Heidelberg/Mannheim Tumor Center.
IBM Scientific Center, Heidelberg.
Members of the APL Club Germany.

Mathematical models for carcinogenesis.
Cooperations:
Institute of Applied Mathematics, University of Heidelberg.
Mathematics Division, University of Mainz.

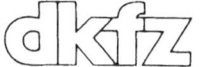

## Spectroscopy Central Working Group

Development of a computer-supported spectroscopic information system.
Cooperations:
Stichting Nederlandse Information Combinatie, Netherlands.

Development of analytical (spectroscopic) methods for investigations on the mechanism of carcinogenesis.
Cooperations:
University of Heidelberg.

## Radiation Protection and Dosimetry Central Facility

Radiation protection dosimetry.
Cooperations:
Institute of Biophysics, University of the Saarland.
Federal Institute for Physics and Technology, Braunschweig.
National Bureau of Standards, Washington D.C., USA.

Dosimetry in radiotherapy and integral dose calculation in radiotherapy patients.
Cooperations:
Department of Neurosurgery, Surgical Hospital, University of Heidelberg.

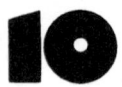

# Organs
# of the Foundation

In the report period, the Foundation Deutsches Krebsforschungszentrum had the following organs in accordance with § 7 Foundation Statutes:

– Board of Trustees
– Management Board
– Scientific Council

## Board of Trustees

In accordance with § 8 Foundation Statutes, the Board of Trustees has the task of supervising the legality, appropriateness and economy of the management of the foundation's business. It decides on the general research objectives and important research policies and financial matters of the foundation. In addition, it adopts the principles of resource management and of checking results, and passes the finance plans over several years, including the extension and investment programs. As a rule, the Board of Trustees meets twice a year.

The Board of Trustees was chiefly concerned with the following tasks in 1983/ 84

– Appointment of Professor Harald zur Hausen as chairman and scientific member of the foundation Management Board (1. 5. 1983)
– discussion and adoption of a new scientific concept for the Institute of Nuclear Medicine
– discussion and adoption of a new scientific concept for the Institute of Documentation, Informatics and Statistics
– foundation of the department "Genome Alteration and Carcinogenesis" as well as the appointment of an acting head for this department

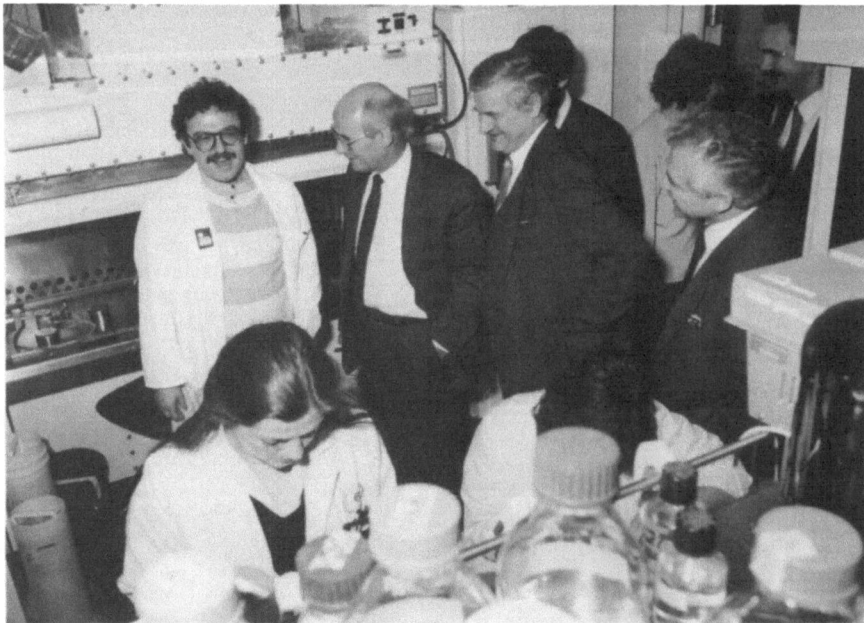

Fig. 152
Secretary of State Hans-Hilger Haunschild and Ministerialdirektor Fritz-Rudolf Güntsch, Chairman of the Board of Trustees of the German Cancer Research Center (both Federal Ministry of Research and Technology), in one of the Laboratories

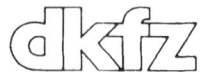

- conclusion of a cooperation agreement between the University of Heidelberg and the Deutsches Krebsforschungszentrum
- foundation of the departments "Biochemistry of Tumours" and "Applied Immunology" in the Institute of Nuclear Medicine with simultaneous dissolution of the departments "Nuclear Medical Diagnosis" and Nuclear Medicine and Special Radiotherapy. Procurement of a Positron Emission Tomograph (PET) as well as a whole-body nuclear Magnetic Resonance Tomograph up to 1.5 Tesla (NMR)
- measures for the reorganization of data processing at the center
- establishment of a project "Cytometry and Chromosome Sorting"
- discussion and application of the results of the appraisal of the Institute of Toxicology and Chemotherapy
- appointment of an administrative member of the Management Board (1. 7. 1984)
- redrafting the agreement on the establishment and operation of the Heidelberg/Mannheim Tumor Center
- foundation of the central facility "Central Data Processing" (ZDV) and appointment of an acting head of this central facility as well as alteration of the field of work of the existing department "Central Data Processing" with simultaneous conferment of a new name "Department of Medical and Biological Informatics"
- discussion and adoption of new project regulations for the center in accordance with § 19 of the Foundation Statutes
- discussion and application of the results of the external expertise on the Institute of Experimental Pathology
- opinion of the Management Board on the report of the Federal Government

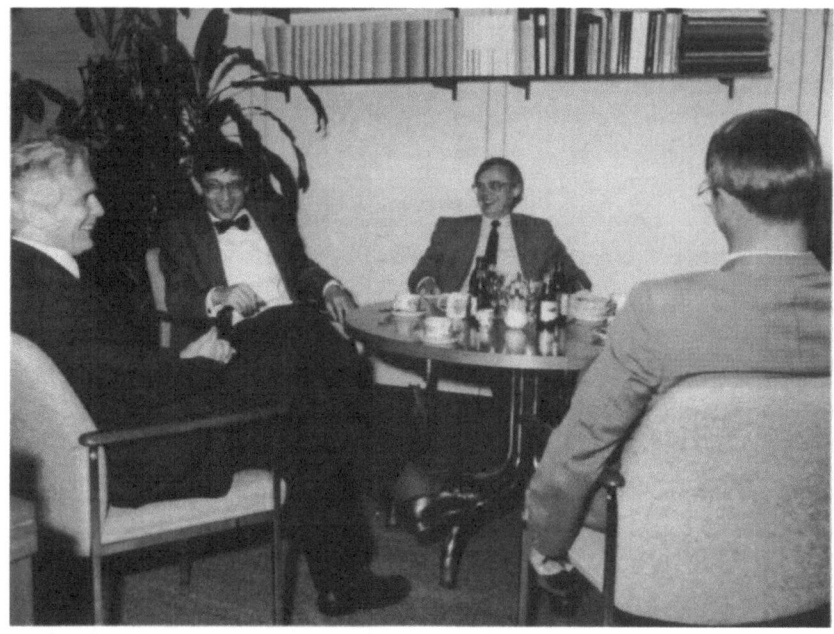

## Management Board of the Foundation

According to § 14.1 of the statutes, the Management Board of the Foundation directs the Foundation. The Management Board of the Foundation consists (§ 15.1) of at least one scientific and one administrative member. The chairman is the scientific representative of the Foundation. The Board of Trustees appoints the members of the Management Board of the Foundation after hearing the Scientific Council (§ 15.2).

Prof. Harald zur Hausen was appointed scientific member and chairman of the Management Board of the Foundation on May 1st, 1983. Dr. Ernst-Lüder Solte (administrative member of the Management Board of the Foundation) left the Deutsches Krebsforschungszentrum on December 31st, 1983 for personal reasons and accepted a new post in the Baden-Württemberg Ministry of Science and Arts. His successor, Dr. Reinhard Grunwald, former managing director the German Primate Center in Göttingen, was appointed on July 1st, 1984.

of April 12th 1984 "Status and perspectives of the large-scale research institutions"

According to the § 10 of the Foundations Statutes, the Scientific Committee of the Board of Trustees has the function of preparing the decisions of the Board of Trustees in all scientific matters. It is responsible in particular for continuous appraisal by scientific experts.

Besides establishing the basis for decisions for the Board of Trustees, the Scientific Committee has to appoint panels of experts consisting of leading international scientists for external appraisal of the institutes of the Deutsches Krebsforschungszentrum. In the report period these appraisals – usually repeated every 5 years – concerned the Institute of

Fig. 153
From the left to the right: Prof. Harald zur Hausen, scientific member of the Management Board of the German Cancer Research Center, Federal Minister of Research and Technology Dr. Heinz Riesenhuber, Ministerialrat Dr. Konrad Buschbeck and Dr. Reinhard Grunwald, administrative member of the Management Board, in discussion

Toxicology and Chemotherapy, the Institute of Experimental Pathology, the Institute of Cell and Tumor Biology as well as the Institute of Virus Research.

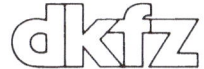

## Scientific Council

The Scientific Council has the task of advising the Board of Trustees and the Management Board in all important matters of a scientific nature. Decisions of the Management Board require the approval of the Scientific Council in these matters.

The Scientific Council is concerned in particular with research projects and research programs, appointments, application of research results, monitoring of results, promotion of the flow of scientific information, collaboration with the university, and other research institutions as well as with budget planning and investment programs.

The Scientific Council consists of 16 members and comprises the executive directors of the eight institutes of the center as well as an equal number of selected representatives of the scientific staff.

In the years 1983/84, the Scientific Council held a total of 23 meetings. After the new elections in late 1983, its third three-year period of office commenced in January 1984.

### Members of the Scientific Council (June 1986)

Priv. Doz. Dr. Angel Alonso
Institute of Experimental Pathology

Prof. Wulf Dröge
Institute of Immunology and Genetics

Prof. Werner Franke
Institute of Cell and Tumor Biology

Prof. Peter Bannasch
Institute of Experimental Pathology

Prof. Erich Hecker (deputy chairman)
Institute of Biochemistry

Prof. Holger Kirchner (Chairman)
Institute of Virus Research

Prof. Walter Lorenz
Institute of Nuclear Medicine

Dr. Hans-Peter Meinzer
Institute of Documentation, Information Science and Statistics

Prof. Klaus Munk
Institute of Virus Research

Prof. Rudolf Preußmann
Institute of Toxicology and Chemotherapy

Dr. Hartmut Richter
Institute of Biochemistry

Prof. Volker Schirrmacher
Institute of Immunology and Genetics

Prof. Dietrich Schmähl
Institute of Toxicology and Chemotherapy

Prof. Günther Schütz
Institute of Cell and Tumor Biology

Prof. Jürgen Wahrendorf
Institute of Documentation, Information Science and Statistics

Dr. Gerhard Wolber
Institute of Nuclear Medicine and Oncological Radiology

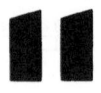

# Staff Council

The Staff Council exercises its rights and duties in accordance with the Staff Representation Law of Baden-Württemberg. In weekly meetings of the Staff Council, all pending problems which are to be treated in the context of codetermination and participation of the Staff Council, are discussed. The Staff Council informs on his work on the bulletin board and at regular staff meetings as well as in smaller meetings on special topics. In addition, the Staff Council has produced an information bulletin since four years.

The Managing Committee of the Staff Council is responsible for current business. Working groups are formed to deal with work arising, for example on questions of pay rates and personnel planning, personnel data protection, security at work, staff training.

Members of the Staff Council
(June 1st, 1985)

Dieter Baumgartl
Helmut Eskerski
Werner Fleischer
Dr. Holger Friesel
Dr. Günther Hartmann, Member of the Managing Committee
Siegfried Herz
Brigitte Hobrecker, Chairman
Jutta Knauft, Member of the Managing Committee
Albert Koch, 1st Deputy Chairman
Sabine Leidig
Christine Martinsohn
Adolf Wesch
Ruth Wittmann, 2nd Deputy Chairman

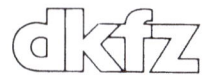

# Administration

## Functions and Organization

As a central service facility, the Administration of the Deutsches Krebsforschungszentrum is responsible for the central administration as well as for the special administration of the institutes and independent facilities. It prepares decisions of the organs of the Foundation, especially of the Management Board, and implements these decisions. Its work is determined by the manifold individual demands from scientists as well as those based upon the numerous federal and Länder laws and regulations resulting from the legal status and matters of financing. In this "field of tension", the Administration endeavors to carry out its work rapidly and unbureaucratically with due consideration of the problems involved. It achieve this

objective, inter alia, by direct and rapid contact with the institutes.

The work of the Administration comprises functions in the departments

- General Administration,
- Personnel and Social Affairs,
- Finance and Accounting,
- Procurement, Material Economy,
- Engineering,
- General Services.

In the report period, the Administration

- was also responsible for drafting a cooperation agreement between the University of Heidelberg and the Deutsches Krebsforschungszentrum;
- instituted measures for the improvement of information and communication by reorganizing data processing in the Administration. These measures, organized in a project, are in-

Fig. 154

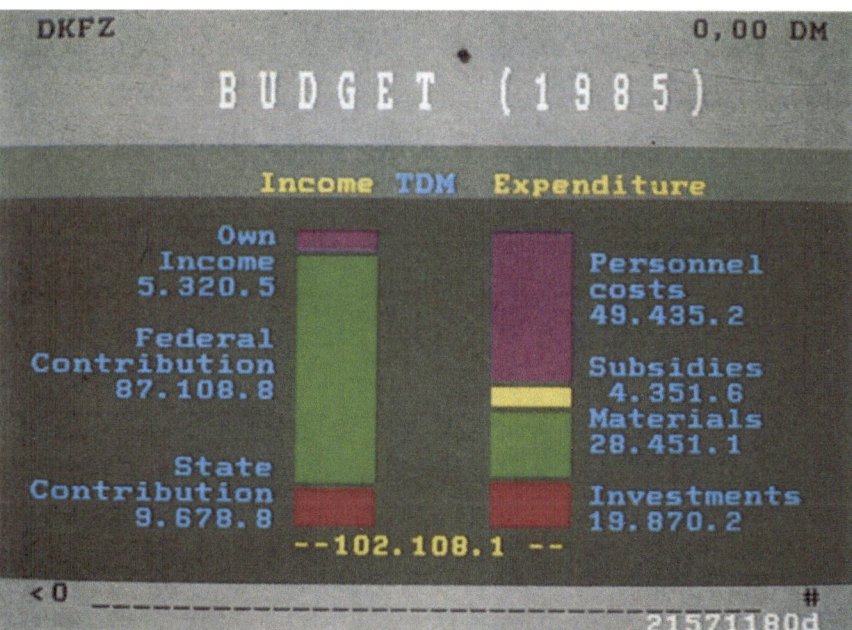

tended to combine the possibilities of applying data processing, which have been developed over the years in the individual departments, and to transfer them into a modern communication system;

– developed and implemented an appropriate distribution of funds in cooperation with the Scientific Council;
– collaborated in the procurement of large-scale medical instruments, including an NMR tomograph, a positron emission tomograph as well as a computer tomograph (SOMATOM DRH 2);
– administered the reorganization of the central animal laboratory. In this connection, containers for animal keeping were procured and allow the animals to be kept in accordance with the most modern scientific principles.

A further important function of the Administration is dealing with legacies. In keeping with the wishes of various testators, legacies are being used directly for certain research projects or also for the award of prizes to scientists with special achievements in the field of cancer research. In this connection, the Meyenburg Prize (25,000 DM), awarded by the Wilhelm and Maria Meyenburg Foundation, and the Walther and Christine Richtzenhain Prize (10,000 DM) are to be specially emphasized.

From the legacy of Mrs. Ilse Blumenthal, a laboratory is at present being equipped in honor of Mrs. Blumenthal's father, Dr. Carl Jacoby, who was murdered in Theresienstadt. The laboratory will bear Dr. Jacoby's name.

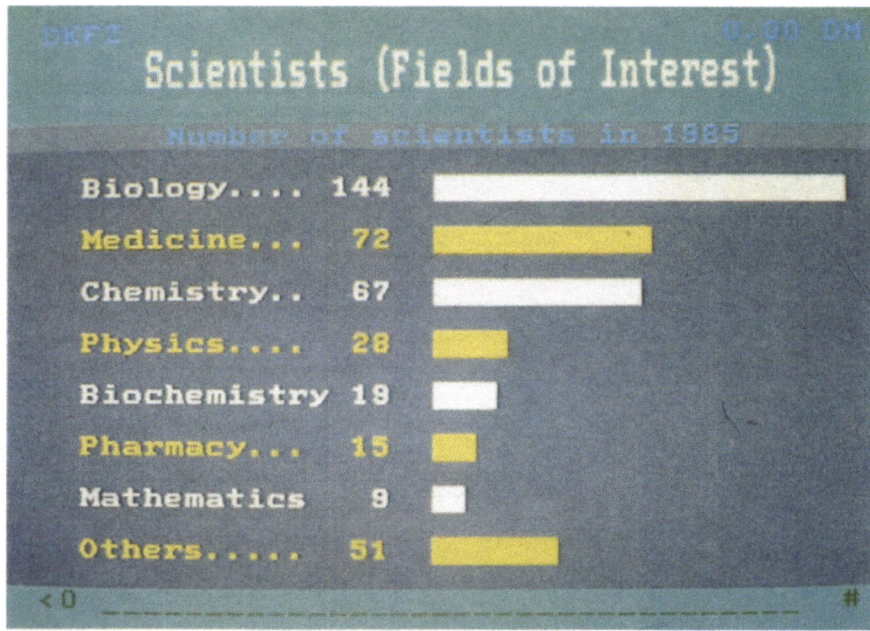

Fig. 155

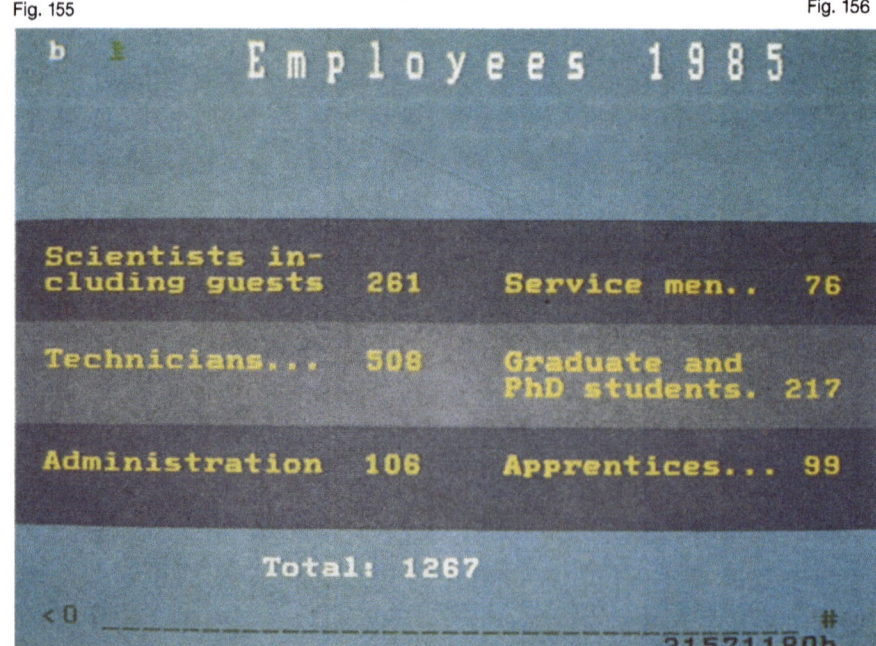

Fig. 156

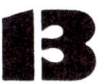

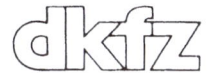

# Teaching, Training, Postgraduate Education

Fostering of up-and-coming scientists is a special concern of the Deutsches Krebsforschungszentrum in order to ensure rapid application of new scientific knowledge in research and clinical practice. The scientists of the Deutsches Krebsforschungszentrum are, therefore, involved in scientific teaching, training and postgraduate education besides their main task of research. From 1983 to 1984 alone, 197 doctoral candidates and diploma candidates carried out research studies at the Cancer Research Center. Fifty-eight dissertations, diploma theses and postdoctoral theses were completed in the same period. In all institutes of the Center, a limited number of places are provided for the performance of scientific work necessary to attain an academic degree.

Fig. 157
Trainees in the teaching laboratory

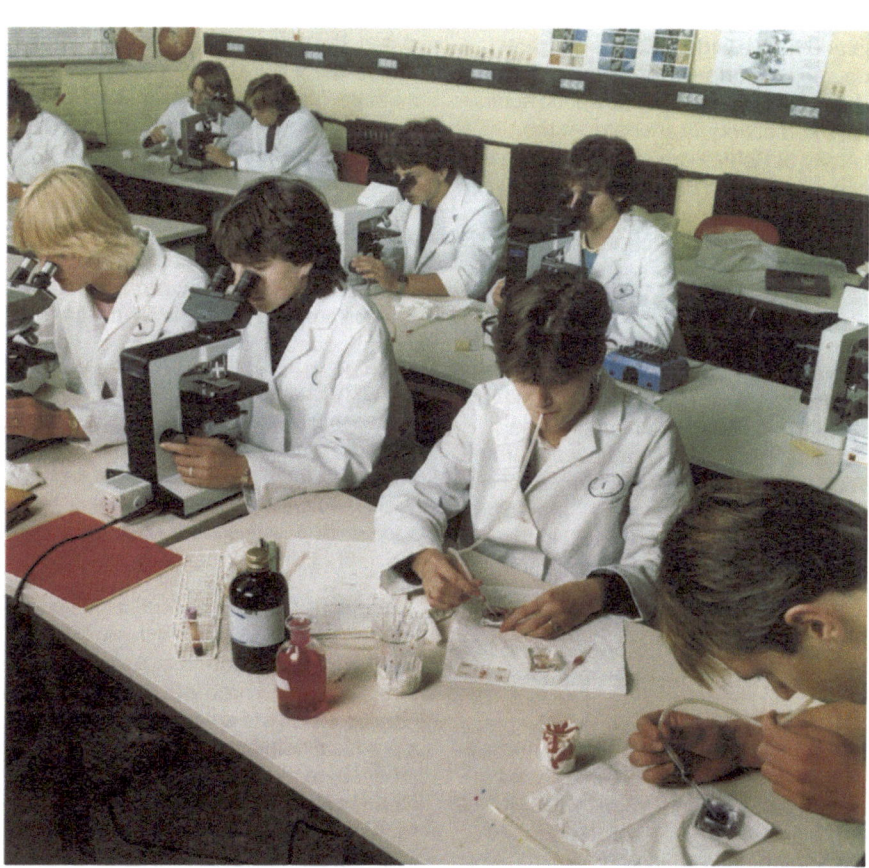

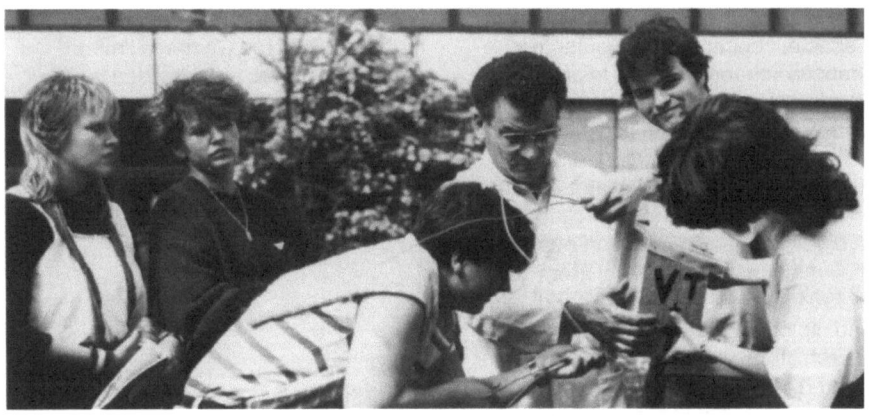

## 13

Fig. 158
Bird protection campaign. The trainees are hanging up self-made bird boxes in the facilities of the Cancer Research Center together with their trainer

In addition, a wide range of practical courses are offered for advanced students, and multifarious scientific seminars and colloquia are held. At the University of Heidelberg and professional schools, around 60 lecture courses are held per term by scientists of the Deutsches Krebsforschungszentrum. In addition, special courses and seminars are held for students in the Center itself.

Since 1981, the Deutsches Krebsforschungszentrum has been able to award its own grants for the promotion of highly qualified young scientists. These scholar ships, which are financed from donation funds, run over a period of six months up to one year and serve to provide young scientists working in the Deutsches Krebsforschungszentrum with special training in novel methods and techniques at home and abroad. In 1983 and 1984, ten up-and-coming young scientists received grants.

The program of colloquia in the Deutsches Krebsforschungszentrum, in which 317 specialist lectures were presented by scientists from 24 countries in 1983 and 1984, serves postgraduate education of the scientists of the Center

as well as interested scientists and physicians of the University of Heidelberg, the Max-Planck Institutes located in Heidelberg and the European Molecular Biology Laboratory.

For the introduction inter techniques and methods, in the development of which working groups of the Cancer Research Center have played a major role, courses are held regularly. Thus the following courses took place:

February 20th to March 2nd 1984: IAEA traineeship at the TRIGA Heidelberg II research reactor, International Atomic Energy Agency (IAEA) as well as two basic medical courses and three courses of postgraduate education in the field of ultrasonography.

In addition, 10 young scientists were appointed in the context of a Junior Scientist Program (project-linked) for two to three years. The promotion of up – and – coming scientists is also the objective of a practical training program in which the students of the Study Foundation of the German Nation can gather experience for four to eight weeks in the Deutsches Krebsforschungszentrum.

This program commenced in 1985 as well as a Trainee Program for postgraduate students of Stanford University (Krupp Foundation).

The Deutsches Krebsforschungszentrum is concerned to extend continuously the number and range of training places for young people. 75 training places have been available each year in 1980 and 1981, 83 places in 1982, 86 places in 1983, 90 places in 1984 and 95 places were available in 1985.

The training places in the various departments of the Deutsches Krebsforschungszentrum are fitted out in such a way that they ensure a comprehensive training, and scientifically trained staff required in research is educated.

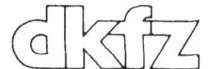

Training for the following occupations is offered at the Center:

In the field of administration:
Doctor's consulting room assistants, office staff, industrial management experts (specialty: public economy);

in the field of engineering:
glass apparatus blowers, precision mechanics, mechanics, joiners, information electronic technicians;

in the laboratory field:
biology laboratory assistants, chemistry laboratory assistants, experimental animal attendants, radiation protection assistants.

The large number of applicants for training places (900) make it necessary to select the trainees by aptitude tests and by demonstration of practical skills. Depending on the occupational objective, a good educational qualification or university entrance qualification is expected.

From 1981 to 1983, more than half of the trainees were able to conclude their training before time with good results in the Chamber of Commerce examinations.

On the basis of a contract with the Baden-Württemberg Ministry of Science and Arts, the Deutsches Krebsforschungszentrum is an official training location for students of the Public Administration Professional School in Stuttgart. Since the beginning of the program in 1979, four subsequent documentation specialists (FH) per year have completed their practical year in the Institute for Documentation, Informatics and Statistics. In addition, radiation protection assistants and radiation protection engineers are trained in the Central Department of Radiation Protection and Dosimetry in collaboration with the Professional Academy in Karlsruhe. Scientists of the Deutsches Krebsforschungszentrum have also been involved in the promotion of young scientific technicians by fulfilling training functions as lecturers at the Heilbronn Professional School and as lecturers at the Training Institute for Medical-Technical Assistants in Heidelberg. Each year, about ten medical technicians and radiological assistants gain practical experience for one year each in the Institute of Nuclear Medicine and Oncological Radiology at the Deutsches Krebsforschungszentrum.

On the basis of a job agreement for postgraduate training at the Deutsches Krebsforschungszentrum, the Deutsches Krebsforschungszentrum has been carrying out an attractive program of postgraduate training since 1981. The program takes into account the needs and justified wishes of the staff and makes an important contribution to the self-realization and further specialization of the staff.

The increasing number of applications for postgraduate training reflects the interest of the staff in postgraduate education. In 1981, 100 members of staff took part in courses, whereas in 1983 more than 500 and in 1984 almost 800 staff members underwent postgraduate training. The internal postgraduate training program ranges from general topics to training in the scientific-technical field for specific occupational groups.

The Deutsches Krebsforschungszentrum also promotes the acquisition of language knowledge with courses carried out at the Center and by individual instruction in external institutions.

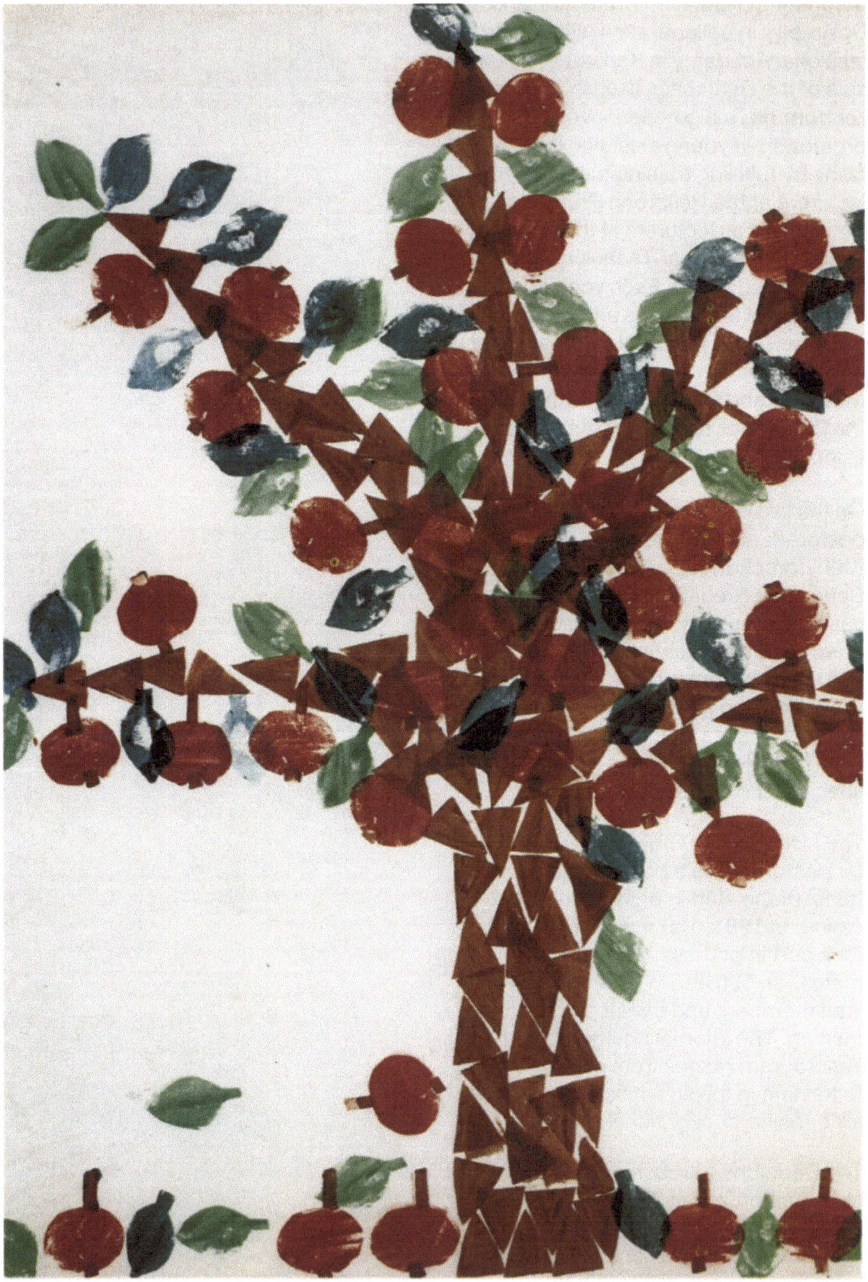

Fig. 159
Heidelberg children created (for the German Cancer Research Center) this picture of an apple tree bearing fruit

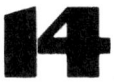

## Statutes

### Statutes and Articles of the Foundation German Cancer Research Center Heidelberg

in the version according to the resolution passed by the Board of Trustees dated 16 December 1982, published in the Legal Gazette Baden-Württemberg on 7 February 1983

## I. General Provisions

### Section 1   Legal Form, Seat

The German Cancer Research Center, a foundation under public law of the Land Baden-Württemberg, has its seat in Heidelberg.

### Section 2   Purpose of the Foundation

(1) It is the purpose of the Foundation to engage in cancer research.
(2) The Foundation may undertake other tasks in this connection, inter alia further education and advanced training.
(3) The research results are to be published.

### Section 3   Non-Profit-Making Institution

(1) As a non-profit-making institution the Foundation shall exclusively and directly serve the public interest, in particular scientific interests according to fiscal regulations.
(2) Any profits made may only be used for the purposes laid down in the Statutes and Articles. The Foundation may not grant benefits to any persons by expenditures which run counter to the purposes of the Foundations or by disproportionately high emoluments.

### Section 4   Assets of the Foundation

The assets of the Foundation shall consist of the goods and titles which have been or are being created or acquired with the aid of the funds placed at its disposal by the Federal Republic of Germany, hereinafter referred to as the Federation, the German Land Baden-Württemberg, hereinafter referred to as the Land, or by third parties. The assets of the Foundation shall be used for the purposes laid down in section 2.

### Section 5   Financing of the Foundation

(1) The Federation and the Land will put up the necessary expenditure of the Foundation in as far as this is not covered by income from other sources or by own or foreign means — with the exception of donations and investment returns therefrom — by allowances according to further agreement.
(2) The means to be put up according to paragraph 1 will be allocated to the Foundation according to the provisions of the budgetary law within the framework of the approved budgets of the Foundation and the budgets of the Federation and the Land.

### Section 6   Budget of the Foundation

(1) The budget of the Foundation must contain any receipts to be expected in the fiscal year, any probable expenses and any probable authorisations to incur liabilities. Receipts and expenditure must be balanced.
(2) The budget will have to be approved by the authority controlling the Foundation.
(3) Grants made to the Foundation are to be recorded in an appendix to the Foundations's accounts.

## II. Organs of the Foundation

### Section 7   Executive Organs

The organs of the Foundation are:
a) the Board of Trustees,
b) the Management Board,
c) the Scientific Council.

### Section 8   Tasks of the Board of Trustees

(1)  The Board of Trustees will supervise the legality, expediency and economy of the conduct of the Foundation's transactions. They will decide on the aims of research and important research policy and financial affairs of the Foundation. They will determine principles of management and those governing efficiency control. They may give directives to the Management Board in special matters of research policy and finance as well as for the implementation of efficiency control.

(2)  The Board of Trustees sets up the annual budgets and the long-term financial plans including the programs for development and investment. They will decide on changes in the Statutes and Articles and on the dissolution of the Foundation as well as on other matters laid down in these Statutes.

(3)  The following matters must be previously approved by the Board of Trustees:

a)  the annual and long-term research programs,

b)  taking up further and discontinuing previous tasks,

c)  the foundation, dissolution and amalgamation of institutes, departments and central installations, the start and termination of projects,

d)  the appointment and recall of the heads of departments, of administrative director as well as of the directors of central installations and projects,

e)  the regulations for institutes and projects,

f)  the regulations for elections and the rules of procedure,

g)  the regulations governing appointments,

h)  principles governing the utilization of the research results of the Foundation,

i)  extraordinary legal transactions and measures exceeding the framework of current business operations which may exert considerable influence upon the position and activity of the Foundation; significant agreements concerning co-operation with other German and foreign undertakings and other institutions; entering into contracts which impose upon the Foundation obligations exceeding a period of one year, inasfar as they are not within the scope of normal business or provided for in the approved budget,

k)  drawing up, changing or terminating employment contracts in excess of or outside the tariff, granting other benefits in excess of or outside the tariff as well as entering into contracts exceeding an amount fixed by the Board of Trustees,

l)  measures of collective tariff commitments or formation and general regulations concerning remuneration and social benefits as well as setting up directives governing the granting of reimbursement of travel and removal costs, of separation allowances and of expenses for the use of motor vehicles.

(4)  For particular types of legal transactions and measures, the Board of Trustees may give its agreement in general.

(5)  In urgent cases it is sufficient to have the prior written consent of the President and the Deputy President of the Board of Trustees. The other members of the Board of Trustees are to be informed by the President immediately.

### Section 9   Composition of the Board of Trustees

(1)  The Board of Trustees consists of at most eighteen honorary members.

(2)  Out of these

a)  four members — one of them being the President — will be delegated and removed from office by the Federation,

b)  two members — one of them being the Deputy President — will be delegated or removed from office by the Land,

c)  three scientists working for the Foundation — at least one of them being head of a department without a seat on the Management Board — will be appointed by the Land in agreement with the Federation from a list of six applicants drawn up by all members of the scientific staff. Further details will be settled by election regulations to be issued by the Management Board in consultation with the Scientific Council and with the consent of the Board of Trustees. If those appointed have seats on the Scientific Council, their membership in the Scientific Council will be terminated upon acceptance of their appointment to the Board of Trustees,

d)  seven external members (mainly specialists) — appointed by the Land in agreement with the Federation upon consultation with the Management Board and the Scientific Council,

e)  Two members as the representatives of the University of Heidelberg, i.e. one proposed jointly by the Faculties of Medicine and Natural Sciences as well as the Rector (President) or a

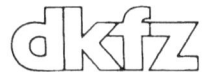

professor charged by the latter — appointed by the Land in agreement with the Federation.

(3) The members referred to in paragraph 2, letters c, d and e will be appointed for a maximum period of three years. Re-appointment is permissible. After expiration of their term of office they will remain in office until the new appointments have been made according to paragraph 2, letters c, d and e. Members may be removed from office for important reasons. Members leaving before their term of office has expired must immediately be replaced from among the non-appointed applicants from the list of suggestions according to paragraph 2, letter c or by a new appointment according to paragraph 2, letter d. Should the list of suggestions be exhausted, the procedure according to paragraph 2, letter c shall be applied. Suggestion and appointment will be valid for the remaining term of office.

## Section 10   Scientific Commitee of the Board of Trustees

(1) The Scientific Commitee prepares the decisions of the Board of Trustees in all scientific matters within the framework of section 8.

(2) The Scientific Commitee bears the responsiblity for the current valuation of the results achieved by the institutes, departments and projects by scientific expertise. As a rule, they set up ad hoc commissions manned by external scientists for this purpose.

(3) The Scientific Commitee of the Board of Trustees consists of the external scientific members of the latter according to section 9, paragraph 2, letter d. From among its members a chairman and a deputy chairman are

elected. The President and the Deputy President of the Board of Trustees may take part in the sessions as guests. The Scientific Commitee may set up standing rules also determining the competence and procedure of the ad hoc commisions in greater detail.

## Section 11   Standing Rules of the Board of Trustees and its Committees

(1) The Board of Trustees may set up standing rules also determining the competence and procedure of the Committees in greater detail. Persons who are not members of the Board of Trustees may also take a seat on the Committee; they will not take part in passing resolutions in Committees granted jurisdiction. A representative of the Federation will take the chair.

(2) The Board of Trustees may set up Committees to prepare their decisions as well as for certain matters to be decided by the Committee itself. At least one member each according to section 9, paragraph 2, letters a to d must have a seat on each Committee.

## Section 12   Meetings of the Board of Trustees and its Committees

(1) The Board of Trustees will be convened by the President once in six months as a rule, but at least once every calendar year.

(2) The members of the Management Board as well as the chairman of the Scientific Council and the chairman of the staff representation or their deputies are entitled to attend the meetings of the Board of Trustees and its Commitees in a consultative capacity, inasfar as the Board of Trustees or the Committee do not decide otherwise.

## Section 13   Resolutions of the Board of Trustees and its Committees

(1) The Board of Trustees will constitute a quorum if two thirds of its members are present or are represented in compliance with paragraph 2.
The President or his deputy must be present. Committees holding power of decision will constitute a quorum if one member each according to section 9, paragraph 2, letters a to c is present or represented.

(2) If unable to attend, the members of the Board of Trustees delegated by the Federation and the Land may arrange to be represented by members of their administration, other members by a member of the Board of Trustees provided with a power of attorney in writing for the individual contingency.

(3) Resolutions of the Board of Trustees are passed with a majority of the valid votes cast. The President and the Deputy President have a double, transferable vote. In case of parity, the President shall have the casting vote. With important questions of research policy, in financial matters, in matters according to section 8, paragraphs 2 and 3 as well as with the appointment of the members and the release of the Management Board, resolutions may not be passed against the votes of members of the Board of Trustees delegated by the Federation or the Land.

(4) Paragraphs 2 and 3 apply to the Committees correspondingly.

(5) In individual cases, the President or, if he is prevented, his deputy may cause resolutions to be passed in writing, by telex of by cable, inasfar as no member of the Board of Trustees registers his immediate protest.

# 14

## Section 14 Functions of the Management Board

(1) The Management Board directs the Foundation.

(2) The Management Board seeks the prior approval of the Scientific Council on the matters set down in section 8, paragraph 3, letters a to g as well as on
— the annual budget and long-term financial plans including the programs for development and investment;
— measures for the implementation of efficiency control of scientific work;
— measures to promote the flow of scientific information within the Foundation (work reports, colloquia, hearings);
— the co-operation with universities other research institutions and international establishments;
— the submission of the scientific progress report to the Board of Trustees.

(3) Inasfar as the Scientific Council's suggestions in these matters should deviate, the Management Board will initiate a renewed joint discussion with the Scientific Council. If agreement cannot be reached, the Management Board will decide. If the Management Board makes a decision which deviates from the recommendations of the Scientific Council, they will have to supply an explanation in writing to the Scientific Council and the Board of Trustees.

## Section 15 Composition of the Management Board, Scope of Authority

(1) The Management Board consists of at least one scientific and one administrative member. The administrative member shall be qualified for employment in the higher administrative service. The term of office for the members of the Management Board is limited and will, as a rule, amount to five years. Re-appointment is permissible. Appointments may be revoked at any time.

(2) The chairman of the Management Board and the other members will be appointed and recalled by the Board of Trustees after consultation with the Scientific Council. The Scienfitic Council has the right of nomination for scientific members and for the chairman.
The members of the Management Board may not at the same time be managing directors of an institute or members of the Scientific Council. The President of the Board of Trustees, who in this capacity represents the Foundation, will enter into, change or terminate contracts with the members of the Management Board.

(3) The chairman of the Management Board will be the scientific representative of the Foundation. Together with the administrative member he will represent the Foundation judicially and extrajudicially. In matters of current administration the administrative member may represent the Foundation on his own.

(4) The Management Board will set up standing rules wich require the approval of the Board of Trustees. The standing rules will also regulate the authority according to paragraph 3, sentences 2 and 3 in the event the authorized representatives are prevented from fulfilling their function.

(5) The administrative member of the Management Board will be in charge of budget affairs in the sense of section 9 of the budget regulations of the Land Baden-Württemberg.

## Section 16 Tasks of the Scientific Council

(1) The Scientific Council advises the Board of Trustees and the Management Board in all significant matters of a scientific nature. In particular, it will proffer advice concerning:

a) the annual and long-term research programs,

b) appointment procedures, in particular the drawing up of appointment lists,

c) the appointment and recall of the heads of departments as well as the directors of central installations and projects,

d) taking up further and discontinuing previous functions,

e) founding, dissolving and amalgamating institutes, departments and central installations, starting and terminating projects,

f) issuing regulations for institutes and projects,

g) the appointments procedure,

h) principles for the utilization of the results of the Foundations's research,

i) the annual budget and long-term financial plans including programs for development and investment,

k) measures for the implementation of efficiency control of scientific work,

l) measures for the promotion of the flow of scientific information within the Foundation (work reports, colloquia, hearings),

m) the co-operation with universities, other research institutions and international establishments, as well as

n) the scientific progress report.
In these matters the Scientific Council, inasfar as this is necessary according to section 13, paragraph 2, will pass

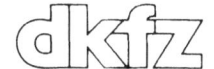

resolutions about their consent with the intended decisions of the Management Board. If agreement cannot be reached, the procedure according to section 13, paragraph 3 will be applied.

(2) The Scientific Council may demand information from the Management Board on scientific matters and matters of research policy.

### Section 17   Composition and Resolutions of the Scientific Council

(1) The Scientific Council consists of at most sixteen members and is composed of

a) at most eight managing directors of an institute,

b) an equal number of representatives of the scientific staff.

(2) Should there be more than eight managing directors of an institute, they will elect their representatives from their midst. The members according to paragraph 1, letter b will be elected for a period of three years by the scientific staff of the Foundation in compliance with an election order. The election order is laid down by the Management Board in consultation with the Scientific Council and with the consent of the Board of Trustees.

(3) The Scientific Council elects from their midst a chairman and a deputy chairman.

(4) The members of the Management Board, the president of the Board of Trustees or a member of the Board of Trustees to be determined by the latter and a member of the staff representation may attend the meetings of the Scientific Council in a consultative capacitiy inasfar as the Scientific

Council does not decide otherwise in any individual instance.

(5) The Scientific Council will constitute a quorum if two thirds of its members including the chairman or the deputy chairman are present. Resolutions require a majority of the valid votes cast.

(6) The Scientific Council in consultation with the Management Board and with the consent of the Board of Trustees will set up standing rules governing the representation of the members.

## III. Institutes, Departments, Projects and Central Installations

### Section 18   Institutes and Departments

(1) Institutes are permanent operational organisational units for the implementation of the scientific work of the Foundation. The institutes consist of departments.

(2) The Management Board will lay down regulations which will, as a rule, provide for an Institute Management Board, an Institute Panel and an Institute Assembly.

(3) The Management Board consists of the heads of departments. It makes decisions about scientific and operational matters concerning the institute. Further details are regulated by the Institute Order to be issued with the consent of the Scientific Council and the Board of Trustees pursuant to paragraph 2.

(4) The Institute Management Board elects from their midst the managing director of the institute and his deputy. The term of office will be three years; re-election is possible.

(5) The Insitute Management Board will be advised by a Panel. The Panel consists of one elected member each of the scientific staff of every department who will be elected by the entire staff of the department in question.

(6) The entire staff of the institute forms the Assembly. It will be informed by the Institute Management Board about essential affairs of the institute and the Foundation.

### Section 19  Projects

(1)  The Foundation may carry out part of the research program in the form of projects. A project is understood to be a research activity largely structured in detail which is temporally and financially limited, bound towards a certain aim and exceeds the framework of an institute.

(2)  The organization and implementation of projects are laid down in a project order which the Management Board will issue with the approval of the Scientific Council and the Board of Trustees.

### Section 20  Central Installations

(1)  Central installations shall serve to fulfil tasks of the entire Cancer Research Center or of several institutes or projects. They are directly responsible to the Management Board.

(2)  The participation of the staff of the central installations in the elections to the Scientific Council is regulated by the Management Board in the respective election orders with the approval of the Board of Trustees and the Scientific Council.

## IV. Administration and Personnel Affairs

### Section 21  Accounting, Auditing and Acceptance of the Accounts

(1)  Accounts must be rendered annually by the Management Board concerning the income and expenditure as well as the assets and liabilities of the Foundation. Notwithstanding the legal auditing rights of the Federal Audit Office and the Audit Office of Baden-Württemberg, the annual accounts must be audited by a chartered accountant or another suitable qualified person or auditing establishment. The Board of Trustees will decide who is to be entrusted with this task.

(2)  At the end of the calendar year a business report and a statement of account is to be submitted to the Board of Trustees, the authority in control of the Foundation and the auditing authorities.

(3)  Section 109, paragraph 3 of the budget regulations of Baden-Württemberg is applicable to the release. Organ for decision making is the Board of Trustees.

### Section 22  Scientific Staff

The scientific staff in the sense of these statutes and articles consists of all coworkers of the Foundation engaged in research activities who are either university graduates or who carry out corresponding activities on the basis of equal abilities and experience and who have entered into an employment contract with the Foundation.

### Section 23  Personnel Affairs

(1)  Prior to the appointment of heads of departments and the employment of scientific staff according to section 8, paragraph 3, letter d, an appointment procedure is to be carried through pursuant to further regulations laid own in an appointment order to be issued by the Management Board in consultation with the Scientific Council and with the consent of the Board of Trustees.

(2)  Decisions concerning the legal status of civil servants employed by the Foundation will be made by the authorities competent according to the legal regulations of the Land on the basis of applications which are decided upon by the competent organs of the Foundation.

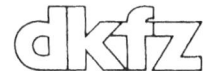

## Section 24 Changes Affecting the Statutes and Articles and Dissolution of the Foundation

Resolutions concerning changes affecting the statutes and articles and the dissolution of the Foundation may not be passed without the votes of the members of the Board of Trustees delegated by the Federation and the Land who have a double vote in such matters. The Management Board and the Scientific Council are to be previously consulted. The resulotions will not take effect until they have been approved by the authority in control of the Foundation.

## Section 25 Accumulation of Assets

(1) In the event of the dissolution of the Foundation, the Foundation's assets will pass to the Federation and the Land proportionate to the value of the grants made by each of them, inasfar as these assets do not exceed the value of the grants awarded and any contributions made in kind at the time of dissolution. Any balance then remaining will, in agreement with the Federation, be used for purposes in the sense of the Public Benefits Decree dated 24 December, 1953 (Federal Legal Gazette I, page 15).

(2) This provision may only be changed with the consent of the members of the Board of Trustees delegated by the Federation and the Land.

## Section 26 Coming into Force and Transitional Provisions

(1) These statutes and articles will come into force on the day following their announcement in the Legal Gazette of Baden-Württemberg.

(2) The Board of Directors in office under the previous statutes and articles will take over the functions of the Management Board according to the provisions of the present statutes and articles on the understanding that the Minister of Education and Culture of the Land Baden-Württemberg in consultation with the Federal Minister for Research and Technology shall provisionally appoint a further member to take charge of the functions of the Administrative Member until the appointment of the latter. For the period up to the provisional appointment the chairman of the Administrative Council will perform the tasks of the Administrative Member. The Management Board will also take over the functions of the Scientific Council until such time as the latter is constituted according to these statutes and articles. The Board of Trustees in office under the previous statutes and articles will take charge of the functions of the Board of Trustees until such time as the latter has been formed and convened for its first meeting; until such time sections 10, paragraph 1, sentence 2 and 12, paragraph 1, sentence 2 do not apply.

(3) The Institute Directors appointed under the provisions of the previous statutes and articles without election will be managing directors of the institutes in question for the period of their activity in the Foundation. They are entitled to waive this privilege.

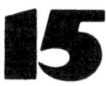
# Register

Additional information of this book

*(Current Cancer Research 1986; 978-3-7985-0712-8)* is provided:

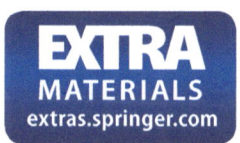

http://Extras.Springer.com